Malignancies of the Nasal Vestibule

Francesco Bussu

Editor

Malignancies of the Nasal Vestibule

A New Perspective on Classification, Staging, and Treatment

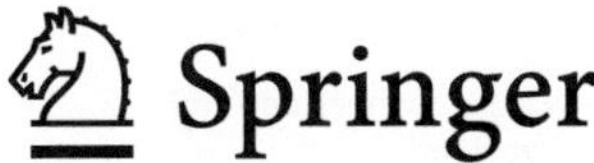

Editor
Francesco Bussu
Department of Medicine, Surgery and Pharmacy
University of Sassari
Sassari, Italy

ISBN 978-3-031-32852-7   ISBN 978-3-031-32850-3   (eBook)
https://doi.org/10.1007/978-3-031-32850-3

This Springer imprint is published by the registered company Springer Nature Switzerland AG
The registered company address is: Gewerbestrasse 11, 6330 Cham, Switzerland

Foreword

A therapeutic paradigm shift is taking place regarding malignant vestibular nasal tumours.

These tumours have long been a neglected entity, whereas in fact they represent the most common nasal and paranasal tumours.

They are completely different neoplasms from those of the ethmoid and maxillary sinus, in terms of clinical behaviour, spreading pattern, and prognostic predictors, in which there is no specific topographical code assigned by the WHO, nor their own classification criteria recognised by the AJCC/UICC staging system.

This book represents an important novelty for the understanding of the specificity of the oncological problems related to these lesions, as it brings together in a sequence of coordinated and very thorough insights the operations related to their treatment.

Particular attention is also paid to the growing evidence on the extreme efficacy of interventional radiotherapy (brachytherapy) as the exclusive treatment of squamous cell carcinomas of the nasal vestibule. This text opens up the possibility of considering brachytherapy of neoplasms of the nasal vestibule as a new standard of therapy for these neoplasms. It also provides potentially very useful technical and practical operative instructions, enriched with new principles for the implantation phase.

I congratulate prof. Francesco Bussu for the above mentioned intuitions and for the effort he has put into compiling and collecting the contributions presented in this book as well as for his competent dedication to treating this particular type of neoplasm with great attention to the multiple needs of patients.

Radiation Oncology
Università Cattolica del Sacro Cuore
Rome, Italy

Vincenzo Valentini

Preface

It has been a long work on a neglected yet extremely relevant subject, a potentially lethal disease affecting the most visible part of the human body.

We have promoted and edited it to spread our knowledge, which we believe can be useful in improving decisively the management of cancers arising in the nasal vestibule.

It has been a team effort, so first and foremost it is incumbent on me to thank all the authors who shaped it by bringing their commitment and expertise to the writing of this volume. We also want to thank Catherine Mazars and all the Springer team who first encouraged and then carefully and patiently supported us in the completion of our effort.

The acquisition of the knowledge and experiences which finally led me to propose and then take care of this book were made possible by mentors and friends, of which some are listed below, who provided their support along with valuable scientific inputs, and to whom my thanks go.

Among these it seems right to me to remember first and foremost who is no longer with us, my first mentor and chairman Professor Maurizio Maurizi.

The one who sensed the new potential of the old therapeutic modality, brachytherapy, which plays a leading role in the present work, was Professor Vincenzo Valentini.

Thanks to Professor Gaetano Paludetti, my chairman for most of my career, who first gave me the great opportunity to acquire all the skills I have and then encouraged me to always move forward.

The expert who retained the skills necessary to perform brachytherapy in years when it seemed to have no future, and trained me in Germany then gave precious advice for all the following years, is Professor George Kovacs. Thanks to Professor Alberto Artuso, the talented surgeon who gave a fundamental contribution to the novel concept and practice of anatomic implantation described in a separate chapter of the present book.

The radiation oncologist colleague who accompanied me on the path of training and growth in brachytherapy, and discovering the extraordinary and probably unhoped-for efficacy on carcinomas of the nasal vestibule of this treatment modality was Dr. Luca Tagliaferri.

And, last but not least, I want to thank Professor Jacopo Galli, who has always accompanied me with benevolence while also participating in the development of many of the useful insights that I believe you will find in this book.

Sassari, Italy   Francesco Bussu

Contents

About the Editor

Francesco Bussu is currently a Professor and Chairman in Otolaryngology and the Head of the ENT Division at the University Hospital of Sassari (Italy). He activated the Residency Program in Otolaryngology in 2023 and the Speech Therapy School in 2020, and he is currently the director of both programs. He is also a member of the Italian commission for National Scientific Qualification for Professorship and the treasurer of the Italian Society of Otorhinolaryngology (SIO).

He has performed about 10,000 surgical procedures as first operator in all the subspecialties of otolaryngology, particularly in head and neck oncology. He introduced the lengthening temporalis myoplasty (Labbè operation) in Italy for long-term facial paralysis rehabilitation, and he has performed more than 100 brachytherapy implants for head and neck malignancies, with more than 50 for nasal vestibule primaries.

He has published over 120 papers in indexed impacted journals, mainly on head and neck surgery and oncology. He contributed to clarifying the oncogenic role of HPV in non-oropharyngeal head and neck malignancies and the clinical limits of the currently employed p16 IHC in the definition of HPV related carcinogenesis in the oropharynx.

Anatomy of the Nose Vestibule

1

Claudio Parrilla, Francesco Bussu, Nicola Turra,
Roberto Gallus, Carla Fonnesu, Nicola Tsatsaris,
and Andrea Montella

1.1 Introduction

Knowledge of anatomy is of utmost importance in medicine, and it is for several reasons (see Chap. 14) one of the main drivers of the new developments in classification and treatment of nose vestibule malignancies we describe in this monograph.

The ultimate knowledge about surgical anatomy is extrapolated from rhinoplasty experience, in the ablative, reconstructive as well as in the cosmetic perspectives. In this book, surgical rhinoplasty anatomy gains further relevance as it is the basis for novel concepts in implantation techniques of plastic tubes for brachytherapy in nose malignancies [1–3].

To properly manage the structures of the nose vestibule it is extremely important for the surgeon to identify all the anatomical components of the nose. All the

C. Parrilla
Department of Otolaryngology, Università Cattolica del S. Cuore, Rome, Italy

F. Bussu
Department of Medicine, Surgery and Pharmacy, University of Sassari, Sassari, Italy

Otolaryngology Division, Sassari University Hospital, Azienda Ospedaliera Universitaria di Sassari, Sassari, Italy

N. Turra (✉) · C. Fonnesu · N. Tsatsaris
Otolaryngology Division, Sassari University Hospital, Azienda Ospedaliera Universitaria di Sassari, Sassari, Italy
e-mail: carla.fonnesu@aouss.it

R. Gallus
Otolaryngology, Mater Olbia Hospital, Olbia, Italy
e-mail: roberto.gallus@materolbia.com

A. Montella
Department of Biomedical Sciences-Human Anatomy, University of Sassari, Sassari, Italy
e-mail: montella@uniss.it

© Springer Nature Switzerland AG 2023
F. Bussu (ed.), *Malignancies of the Nasal Vestibule*,
https://doi.org/10.1007/978-3-031-32850-3_1

structures constituting the rigid framework of the nose tip, cartilages, bones and ligaments, should be exploited in reconstructive surgery, but also, even more, for the correct positioning of the catheters used in brachytherapy, taking advantage of their ability to block the disease as well as direct its spread. Conversely, if unnecessarily damaged, they could represent a way of tumor spreading or spillage, making it somehow unpredictable and putting it out of control particularly in post-surgical recurreces.

1.2   Osteocartilaginous Framework and Nose Vestibule

The nasal pyramid is formed, from top to bottom, by the following structures:

- nasal bones,
- ascending processes of the maxilla,
- superior margin of septal cartilage,
- upper lateral cartilage,
- lower lateral cartilage (major alar cartilage),
- minor alar cartilages, and
- fibro-fatty tissue (Fig. 1.1).

The medial surface of the frontal process of the maxilla contributes to form the piriform aperture, while its upper portion articulates with the ethmoid [4–6].

Blood supply and innervation are shown in Tables 1.1 and 1.2.

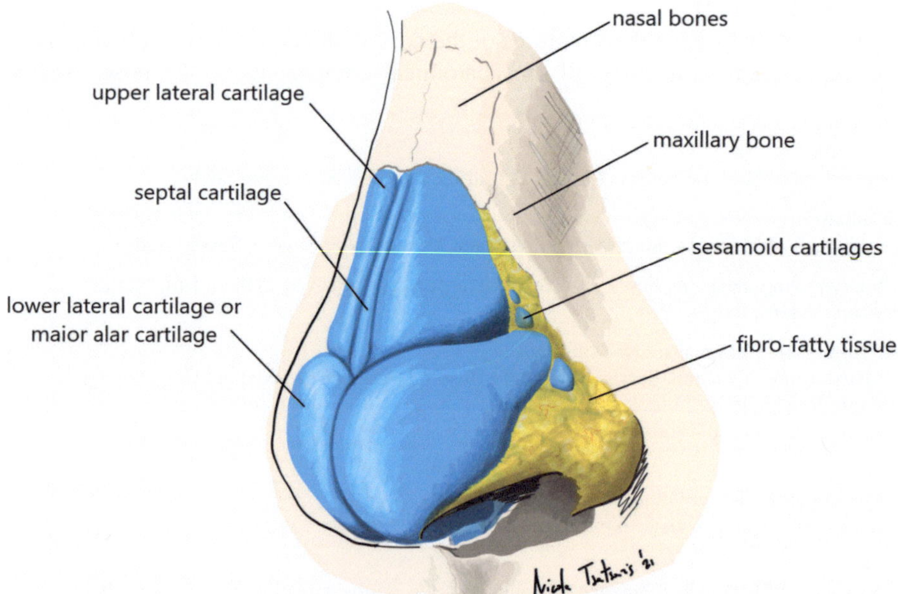

Fig. 1.1 Main structure, with the rigid framework in evidence, of the nose tip

Table 1.1 External nose (EN) nerve and blood supply

	Arterious vessels	Sensory nerve supply
Upper EN	Angular artery Dorsal branches of the ophthalmic artery	Infratrochlear branch of the ophthalmic nerve (1 V)
Middle EN	Angular artery Branches (dorsum)	Infraorbital branch of the maxillary nerve (2 V)
Lower EN	Superior labial artery (columella) Superior and inferior alar arteries (lobules)	External branches of the ethmoidal nerve (1 V)

Table 1.2 Internal nose (IN) blood supply

Ophthalmic artery	Posterior ethmoidal AA.	Posterior ethmoidal cells Posterior nasal septum
	Anterior ethmoidal AA.	Anterior ethmoidal cells Anterior nasal septum Lateral nasal wall
Maxillary artery	Descending palatine A.	Lower nasal septum
	Sphenopalatine A.	Posterior nasal septum
Facial artery	Superior labial A.	Anterior nasal septum
	Lateral nasal branches	

The nasal vestibule is a sagittally elongated aperture, and it has a lower orifice, and an upper one, in continuity with the proper nasal cavity. It is bounded laterally by the ala and lateral part of the major alar cartilage and medially by the medial crus or septal process of this cartilage. The vestibule extends as a small recess toward the apex of the nose. Its lumen is lined with the skin, the inferior region bearing sebaceous and sweat glands, and coarse hairs (vibrissae) curving toward the naris and helping to arrest the passage of particles in inspired air (Fig. 1.2). In males, after middle age, these hairs increase considerably in size. The vestibule is classically considered limited above and behind by a curved ridge, the limen nasi or nasal valve, corresponding to the lower margin of the upper lateral cartilage anteriorly and the pyriform nasal aperture posteroinferiorly [7]. At this demarcation, the skin of the vestibule is continuous with the nasal mucosa.

We propose, for oncological reasons, considering the pattern of tumor spread and the potential indication to brachytherapy treatment, to consider the nose vestibule as a subsite of the nasal cavity with a clear posterior limit, identified radiologically and by palpation, which is the pyriform aperture [2, 3]; it means that the "nose vestibule" subsite does not end superiorly at the lower margin of the upper lateral cartilage but about 1.5 cm behind and above (Fig. 1.3). The radiological landmark separating the nose vestibule from the nasal cavity proper would simply be the tangential plane to the bony piriform opening (Fig. 1.4).

The nose vestibule would be therefore the nasal cavity subsite corresponding to the "so-called" nose tip, that is, the "soft part" of the nasal pyramid, with a

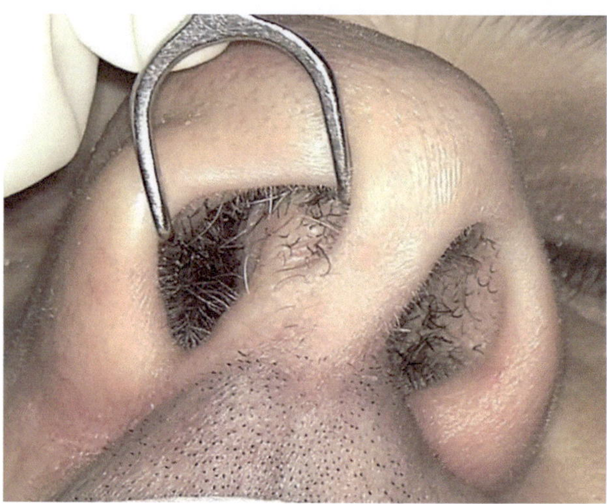

Fig. 1.2 Anterior nares: lumen is lined with the skin, sebaceous and sweat glands, and vibrissae, which act like a filter

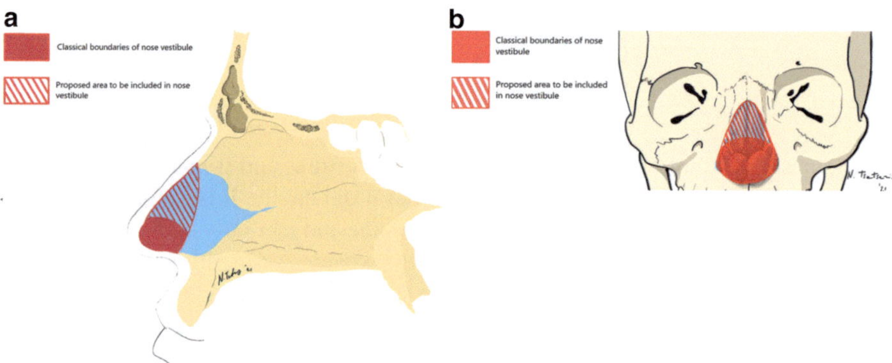

Fig. 1.3 The inclusion of a wider area in the subsite "nose vestibule" is proposed basing upon anatomical and oncological criteria (in **a** and **b,** respectively, sagittal and frontal views are displayed)

cartilaginous framework and an external covering, which is the surface of the nose tip with a variable thickness of the skin.

The lining of the anterior part of the nasal cavity and vestibule is continuous with the skin and consists of keratinized stratified squamous epithelium overlying a connective tissue lamina propria. Further posteriorly, at the limen nasi, this grades into a mucosa lined at first by non-keratinizing stratified squamous epithelium, then by pseudostratified ciliated (respiratory) epithelium with numerous goblet cells.

As the nose vestibule section is crossly triangular, we identify three walls, a lateral one below the nose ala and the lateral cartilage, a medial one, along the anterior part of the nose septum and columella, and an inferior one (the shortest) along the most anterior part of the nasal floor from the inferior side of the pyriform opening to the superior lip.

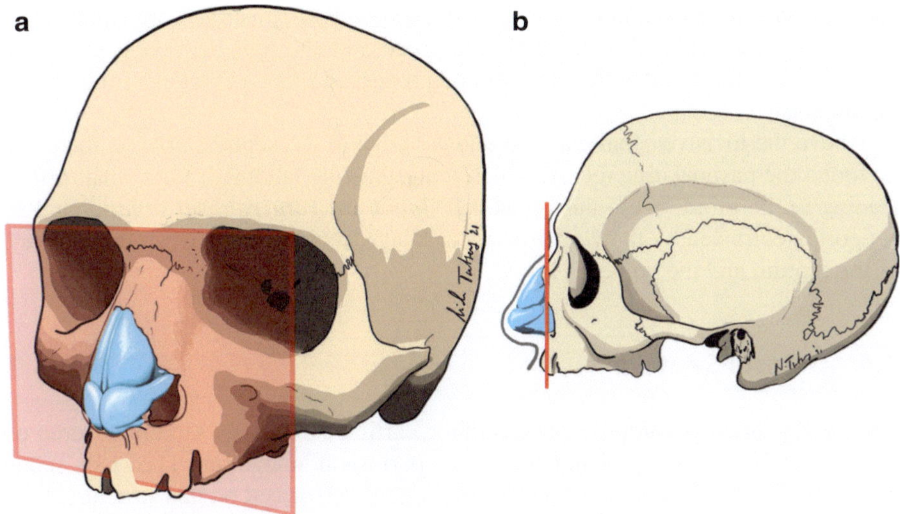

Fig. 1.4 Tangential plane to the piriform opening as radiological landmark separating nose vestibule from nasal cavity proper (tridimensional, **a**, and sagittal, **b**, representation)

1.3   Cartilaginous Pyramid (Nose Vestibule Framework)

It is crucial to keep in mind that the lower third of the nasal pyramid is exclusively made out of cartilage and fibro-fatty tissue.

At this level, we find the ***nasal valve area***, which is formed by the joint between the upper lateral cartilages and the nasal septum, and this is the area where the change from keratinized squamous epithelium to nasal mucosa occurs.

The areas occupied by loose tissue contain sesamoid cartilages, which offer additional support to the lower third of the nasal pyramid. In addition to that, other support structures for the tip of the nose are: the membranous and cartilaginous septum, the anterior nasal spine, the ligaments that connect the skin to the interdomal region [8–10].

A fat pad is enclosed in the interdomal space, of varying sizes, and fatty (bulbous) noses present larger fat pads.

The ***upper lateral cartilage*** articulates superiorly with the lower margin of the nasal bone and with the frontal process of the maxilla: it has a triangular shape, with a posterosuperior base and an anteroinferior apex. The medial side of this cartilage is located in continuity with the upper edge of the septal cartilage. Its lower margin is articulated, instead, both with the sesamoid cartilages contained in the alar tissue and with the greater alar cartilage.

The ***lower lateral (major alar) cartilage*** is V-shaped, with the medial branch of shorter length than the lateral one. Due to its conformation, this cartilage contributes to form both the medial and lateral walls of the nasal vestibule and the tip of the nose. The medial wall (*crus mediale*) connects with the contralateral: the nasal septum is interposed between them.

The ***minor alar cartilages***, also known as *sesamoid cartilages*, are small structures that are articulated with the frontal process of the maxilla, connected to the major alar cartilage and to the same frontal process through a thin but strong fibrous membrane.

Above the incisive canal and at the lower edge of the septal cartilage, there can be found the nasopalatine recess, which represents the landmark for a small orifice leading to the blind recess known as the "***Jacobson vomeronasal organ***," and its support is entrusted by the vomeronasal cartilage, which lies between the cartilage of the septum and the vomer [11].

1.4   Nasal Septum

The nasal septum is composed of a midline cartilage and bony septum covered on either side by a mucoperichondrial–mucoperiosteal membrane [12, 13]; septal hematoma is often the result of trauma or surgery performed on this structure.

The bony and cartilaginous structures of the nasal septum, although having a different embryological origin, are both covered, besides mucoperiosteum and mucopericondrium, by a thick, pseudostratified respiratory epithelium. Nevertheless, the subperichondreal and subperiosteal planes are discontinuous at the junction point between the cartilaginous septum and the vomer bone (this represents, in fact, an area of weakness with a higher risk of damage during surgery and perforations).

As previously said, it is extremely important to keep the mucoperiosteum and mucoperichondrium intact as far as possible, periosteum being a fibrous membrane that covers the surface of the bones and mucoperichondrium being a structure formed by mucosal tissue and the perichondrium itself. Furthermore, as long as the tumor is confined to the lamina propria, the two mucoperichondrial layers and the cartilage of the septum work as barriers against tumor spread. Several studies in the scientific literature show that maintaining the integrity of these structures is associated not only with a lower risk of recurrence but also with shorter times of re-epithelialization and repair of the overlying tissues.

The nasal septum consists of the perpendicular lamina of the ethmoid, the vomer bone, and the cartilage of the septum. Irregularities are frequently observed, since the septal cartilage might be deflected, even at the point of reaching the lateral wall of the nasal cavity. The cartilage of the septum presents in a quadrangular shape that posteriorly arises to fill the gap between the perpendicular lamina of the ethmoid and the vomer bone.

The nasal septum is abundantly vascularized by six arteries:

- upper labial arteries,
- lateral nasal arteries,
- posterior septal artery (branch of the sphenopalatine artery),
- anterior and posterior ethmoid arteries, and
- major palatine artery.

In the anterior third of the septum, these arteries form a dense anastomotic network, with capillaries, which push close to the epithelium, known as the **_Kiesselbach's area_**. The deep branches of these arteries are located near the periosteum.

The **_nasal columella_** (also known as sub-septum) [14–16] is the tissue that connects the nasal tip to the nasal base, separating the nares. The dermocartilaginous ligament of the nose is a narrow, central, fibrous, white structure in the center of the nasal _dorsum_, which was first described by Pitanguy. This structure was initially believed to connect the dermis of the upper third of the nose, _medial crura_, and subseptum. However, in a recent study, no direct connection was found between it and dermal tissue, arguing that this ligament cannot be considered as a stand-alone structure. This structure originates from the transverse nasalis muscular tissue and terminates at the caudal edge of the septal cartilage and _orbicularis oris muscle_ in some cases. Histologic findings are also incompatible with the term ligament and demonstrate that it is in fact a fascia.

According to some authors, [17] nasal columella should be considered separate from nose vestibule; we consider it the most caudal part of the medial wall of the nose vestibule.

1.5 Muscles and Ligaments

The muscular apparatus is represented by:

- angular head of the square muscle of the upper lip (levator labii superioris alae-que nasi muscle),
- depressor septi nasi muscle,
- nasalis muscle.

The **_nasalis muscle_** consists of two parts: _compressor naris_, which arises from the maxilla and reaches the aponeurosis of the procerus muscle, and _dilator naris_, which inserts on the major alar cartilage. At the root of the nose, the frontal muscle is inserted. Loose connective tissue separates the nose skin from the underlying bone structures.

The preservation of the intercartilaginous ligaments of the lower third of the nose is extremely important, not only to avoid the spread of the underlying malignant pathology but also for purely aesthetic reasons (projection of the tip of the nose, rotation, and position) [18–20].

The **_interdomal ligament_** connects the two medial crura of the major wing cartilages, is a rigid structure, and can be easily identified during the dissection of the nose. To be precise, it is located at the point of maximum curvature of the major wing cartilages, in a more posterior and cephalic position than the nasal dome.

The **_footplate ligament_** is an important fibrous pillar that supports the tip of the nose. It is located superiorly to the interdomal ligament, its larger diameter is transversal, and its length is inversely proportional to the width of the base of the nasal columella [21].

Sesamoid ligaments are circular fibrous structures that incorporate the homonymous cartilages and attach them to the pyriform aperture.

The ***pyriform ligament*** is a structure located at the level of the bones that frame the pyriform opening, but it does not seem, from what emerges from the most recent studies, to represent real ligamentous support to the other structures of the nasal pyramid.

The ***Pitanguy ligament*** (see Sect. 1.4).

1.6 Conclusions

The perfect knowledge of soft and rigid structures of the nose and in particular of the tip should lead to an adequate definition of the nose vestibule malignancies for a proper planning and correct accomplishment of the therapeutic procedures [22–24], because through the preservation of those anatomical structures, especially the cartilaginous and ligamentous ones, we can achieve the best treatment, prevent the spread of the tumor, and preserve cosmesis of the most exposed part of the human body, the nose tip, at the same time.

References

1. Tagliaferri L, Fionda B, Bussu F, et al. Interventional radiotherapy (brachytherapy) for squamous cell carcinoma of the nasal vestibule: a multidisciplinary systematic review. Eur J Dermatol. 2019;29:417–21.
2. Bussu F et al. New standards for the management of nose vestibule malignancies Acta Oto-Laryngologica. 2023;143(3):215–22. https://doi.org/10.1080/00016489.2023.2179662.
3. Bussu F, Tagliaferri A, Piras D, Rizzo N, Tsatsaris E, De CC, Parrilla GP. Multidisciplinary approach to nose vestibule malignancies: setting new standards Approccio multidisciplinare ai tumori maligni del vestibolo del naso: verso la definizione di nuovi standard Acta Otorhinolaryngologica Italica. 2021;41(Suppl. 1):S158–S165. https://doi.org/10.14639/0392-100X-suppl.1-41-2021-16.
4. Freeman M, Gurrola J, Payne SC. Rhinologic evaluation of patients undergoing transsphenoidal surgery. Transsphenoidal Surg. 2017;87–94.
5. Nguyen PS, Bardot J, Duron JB, Jallut Y, Aiach G. Surgical anatomy of the nose. Ann Chir Plast Esthet. 2014;59:380–6.
6. Weeden AM, Degner DA. Surgical approaches to the nasal cavity and sinuses. Vet Clin North Am Small Anim Pract. 2016;46:719–33.
7. Standring S. Gray's anatomy: the anatomical basis of clinical practice. Gray's anatomy. London: Churchill Livingstone Elsevier; 2020.
8. Han S-K, Jeong S-H, Lee B-I, Kim W-K. Updated anatomy of the dermocartilaginous ligament of the nose. Ann Plast Surg. 2007;59:393–7.
9. Parrilla C, Artuso A, Gallus R, Galli J, Paludetti G. The role of septal surgery in cosmetic rhinoplasty. Acta Otorhinolaryngol Ital. 2013;33:146–53.
10. Molumi CP, Dubey SP, Apaio ML. Preservation of palatal mucoperiosteum for oronasal separation after total maxillectomy. Indian J Cancer. 2012;49:209–14.

11. Bhatnagar KP, Smith TD, Winstead W. The human vomeronasal organ: part IV. Incidence, topography, endoscopy, and ultrastructure of the nasopalatine recess, nasopalatine fossa, and vomeronasal organ. Am J Rhinol. 2002;16:343–50.
12. Bussu F, Tagliaferri L, Mattiucci G, et al. HDR interventional radiotherapy (brachytherapy) in the treatment of primary and recurrent head and neck malignancies. Head Neck. 2019;41:1667–75.
13. Nease CJ, Deal RC. Septoplasty in conjunction with cosmetic rhinoplasty. Oral Maxillofac Surg Clin North Am. 2012;24:49–58.
14. Bussu F, Tagliaferri L, Mattiucci G, et al. Comparison of interstitial brachytherapy and surgery as primary treatments for nasal vestibule carcinomas. Laryngoscope. 2016;126:367–71.
15. Shah J, Roxbury CR, Sindwani R. Techniques in septoplasty: traditional versus endoscopic approaches. Otolaryngol Clin North Am. 2018;51:909–17.
16. Most SP, Rudy SF. Septoplasty: basic and advanced techniques. Facial Plast Surg Clin North Am. 2017;25:161–9.
17. Dias FL. Rhinectomy. Master Techniques in Otolaryngology-Head Neck Surgery: Larynx, Hypopharynx, Oropharynx, Oral Cavity and Neck. 2013;1:183–90.
18. Simons RL, Greene RM. Rhinoplasty5 pearls: value of the endonasal approach and vertical dome division. Clin Plast Surg. 2010;37:265–83.
19. Palma P, Khodaei I. Hybrid rhinoplasty: the 21st century approach to remodeling the nose. Arch Facial Plast Surg. 2010;12:412–4.
20. Tebbetts JB. Rethinking the logic and techniques of primary tip rhinoplasty. Clin Plast Surg. 1996;23:245–53.
21. Rohrich RJ, Muzaffar AR, Janis JE. Component dorsal hump reduction: the importance of maintaining dorsal aesthetic lines in rhinoplasty. Plast Reconstr Surg. 2004;114:1298–308; discussion 1309–12.
22. Dobratz EJ, Tran V, Hilger PA. Comparison of techniques used to support the nasal tip and their long-term effects on tip position. Arch Facial Plast Surg. 2010;12:172–9.
23. Stevens MR, Emam HA. Applied surgical anatomy of the nose. Oral Maxillofac Surg Clin North Am. 2012;24:25–38.
24. Apaydin F. Septal surgery challenges in rhinoplasty. Facial Plast Surg. 2016;32:351–60.

Histology of Nose Vestibule Malignancies

2

Giulia Scaglione, Laura Maria De Luca,
Francesco Giuseppe Riu, Paolo Fois, Claudia Crescio,
and Valerio Gaetano Vellone

2.1 Normal Histology

Before systematically treating the malignant neoplasms of the nasal vestibule, it is necessary to keep in mind some notions of normal tissue histology. For long decades, pathologists have speculated about the tissue origin of the observed neoplasm. However, today, it is more appropriate to think about its differentiation, taking into account the concept of neoplastic staminality.

Nasal cavities are separated by the nasal septum. The nasal vestibules are the most anterior parts of the nasal cavities corresponding on the cutaneous surface to the nose tip. The hard framework of nasal vestibule/nose tip, as that of the nasal septum is composed of hyaline cartilage. The openings of the nasal vestibules and its anterior boundaries, the nares, are further divided by a vertical soft structure in continuity with the septum called columella, completely covered by skin.

The nasal cavity as a whole extends from the nares anteriorly to the choanae posteriorly.

A ridge (limen nasi) on the lateral/medial wall separates the vestibule from the rest of the nasal cavity (nasal cavity proper). The olfactory region occupies the

G. Scaglione
Department of Integrated Surgical and Diagnostic Sciences (DISC), University of Genoa, Genoa, Italy

L. M. De Luca (✉) · F. G. Riu · P. Fois · C. Crescio
Otolaryngology Division, Azienda Ospedaliera Universitaria di Sassari, Sassari, Italy
e-mail: francesco.riu@aouss.it; paolo.fois@aouss.it; claudia.crescio@aousassari.it; ccrescio1@uniss.it

V. G. Vellone
Department of Integrated Surgical and Diagnostic Sciences (DISC), University of Genoa, Genoa, Italy

Anatomic Pathology University Unit, IRCCS Ospedale Policlinico San Martino, Genoa, Italy
e-mail: valeriovellone@gaslini.org

© Springer Nature Switzerland AG 2023
F. Bussu (ed.), *Malignancies of the Nasal Vestibule*,
https://doi.org/10.1007/978-3-031-32850-3_2

upper part of each nasal cavity proper. The rest of the cavity consists of the respiratory region. On the lateral wall of each nasal fossa, there are the superior/middle and inferior turbinates.

A fourth supreme turbinate may be present at the uppermost lateral nasal wall. The scroll-shaped turbinates hang over the corresponding funnel passages, or meatuses, into which the various paranasal sinuses open.

The lining of the nasal cavity gradually changes at the level of limen nasi, from keratinizing squamous epithelium to non-ciliated cuboidal or columnar epithelium and then to ciliated respiratory-type epithelium. The ciliated respiratory-type epithelium lines most of the nasal cavity and all the paranasal sinuses, except for the roof.

The olfactory epithelium is predominantly made of columnar non-ciliated sustentacular cells, with scattered bipolar sensory neurons and basal cells.

The lamina propria of the nasal epithelia contains several seromucous glands, lymphocytes, monocytes, and a well-developed vascular network, particularly in the inferior and middle turbinate. The olfactory epithelium is predominantly made of columnar non-ciliated sustentacular cells, with scattered bipolar sensory neurons and basal cells [1].

2.2 Malignancies of the Nasal Vestibule

Carcinomas of the nasal vestibule are often accounted as sinonasal, although they are anatomically different entities. They are usually considered rare malignancies, however their incidence is probably underestimated and some authors even consider them the most common nasal malignancies [2].

Carcinoma of the nasal vestibule consists of a very heterogeneous pathology, extremely difficult to be diagnosed, because of the absence of specific symptoms, and the common misdiagnosis with benign conditions, as vestibulitis, or with non melanoma skin cancers, because of the early invasion of the skin (see Chap. 3 [3, 2]). Thus, a delay of the correct diagnosis is observed in clinical practice, nasal vestibule carcinoma is often misdiagnosed, and the median time interval from the first symptoms to diagnosis ranges approximately from 5 to 6 months [4–6]. This delay is due to nonspecific symptoms including obstruction, rhinorrhea, epistaxis, and pain and to the lack of awareness about this *not so uncommon* and ofter devastating disease.

Nasal vestibule carcinoma occurs more frequently in men, and it affects a wide age range from 40 to 90, with cases also under 30. The most anterior part of the nasal cavity is lined with keratinizing squamous epithelium and contains other elements as skin-bearing hair follicles, sebaceous glands, and sweat glands.

The vast majority of nose vestibule malignancies are squamous cell carcinomas (SCCs), followed by adenocarcinomas and melanoma [7]. The markedly higher prevalence of SCCs than other histotypes has to be emphasized, because it is another key difference from the other nose and paranasal subsites, where a markedly higher histopathological variability is observed. This brings fundamental clinical implications, making nose vestibule malignancies more similar to the other head and neck mucosal sites (oral cavity, pharynx, and larynx) whose most common malignancy is SCC as well. Consequently, as "mucosal" head and neck SCCs, and differently from the other nose/paranasal subsites, nose vestibule SCCs are characterized by the rarity of distant metastases and by nodal relapse as the most common pattern of failure.

In fact, nasal vestibule carcinomas are associated to the development of ipsilateral or contralateral lymph nodes metastases. Lymphatic drainage leads primarily to the submental and submandibular nodes, then facial, superficial parotid, and deep cervical lymph node groups (see Chap. 14).

Therefore, even if in nose vestibule carcinomas, upfront neck treatment is indicated only in high-stage tumors, and clinically suspicious lymph nodes [8], a careful diagnostic work-up and close follow-up of the neck are always mandatory.

Most patients show a limited neoplasia at the time of diagnosis (stage I or II), without cartilage or bone invasion (see Chaps. 3, 5).

2.2.1 Squamous Cell Carcinoma

Squamous cell carcinoma (SCC) is the most common malignancy of nasal vestibule [9]. It is the predominant histology dealt in this book, and in the following chapters, malignancies should be considered by default SCC unless otherwise specified.

Nasal vestibule SCC etiology still remains unclear; it has been associated with leather, nicotine, and nickel exposure. As well, in the last few years, human papillomavirus (HPV) has been shown to be an important risk factor in carcinomas of the head and neck, especially in the oropharynx, but its role in SCC of the nasal cavity as in other non-oropharyngeal head and neck subsites is not certain yet [10, 11–16].

SCC arises from the surface squamous epithelium lining nasal vestibule.

Gross Findings: SCC appears similar to skin cancers, both exophytic and endophytic, with a various aspects, papillary or ulcerated with necrosis and hemorrhages [17].

The majority of vestibule cancers are well to moderately differentiated and closer to skin cancer than to sinonasal SCC for their natural history and better prognosis [18].

Generally, SCC occurs as localized disease at first, with small-medium-sized, T1/T2 stage without cartilage invasion. The most frequent histotypes are conventional keratinizing or non-keratinizing type, but different variants may occur as exophytic squamous carcinoma, verrucous, spindle cells, helpful to stratify the prognostic risk and specific treatment of certain histological subtypes.

Fig. 2.1 (Hematoxylin/eosin 100×). Well-differentiated squamous cell carcinoma (G1) with focal keratin pearl formation

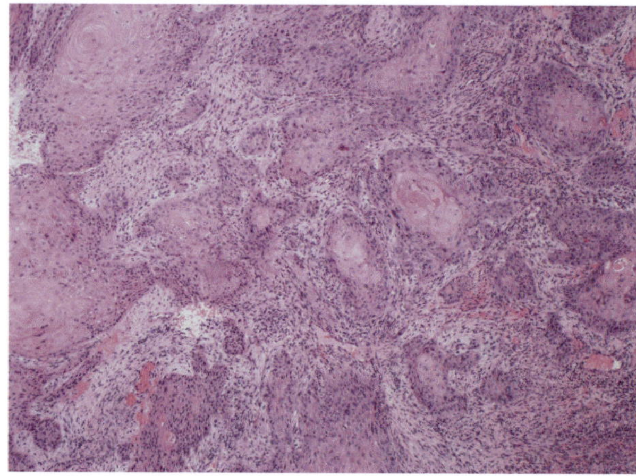

Fig. 2.2 (Hematoxylin/eosin 400×). Poorly differentiated carcinoma (G3) constituted by chords and sheets of cells with marked atypia

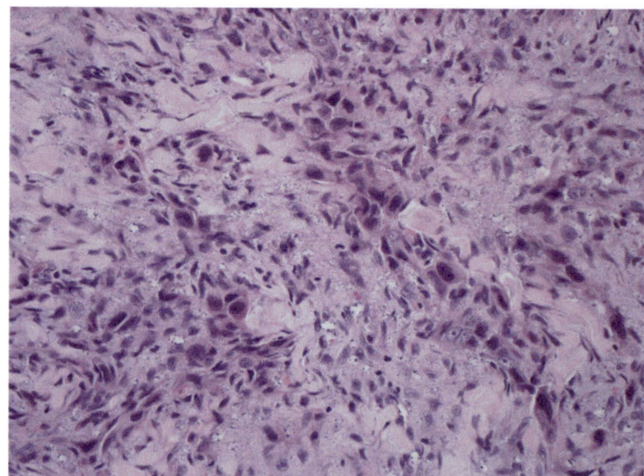

2.2.1.1 Keratinizing Squamous Cell Carcinoma of Nasal Vestibule

Keratinizing squamous carcinoma is the most common SCC of the nasal vestibule, showing the same histological features of other head and neck SCCs.

It is characterized by an irregular proliferation in sheets (Fig. 2.2), islands, and nests of large cells containing keratin, keratin pearls, dyskeratosis, and intercellular bridges. Tumor cells are polygonal with distinct borders and wide eosinophilic cytoplasm, pleomorphic and occasionally bizarre nuclei, with prominent nucleoli and irregular chromatin. Stromal invasion shows cohesive nests or cords of malignant cells with desmoplasia, collagen deposition, and chronic inflammatory infiltrate.

Malignancy is graded according to the degree of differentiation, cellular pleomorphism, and mitotic activity. Grades include well (Fig. 2.1), moderately, and poorly differentiated (Figs. 2.2 and 2.3).

Fig. 2.3 (Hematoxylin/ eosin 100×). Poorly differentiated carcinoma (G3) infiltrating the superficial layers of the nasal cartilage

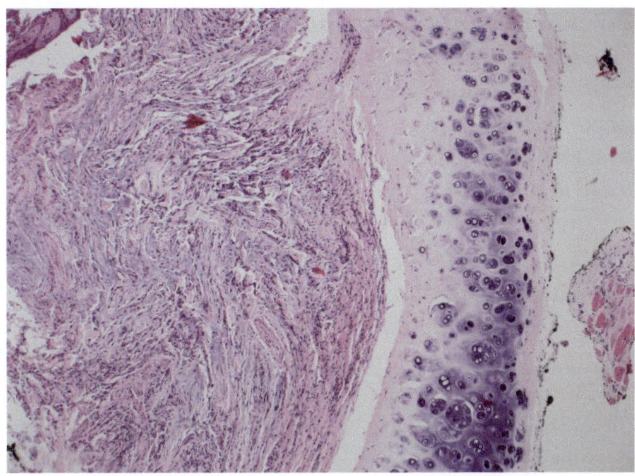

The lymph vascular invasion and perineural spread have been considered as adverse prognostic factors, and they have to be underlined in the pathological report [19].

There is no significant differential diagnosis for keratinizing SCC; indeed, morphological features are characteristic, even in poorly differentiated form.

2.2.1.2 Non-Keratinizing Squamous Cell Carcinoma of Nasal Vestibule

Non-keratinizing squamous cell carcinoma is less frequent than its keratinizing counterpart. According to some authors these tumors arise from a high-risk HPV infection. Moreover, some sinonasal papillomas progress to malignant transformation.

Non-keratinizing SCC is characterized by a ribbon-like growth pattern without keratinization or limited cellular maturation. Cells present an increased nuclear-cytoplasmic ratio and nuclear irregularities. The neoplasia shows pushing borders, peripheral palisading, and minimal desmoplasia.

Nuclear atypia is variable, but mitotic figures are numerous. Tumor grading has no certain usefulness.

Differential Diagnoses

Differential diagnosis for non-keratinizing SCC should be searched in "round blue cells tumors family," such as neuroendocrine carcinoma, NUT-midline carcinoma, neuroblastoma, Ewing sarcoma, lymphoma, alveolar rhabdomyosarcoma, melanoma, and sinonasal undifferentiated carcinoma.

A background of squamous carcinoma in situ may assist the diagnosis of non-keratinizing SCC.

Furthermore, the use of immunohistochemistry improves the diagnostic accuracy, particularly cellular expression of antibodies such as p63, p40, and Citokeratins, typically squamous lineage markers, focuses on a squamous carcinoma [20].

2.2.1.3 Basaloid Squamous Cell Carcinoma

Basaloid squamous cell carcinoma is characterized by basaloid, hyperchromatic cells with round nuclei arranged in lobules and nests with peripheral palisading and lined by hyalinized material. Necrosis and high mitotic range are observed. Then, basaloid neoplasia shows a squamous phenotype, expressing squamous immunohistochemical markers as p63 and keratin 34βE12 and pankeratin AE1/AE3 [21].

2.2.1.4 Spindle Cell Carcinoma

Spindle cell carcinoma is an unusual variant of squamous cell carcinoma. This neoplasia consists of predominant spindle and pleomorphic cells arranged in fascicular or storiform pattern with sarcomatous appearance.

The differential diagnosis includes mesenchymal tumors; however, most of spindle cell SCCs present a recognizable squamous neoplasia component or squamous dysplasia. If only the sarcomatous component occurs, immunohistochemistry for epithelial markers, such as p63, p40 and cytokeratins, is mandatory in order to make the diagnosis. A further aid is given by the lack of any specific sarcomatous pattern [22].

2.2.1.5 Verrucous Carcinoma

Verrucous squamous cell carcinoma is a rare well-differentiated variant of SCC, frequent in elderly male. Histopathological findings are typical in all sites of occurrence.

Verrucous carcinoma shows a complex exophytic and endophytic architecture, with hyperkeratosis, acanthosis, and intradermal growth with pushing borders. Cytologic atypia is minimal, and the associated stroma can be rich in inflammatory cells.

The diagnosis can be challenging especially to a reactive process, due to its lack of atypia.

Usually surgical excision is curative, but local recurrences may be observed [23].

2.2.1.6 Adenosquamous Carcinoma

In exceptional cases, some squamous carcinomas may present variable areas of glandular differentiation, as reported in other areas of the nasal cavities. Adenosquamous carcinoma (ASC) of the head and neck region is a controversial tumor, since until some years ago, it was considered to be the same entity as salivary gland mucoepidermoid carcinoma. Evidence of origin from salivary or seromucinous glands should be excluded, and mucin stain positive immunoreactivity for CEA, CK7, and CAM5.2 helps to identify the glandular component [24].

2.2.2 Malignant Melanoma

Malignant melanomas of the nasal cavity are extremely rare, accounting for about 1% of all melanomas and less than 4% of sinonasal tumors.

Patient age range of onset is wide, with an incidence increase in late adulthood.

Reviews of mucosal malignant melanoma, especially sinonasal, reported high rates of local recurrence, distant metastasis, and low survival rates [25–27].

On clinical examination, a malignant melanoma frequently appears as a polypoid nodule and occasionally friable and hemorrhagic. It can be pigmented with irregular black-brown macules.

Histological examination reveals solid sheets or nests of atypical epithelioid melanocytes, proliferating within the mucosal epithelium, even with superficial spreading and infiltrating the submucosal, with or without surface ulceration.

Cellular morphology is extremely variable, ranging from epithelioid, spindle, plasmacytoid to undifferentiated shape, with prominent nucleoli and nuclear inclusion. The presence of melanin pigment makes differential diagnostics less challenging, although roughly half of the lesions are amelanotic resulting in a broader differential diagnosis at this site, including small blue cell tumors, high-grade carcinomas, and neuroendocrine carcinomas. Immunohistochemistry is necessary for the diagnosis, and the expression of s100 and melanocytic markers (Melan—A, SOX.10 and HMB.45) leads to the diagnosis of melanocytic lesion.

Finally, mucosal melanomas show a high rate of KIT mutations, followed by NRAS and BRAF mutations, unlike cutaneous melanomas [28].

2.2.3 Merkel Cell Carcinoma

Merkel cell carcinoma (MCC) is a rare, aggressive cutaneous malignancy that accounts for less than 1% of cutaneous tumors. The risk of MCC is linked to sun exposure and immunocompromised state. It is more common in middle-aged Caucasian males.

Studies illustrate that Merkel cells originate from neural crest, and MCC can be described as cutaneous neuroendocrine carcinoma [29].

On clinical examination, Merkel cell carcinoma appears as a single painless lump on sun-exposed skin.

Histologically MCC grows in sheets, with geographical necrosis, solid nests, and trabeculae separated by fibrovascular septa.

Neoplastic cells are medium-sized with high nuclear/cytoplasmic ratio, scant cytoplasm, nuclei with dispersed salt-and-pepper chromatin, and inconspicuous nucleoli.

Differential diagnosis includes basal cell carcinoma, poorly differentiated squamous cell carcinoma, and melanoma, but also metastatic neuroendocrine carcinomas.

Therefore, immunohistochemical staining is used to confirm the diagnosis of MCC.

Merkel tumor usually shows diffuse expression of Citokeratins, especially pan-cytokeratins and Ck20, in perinuclear dots. Neuroendocrine markers such as Chromogranin-A, Synaptophysin, and CD56 are positive, whereas TF-1 and Ck7 are usually negative [30].

Prognosis is thought to be poor, although a prompt and radical surgery could ameliorate the life expectancy [31].

2.2.4 Adenocarcinoma

Nasal vestibule adenocarcinoma is a rare entity. In the sinonasal cavity, three histological types have been identified: intestinal, non-intestinal, and salivary type. However, only salivary-type adenocarcinomas have been reported in nasal vestibule. The most common malignant salivary gland tumor in the nasal tract is adenoid cystic carcinoma, followed by mucoepidermoid and acinic cell carcinoma. Macroscopically salivary glands carcinomas are described as exophytic or polypoid lesions. The pathogenesis is not known; therefore, some studies have found that tobacco, alcohol, and previous radiation might increase the risk of adenocarcinoma.

2.2.4.1 Adenoidcystic Carcinoma

Adenoid cystic carcinoma represents the 5% of sinonasal malignancy, and the most common site involved is the maxillary sinus and then nasal cavity. Typically, it occurs in adults.

Grossly, adenoid cystic carcinoma is variably encapsulated, polylobate, gray lesion. Histological characteristics overlap adenoid cystic carcinoma of more common sites. This neoplasia shows a classic cribriform pattern, less frequently tubular, solid or mixed, and it consists of epithelial and myoepithelial elements. Cribriform pattern demonstrates a "Swiss cheese" configuration with circular spaces, containing basophilic mucinous substance or hyalinized eosinophilic material. Cells are generally small with eosinophilic to clear cytoplasm, nuclei hyperchromatic, oval, angulated with small nucleoli. Mitotic figures, necrosis, and atypia are rare. The main differential diagnosis is to be found in other salivary gland tumors, adenocarcinomas, or metastasis. Immunophenotype is not useful, because salivary gland neoplasia often shows overlapped expression of Citokeratin, p40, and p63. However, many adenoid cystic carcinomas have chromosomal translocation resulting in MYB- NFIB fusion or EWSR1–ATF-1 fusion [32].

Adenoid Cystic carcinoma has usually good short-term prognosis and poor long-term survival [33].

2.2.4.2 Mucoepidermoid Carcinoma

Mucoepidermoid carcinomas (MEC) of the nasal vestibule are extremely rare, and they represent less than 1% of all malignancies of the head and neck. MEC occurs in adults in the fourth and fifth decades, with females affected more than males. This neoplasia generally arises from major and minor salivary glands, and the parotid is more commonly involved. It presents various spectra of behaviors with occasionally local and distant aggressiveness, which lies in the histopathological grading [34].

Macroscopically, a low-grade tumor comes as a well-circumscribed lesion, gray-white, and partially mucin-filled cyst; otherwise, a high-grade one is less defined and solid.

Microscopically, mucoepidermoid carcinoma is characterized by cords, sheets, and nest of squamous, mucinous-producing, intermediate-type, or clear cells in a cystic or solid growth pattern. Mucicarmine staining and periodic acid–Shiff (PAS) stain allow to demonstrate mucin presence in the cytoplasm.

Low-grade MEC is generally mucin-rich, cystic, and well circumscribed, while intermediate grade is more solid until it reaches high grade with necrosis, atypia, increased mitotic index, and perineural, lymph vascular or bony invasion.

In high-grade tumors, the diagnosis can be challenging, due to the presence of squamous aspects and cell pleomorphism. Skin cancer must be excluded searching for low- or intermediate-grade foci in the neoplasia. In most of MECs, translocation (11;19)(q21;p13) and CRTC1-MALM2 gene fusion have been observed.

Low-grade tumor usually presents a favorable outcome, even if local lymph nodes metastasis can be rarely observed. High-grade variant is aggressive locally, with local recurrence and regional lymph node spread [35].

2.2.4.3 Acinic Cell Carcinoma

Acinic cell carcinoma arising in the nose is exceptionally rare, and few reports are present in the literature; actually 95% of acinic cell carcinoma occurs in the parotid gland. The mean presentation age is approximately 50 years [36].

ACC is typically a well-circumscribed, low-growing mass characterized by acinar and ductal cells, vacuolated, clear or oncocytic with a microcystic, follicular or solid pattern. These tumors may have a various pattern presentations; however, acinic cells are generally large, polygonal cells, with basophilic granular cytoplasm and round eccentric nuclei. The predominant variant is the solid growth pattern. Mitosis, necrosis, or pleomorphism is barely observed; however, neural invasion is associated with aggressive behavior [37].

Acinic cell carcinoma can be considered as a low/intermediate-grade malignancy, and local relapse is generally reported as the most frequent type of recurrence [38].

2.2.5 Mesenchymal Tumors

Rhabdomyosarcoma is a malignant mesenchymal tumor with skeletal muscle differentiation. It is the most common sinonasal sarcoma in children, and some cases have been described in nasal vestibule. Macroscopically, it is characterized by a fleshy and gelatinous polypoid mass.

Pathological subtypes are: embryonal variant, with good prognosis and submucosal location; alveolar variant, with poor prognosis and metastatic spread; pleomorphic, more common in adults and with poor outcome.

In the sinonasal tract, embryonal rhabdomyosarcoma is the most common histological subtype. It consists of a moderately cellular sheet proliferation of small, round, undifferentiated cells with skeletal muscle differentiation.

Sinonasal alveolar rhabdomyosarcoma is more frequent in adults. This neoplasia is characterized by a densely cellular proliferation of undifferentiated, dyscohesive round elements, with scant cytoplasm and hyperchromatic nuclei, organized in lobules with necrosis.

Immunohistochemically, most useful markers are desmin and myogenin, practically expressed in all subtypes. Other skeletal muscle markers such as MYOD1, myoglobin, and MSA are variably expressed.

Most alveolar rhabdomyosarcomas harbor a PAX3-FOXO1 fusion or, less frequently, PAX7-FOXO1 fusion. The finding of this molecular alteration can be used also in a diagnostic setting in rare unusual cases [39].

2.2.6 Hematolymphoid Tumors

Lymphoid tumors arising from the nasal cavity account for 12–15% of all head and neck cancers. It is the third most common sinonasal malignancy, and also nasal vestibule localization is reported.

In lymphoid nasal tumors, symptoms overlap clinical manifestations of all other nasal tumors, such as obstruction and epistaxis, but about 10–20% of cases show B symptoms (fever, night sweats, and weight loss).

Diffuse large B-cell lymphoma (DLBCL) is the most commonly observed type of non-Hodgkin lymphoma, and it can be present at various extranodal sites. DLBCL is followed by extranodal NK/T-cell lymphoma, Burkitt lymphoma, Malt lymphoma, plasmacytoma, and histiocytic neoplasm.

2.2.6.1 Diffuse Large B-Cell Lymphoma

Diffuse large B-cell lymphoma is a neoplasm of medium-large B lymphoid cells with a diffuse growth pattern. Morphologically and biologically, clinical studies divided DLBCL into different subtypes and distinct disease entities, but it still represents an aggressive neoplasm.

It affects elderly individuals with a median age of 70; however, it can occur also in young adults.

Histologically, we observe a diffuse proliferation of medium/large lymphoid cells.

In immunohistochemistry, the expression of pan-B cell markers can help the diagnosis, such as CD20, CD79a, PAX5, while Citokeratins and T-cell markers are negative. On Ki-67 staining, the proliferative index is always high.

2.2.7 Rare Entities

Here follow some entities seldom reported as primary not arising in the nasal vestibule but can secondary involve this structure.

2.2.7.1 Sinonasal Undifferentiated Carcinoma (SNUC)

SNUC arises usually in older patients, with a rapid onset of obstructive/destructive symptoms.

It consists of a proliferation of atypical and pleomorphic cells in a lobular, nested pattern with high mitotic index and necrosis. A neuroendocrine differentiation can be present. SNUC expresses cytokeratins, without expression of epithelial markers, such as p40.

2.2.7.2 NUT Carcinoma

NUT midline carcinoma (NMC) is a rare, highly aggressive carcinoma of the midline axis, in young adults, especially females, and defined by the translocations involving the NUT gene on chromosome 15q14.

NMC involves midline structures including sinonasal tract. Usually, NMC is associated with obstructive symptoms, caused by the aggressive behavior and rapid growth of this neoplasia. Prognosis is poor and usually at an advanced stage at the time of diagnosis, due to an early disease spread. Approximately half of NMCs present lymph node involvement or distant metastasis.

The NMC is an undifferentiated carcinoma characterized by sheets of cells with round, large nuclei, distinct nucleoli, and cytoplasm scant to moderate. High mitotic rate and necrosis are observed.

NMC differential diagnosis is poorly differentiated squamous cell carcinoma, sinonasal undifferentiated carcinoma, and Ewing' sarcoma, due to its nonspecific morphology.

Immunohistochemical markers commonly positive in NMC are p63, p540, and Citokeratins. NUT carcinoma is genetically defined by rearrangements of NUT gene (NUTM1); hence, the analysis with immunohistochemical probes or molecular genetics is essential for diagnosis.

References

1. Balogh KM. Nose, and paranasal sinuses. In: Mills S, editor. Histology for pathologists. 3rd ed. Philadelphia, PA: Lippincott Williams & Wilkins; 2007.
2. New standards for the management of nose vestibule malignancies Acta Oto-Laryngologica. 2023;143(3):215–222. https://doi.org/10.1080/00016489.2023.2179662.
3. Francesco BL, Tagliaferri A, Piras D, Rizzo N, Tsatsaris E, De CC, Parrilla GP. Multidisciplinary approach to nose vestibule malignancies: setting new standards Approccio multidisciplinare ai tumori maligni del vestibolo del naso: verso la definizione di nuovi standard Acta Otorhinolaryngologica Italica. 2021;41(Suppl. 1):S158–S165. https://doi.org/10.14639/0392-100X-suppl.1-41-2021-16.
4. Daele JJ, Vander Poorten V, Rombaux P, Hamoir M. Cancer of the nasal vestibule, nasal cavity and paranasal sinuses. B-ENT. 2005;Suppl 1:87–94; quiz 95–6.
5. Kim SJ, Byun SW, Lee S-S. Various tumors in the nasal vestibule. Int J Clin Exp Pathol. 2013;6:2713–8.
6. Ho YM, Coman WB. Nasal septum malignancy. ANZ J Surg. 2011;81:533–6.
7. Kuijpens JLP, Louwman MWJ, Peters R, Janssens GORJ, Burdorf A, Coebergh JWW. Trends in sinonasal cancer in The Netherlands: more squamous cell cancer, less adenocarcinoma: a population-based study 1973–2009. Eur J Cancer. 2012;48:2369–74.
8. Scurry WC Jr, Goldenberg D, Chee MY, Lengerich EJ, Liu Y, Fedok FG. Regional recurrence of squamous cell carcinoma of the nasal cavity: a systematic review and meta-analysis. Arch Otolaryngol Head Neck Surg. 2007;133:796–800.
9. Pantelakos ST, McGuirt WF, Nussear DW. Squamous cell carcinoma of the nasal vestibule and anterior nasal passages. Am J Otolaryngol. 1994;15:33–6.

10. Ang KK, Harris J, Wheeler R, et al. Human papillomavirus and survival of patients with oropharyngeal cancer. N Engl J Med. 2010;363:24–35.
11. Accuracy of p16 IHC in Classifying HPV-Driven OPSCC in Different Populations Cancers. 2023;15(3):656. https://doi.org/10.3390/cancers15030656.
12. Prevalence of HPV Infection and p16INK4a Overexpression in Surgically Treated Laryngeal Squamous Cell Carcinoma Vaccines. 2022;10(2):204. https://doi.org/10.3390/vaccines10020204.
13. Bussu FM, Sali R, Gallus VG, Vellone GF, Zannoni R, Autorino N, Dinapoli R, Santangelo R, Martucci C, Graziani F, Miccichè G, Almadori J, Galli G, Delogu M, Sanguinetti G, Rindi V, Valentini G, Paludetti. HPV infection in squamous cell carcinomas arising from different mucosal sites of the head and neck region. Is p16 immunohistochemistry a reliable surrogate marker? British Journal of Cancer. 2013;108(5):1157–1162. https://doi.org/10.1038/bjc.2013.55.
14. Boscolo-Rizzo PF, Bussu. Beware of the dangers along the path towards the diagnosis of HPV-driven oropharyngeal squamous cell carcinoma Attenzione alle insidie riservate dalla diagnosi del carcinoma squamocellulare orofaringeo HPV-relato Acta Otorhinolaryngologica Italica. 2017;37(1):63–64. https://doi.org/10.14639/0392-100X-1323.
15. Francesco BM, Sali R, Gallus G, Petrone R, Autorino R, Santangelo M, Pandolfini F, Miccichè G, Delogu G, Almadori J, Galli M, Sanguinetti G, Rindi M, Tommasino V, Valentini GP. HPV and EBV Infections in Neck Metastases from Occult Primary Squamous Cell Carcinoma: Another Virus-Related Neoplastic Disease in the Head and Neck Region Annals of Surgical Oncology. 2015;22(S3):979–984. https://doi.org/10.1245/s10434-015-4808-5.
16. Bussu F, Ragin C, Boscolo-Rizzo P, Rizzo D, Gallus R, Delogu G, Morbini P, Tommasino M. HPV as a marker for molecular characterization in head and neck oncology: Looking for a standardization of clinical use and of detection method(s) in clinical practice. Head Neck. 2019;41(4):1104–1111. https://doi.org/10.1002/hed.25591.
17. Zaoui K, Plinkert PK, Federspil PA. Primary surgical treatment of nasal vestibule cancer—therapeutic outcome and reconstructive strategies. Rhinology. 2018;56:393–9.
18. Mendenhall WM, Stringer SP, Cassisi NJ, Mendenhall NP. Squamous cell carcinoma of the nasal vestibule. Head Neck. 1999;21:385–93.
19. Martínez-Gimeno C, Rodríguez EM, Vila CN, Varela CL. Squamous cell carcinoma of the oral cavity: a clinicopathologic scoring system for evaluating risk of cervical lymph node metastasis. Laryngoscope. 1995;105:728–33.
20. Kanaya H, Akutsu M, Kashiwagi T, Tsunemi Y, Haruna S-I. A rare case of squamous cell carcinoma arising from nasal vestibule. Otolaryngol Case Rep. 2020;14:100145.
21. Ereño C, Gaafar A, Garmendia M, Etxezarraga C, Bilbao FJ, López JI. Basaloid squamous cell carcinoma of the head and neck: a clinicopathological and follow-up study of 40 cases and review of the literature. Head Neck Pathol. 2008;2:83–91.
22. Lewis JS Jr. Sinonasal squamous cell carcinoma: a review with emphasis on emerging histologic subtypes and the role of human papillomavirus. Head Neck Pathol. 2016;10:60–7.
23. Durden FL Jr, Moore CE, Muller S. Verrucous carcinoma of the paranasal sinuses: a case report. Ear Nose Throat J. 2010;89:E21–3.
24. Alos L, Castillo M, Nadal A, Caballero M, Mallofre C, Palacin A, Cardesa A. Adenosquamous carcinoma of the head and neck: criteria for diagnosis in a study of 12 cases. Histopathology. 2004;44:570–9.
25. Loree TR, Mullins AP, Spellman J, North JH Jr, Hicks WL Jr. Head and neck mucosal melanoma: a 32-year review. Ear Nose Throat J. 1999;78:372–5.
26. Prasad ML, Busam KJ, Patel SG, Hoshaw-Woodard S, Shah JP, Huvos AG. Clinicopathologic differences in malignant melanoma arising in oral squamous and sinonasal respiratory mucosa of the upper aerodigestive tract. Arch Pathol Lab Med. 2003;127:997–1002.
27. Mendenhall WM, Amdur RJ, Hinerman RW, Werning JW, Villaret DB, Mendenhall NP. Head and neck mucosal melanoma. Am J Clin Oncol. 2005;28:626–30.

28. Thompson LDR, Wieneke JA, Miettinen M. Sinonasal tract and nasopharyngeal melanomas: a clinicopathologic study of 115 cases with a proposed staging system. Am J Surg Pathol. 2003;27:594–611.
29. Khatchaturian EM, Zohrabian N. A novel report of a primary Merkel cell carcinoma lesion in the nasal vestibule. Clin Case Rep. 2018;6:2033–6.
30. Becker JC, Kauczok CS, Ugurel S, Eib S, Bröcker EB, Houben R. Merkel cell carcinoma: molecular pathogenesis, clinical features and therapy. J Dtsch Dermatol Ges. 2008;6:709–19.
31. Jiang P, Lai J. Merkel cell carcinoma clinically mimicking a traumatic suture scar in the nasal vestibule: earlier diagnosis for better prognosis. Anticancer Res. 2020;40:1123–6.
32. Bussu F, Tagliaferri L, Crescio C, Rizzo D, Gallus R, Parrilla C, Fionda B, Lancellotta V, Mattiucci GC, Galli J. New standards for the management of nose vestibule malignancies. Acta Otolaryngol. 2023;143(3):215–22. https://doi.org/10.1080/00016489.2023.2179662.
33. Bussu F, Tagliaferri L, Piras A, Rizzo D, Tsatsaris N, De Corso E, Parrilla C, Paludetti G. Multidisciplinary approach to nose vestibule malignancies: setting new standards. Approccio multidisciplinare ai tumori maligni del vestibolo del naso: verso la definizione di nuovi standard. Acta Otorhinolaryngol Ital. 2021;41(Suppl. 1):S158–65. https://doi.org/10.14639/0392-100X-suppl.1-41-2021-16.
34. Gallus R, Nauta IH, Marklund L, Rizzo D, Crescio C, Mureddu L, Tropiano P, Delogu G, Bussu F. Accuracy of p16 IHC in classifying HPV-driven OPSCC in different populations. Cancers. 2023;15(3):656. https://doi.org/10.3390/cancers15030656.
35. Gallus R, Gheit T, Holzinger D, Petrillo M, Rizzo D, Petrone G, Miccichè F, Mattiucci GC, Arciuolo D, Capobianco G, Delogu G, Valentini V, Tommasino M, Bussu F. Prevalence of HPV infection and p16^{INK4a} overexpression in surgically treated laryngeal squamous cell carcinoma. Vaccines. 2022;10(2):204. https://doi.org/10.3390/vaccines10020204.
36. Bussu F, Sali M, Gallus R, Vellone VG, Zannoni GF, Autorino R, Dinapoli N, Santangelo R, Martucci R, Graziani C, Miccichè F, Almadori G, Galli J, Delogu G, Sanguinetti M, Rindi G, Valentini V, Paludetti G. HPV infection in squamous cell carcinomas arising from different mucosal sites of the head and neck region. Is p16 immunohistochemistry a reliable surrogate marker? Br J Cancer. 2013;108(5):1157–62. https://doi.org/10.1038/bjc.2013.55.
37. Boscolo-Rizzo P, Bussu F. Beware of the dangers along the path towards the diagnosis of HPV-driven oropharyngeal squamous cell carcinoma. Attenzione alle insidie riservate dalla diagnosi del carcinoma squamocellulare orofaringeo HPV-relato. Acta Otorhinolaryngol Ital. 2017;37(1):63–4. https://doi.org/10.14639/0392-100X-1323.
38. Bussu F, Sali M, Gallus R, Petrone G, Autorino R, Santangelo R, Pandolfini M, Miccichè F, Delogu G, Almadori G, Galli J, Sanguinetti M, Rindi G, Tommasino M, Valentini V, Paludetti G. HPV and EBV infections in neck metastases from occult primary squamous cell carcinoma: another virus-related neoplastic disease in the head and neck region. Ann Surg Oncol. 2015;22(S3):979–84. https://doi.org/10.1245/s10434-015-4808-5.
39. Bussu F, Ragin C, Boscolo-Rizzo P, Rizzo D, Gallus R, Delogu G, Morbini P, Tommasino M. HPV as a marker for molecular characterization in head and neck oncology: looking for a standardization of clinical use and of detection method(s) in clinical practice. Head Neck. 2019;41(4):1104–11. https://doi.org/10.1002/hed.25591.

Peculiar Patterns of Spread of Nose Vestibule Malignancies

3

Francesco Bussu, Davide Rizzo, Pierangela Tramaloni, Mario Rigante, Nicola Tsatsaris, Massimo Ralli, Roberto Gallus, and Livio Presutti

F. Bussu · D. Rizzo (✉)
Otolaryngology Division, Azienda Ospedaliera Universitaria di Sassari, Sassari University Hospital, Sassari, Italy

Department of Medicine, Surgery and Pharmacy, University of Sassari, Sassari, Italy
e-mail: fbussu@uniss.it; davide.rizzo@aouss.it; drizzo@uniss.it

P. Tramaloni
Otolaryngology Division, Azienda Ospedaliera Universitaria di Sassari, Sassari University Hospital, Sassari, Italy
e-mail: pierangela.tramaloni@aouss.it

M. Rigante
Unit of Otorhinolaryngology, "A. Gemelli" University Hospital Foundation, IRCCS, Rome, Italy

N. Tsatsaris
Medicine Faculty, University of Sassari, Sassari, Italy

M. Ralli
Dipartimento di Organi di Senso, Sapienza Università di Roma, Rome, Italy
e-mail: massimo.ralli@uniroma1.it

R. Gallus
Otolaryngology Division, Mater Olbia Hospital, Olbia, Italy
e-mail: roberto.gallus@materolbia.com

L. Presutti
Department of Specialist, Diagnostic and Experimental Medicine, University of Bologna, Bologna, Italy
e-mail: livio.presutti@unibo.it

© Springer Nature Switzerland AG 2023
F. Bussu (ed.), *Malignancies of the Nasal Vestibule*,
https://doi.org/10.1007/978-3-031-32850-3_3

3.1   Introduction

The nose vestibule is defined as that part of the anterior nasal cavity that is lined by squamous epithelium up to the limen nasi, which is the muco-cutaneous junction [1]. The framework of the nose vestibule is given mostly by the cartilages of the nose tip (see Chap. 1). The section of the nose vestibule, both in the coronal and in the axial plane, is triangular (Fig. 3.1), so that three walls can be easily identified,

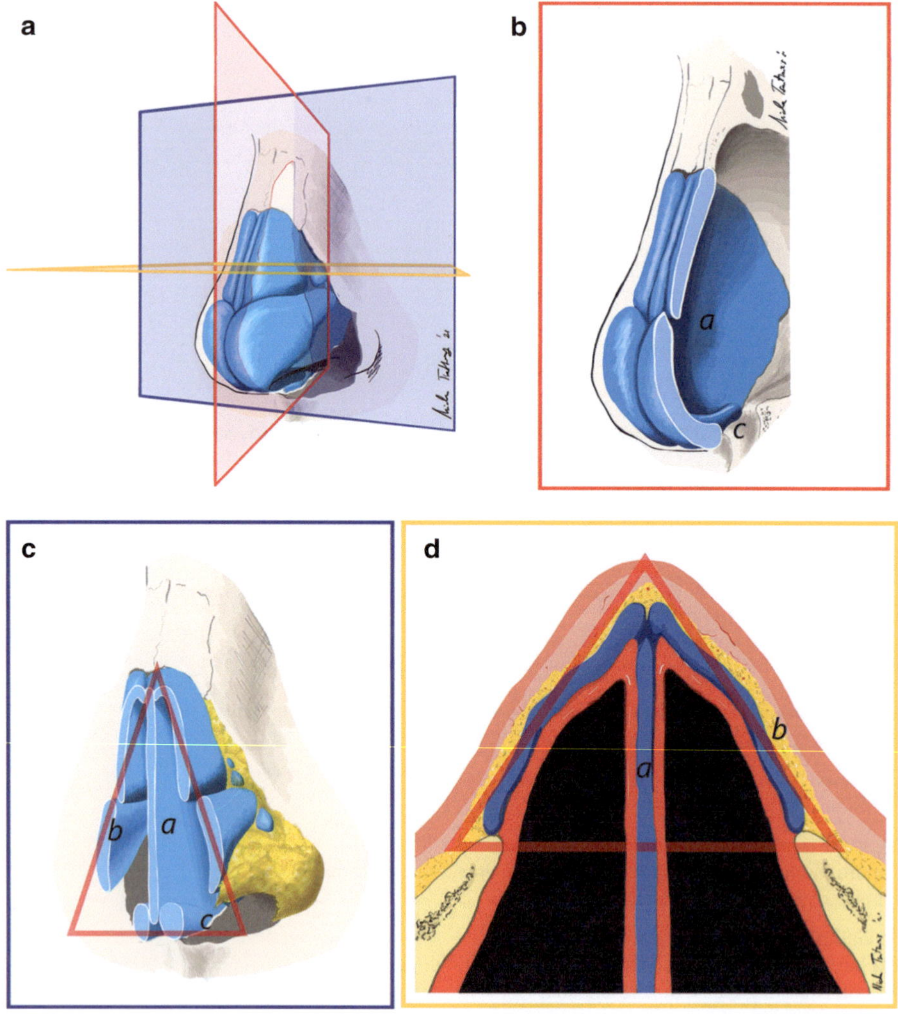

Fig. 3.1 Nose vestibule along the three planes (**a**), and in particular sagittal (**b**), coronal (**c**), and axial (**d**). The three layers of the nasal wall are evident (mucosa in red, cartilage in blue, skin and subcutaneous in pink/yellow) (**d**)

and namely the "columella/septum" (a), the "ala/limen nasi"(b), the "floor of nasal cavity/superior lip" (c) [2].

With the novel boundaries proposed for the nose vestibule (see Chap. 1, Fig. 3.2), medial and lateral wall areas are much larger than with the previous anatomical boundaries, while the inferior wall (floor of nasal cavity) still has almost no antero-posterior extension (Fig. 3.2).

The patterns of spread of primary tumors, and in particular carcinomas, arising in and/or involving each given nose vestibule wall are pretty typical and can be understood and predicted through the knowledge of anatomy and histology of the area. To this aim, the clinician should consider the anatomy of the nose tip tridimensionally with a clear knowledge of each tissue comprised and of its features, ultrastructure, and mutual relationships, as critical determinants of tumor spread.

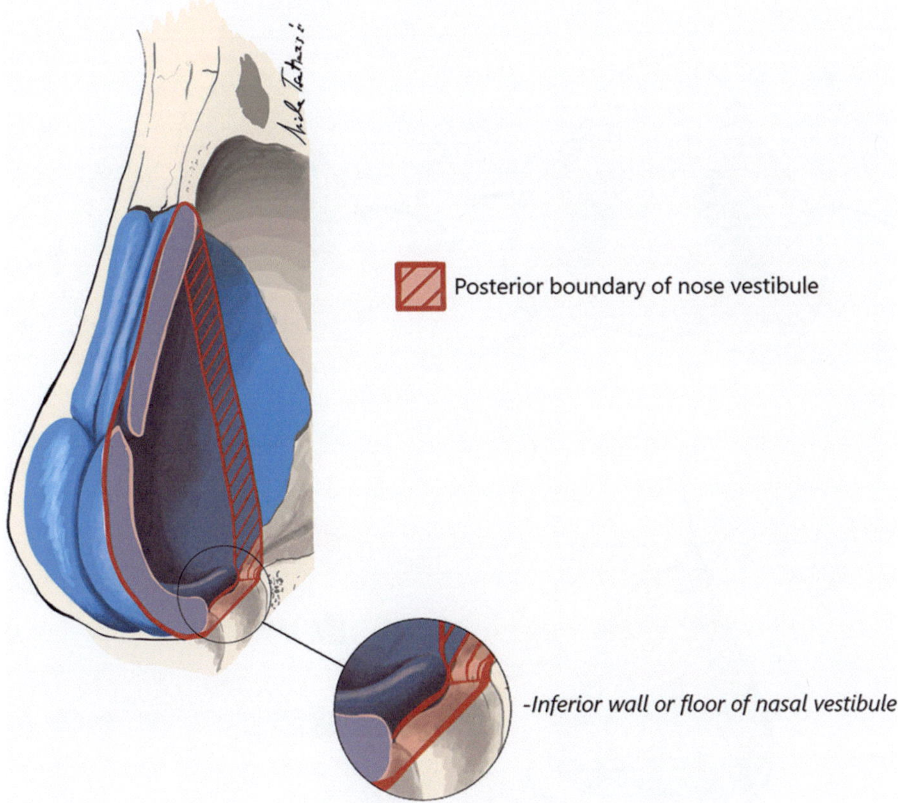

Fig. 3.2 Inferior wall of the nose vestibule is the smallest and is in continuity with the floor of nasal cavity proper posteriorly and with the filter and superior lip anteriorly

3.2   Determinants of Tumor Spread from the Nose Vestibule

In fact, every structure in the nose tip has its own histology with typical features in terms of vascularization patterns, consistency, and contribution to the function and appearance of the nose and, most of all, resistance to tumor spread and infiltration. In turn tumor spread results from tridimensional anatomy and mutual relationship (morphology) of such structures and from their own peculiar histologic features. The structures that make up the nose tip are: cartilages, internal lining (from which nose vestibule primaries arise), which includes the respiratory mucosa, transition area, and skin, "external" skin, and connective tissue.

Three main cartilages can be identified, one median (in common with the two nostrils), the septal cartilage, two lateral and paired, the alar and the lateral cartilages (Fig. 3.3). Cartilages are connected by fibrous tissue, mutually and with nasal and maxillary bones at the level of the pyriform aperture (posterior border of the

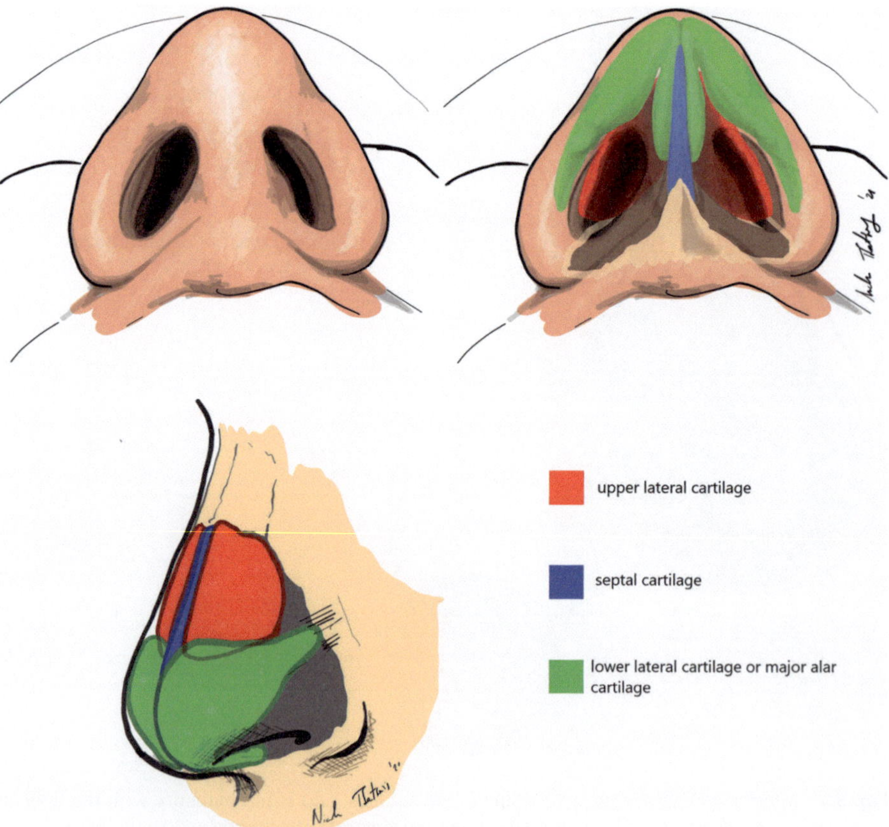

Fig. 3.3 Cartilages of the nose tip

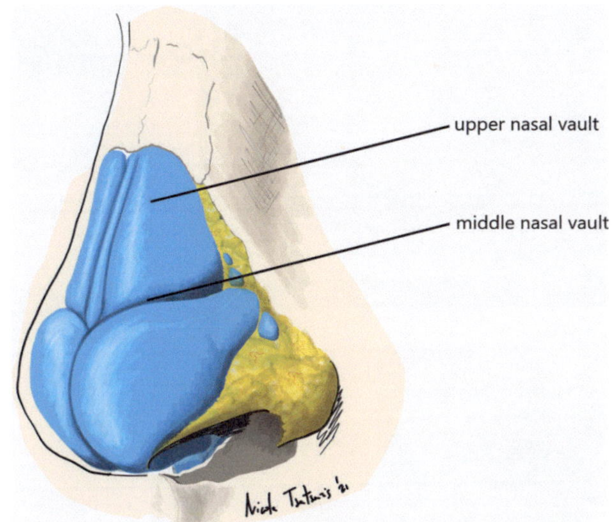

Fig. 3.4 Hard external framework of the nose

nose vestibule itself) and more posteriorly with vomer and ethmoid bone. Cartilages and bones make up the external "hard framework" of the nose (Fig. 3.4), mostly accounting, as nose surgeons know well, for its complex tridimensional shape with a number of typical small hollows and relieves. The hard framework is covered externally by thin skin, internally by the internal lining with its transition from the skin to respiratory mucosa.

It is well known also from laryngeal oncology [3] that cartilage itself is particularly resistant to tumor invasion also because it is devoid of blood vessels and fed through the interstitium by direct diffusion from vascularized perichondrium [4]. In fact, as blood vessels are brought in by ossification, the probability of invasion drastically increases. Nose cartilages, differently from laryngeal ones, and thyroid cartilage in particular, do not usually get ossified even in the elderly, and in fact, direct invasion is very late in nose vestibule SCCs. Cartilages can be surrounded by malignant growth before being disrupted or even infiltrated, and the destruction of cartilage is probably most often caused by the extensive invasion of perichondrium and interruption of perichondral feeding, more than by cancer invasion itself. This fact together with the resistance of nose cartilages to irradiation [2, 5–9] contributes to the possibility to restore the cosmetic appearance after radiotherapy (and especially brachytherapy) for NV malignancies, even when the framework of the tip appears surrounded by tumor growth, through "selective" preservation of cartilages (Fig. 3.5).

This also implies that preferential patterns of spread of nose vestibule SCC follow cartilagineous surfaces, practically sliding along them.

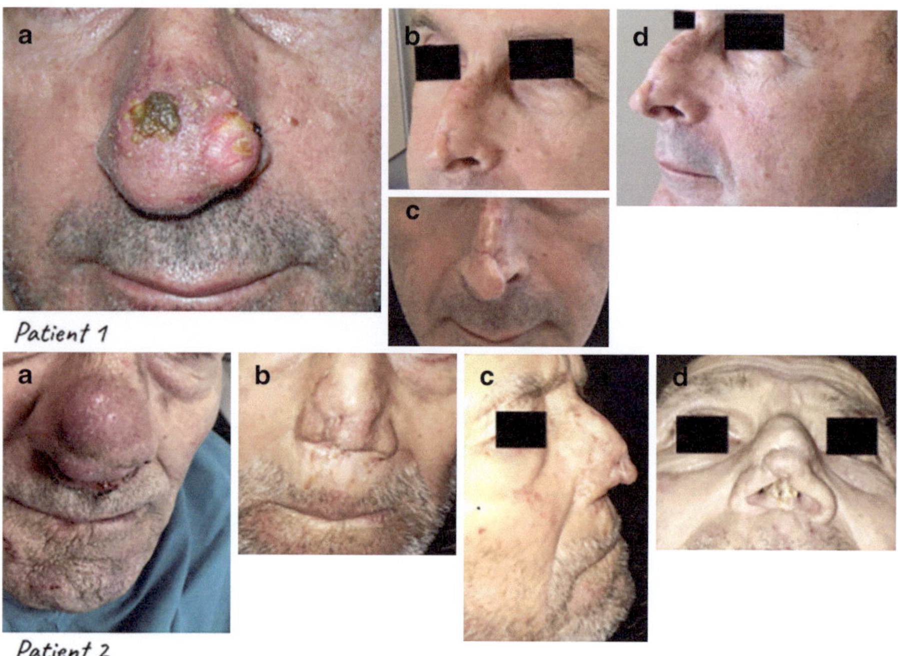

Fig. 3.5 Two patients before and after brachytherapy. Patient 1 and Patent 2: (**a**) before brachiteraphy and (**b, c, d**) after brachiteraphy. In patient 1, the cartilage scaffold is preserved despite the massive tumor growth, in patient 2 tumor destroyed part of the septal and alar cartilages, but irradiation through plastic tubes did not cause any additional destruction to the framework

3.3 Typical Patterns of Spread from the Lateral Wall

Tumors of the lateral wall of the nose vestibule arise from the internal lining (Fig. 3.6) of the fibroareolar "soft" tissue of the ala (a), of the crus lateralis of the alar cartilage (b), of the upper lateral cartilage (c).

The fibroareolar soft tissue of the ala is "de facto" subcutaneous tissue, so that there are no barriers to the external skin, which has to be considered always involved if the primary lesion arises at this level (a very rare event) (the fibroareolar soft tissue is marked by an italic *a* in the panel A of Fig. 3.6).

Most frequently, the primary tumors of the lateral wall of the vestibule arise in correspondence of the alar cartilages (marked by an italic b in the panel A of figure Fig. 3.6 and clearly evident in the case showed in Fig. 3.7); in these cases, they tend to slide along the deep surface of the crus lateralis up to the nasal valve, which is the junction between the alar and lateral cartilages, where nose surgeons perform the intercartilagineous incision in rhinoseptoplasty. As surgeons know well and experience in their daily practice when performing their intercartilagineous incisions, the upper border of the alar cartilage lies superficial to the inferior border of the lateral

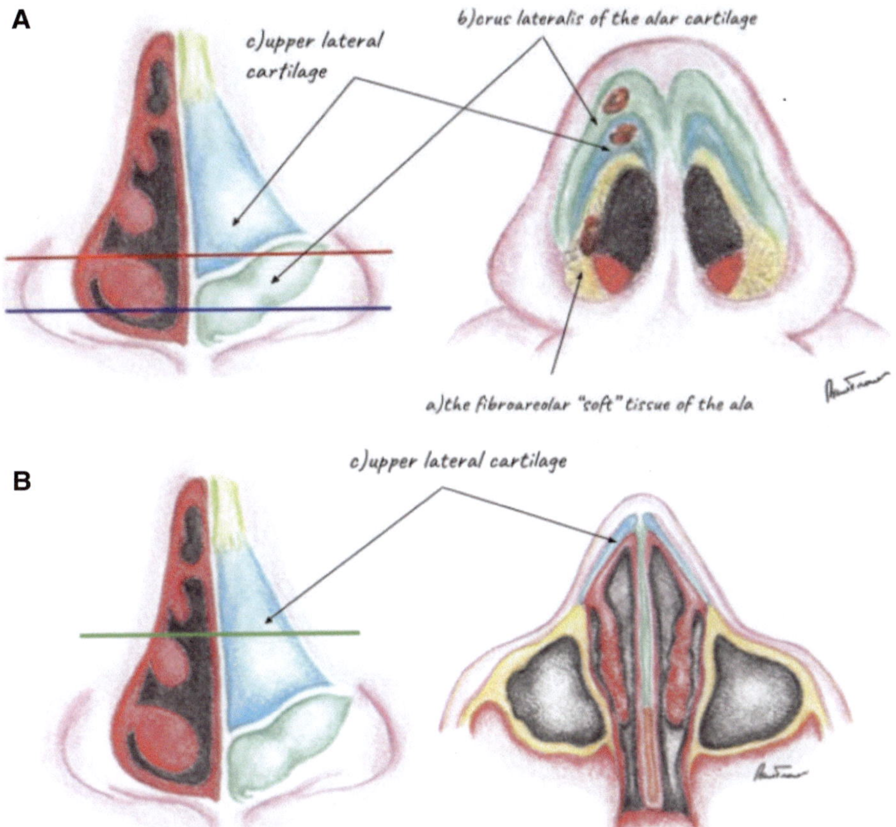

Fig. 3.6 (**A**) Inferior view from the nostrils of different areas in the lateral wall of the nose vestibule. (**B**) Sectional view at the level of lateral cartilage of the upper part of the nasal vestibule

cartilage, allowing easy access to the surface of middle and upper nasal vault (Figs. 3.4 and 3.7).

Less frequently, primary vestibular lesions arise more cranially from the internal lining of the lateral alar cartilage (c) upper lateral cartilage in Fig. 3.6); also in these cases, the tumors run upward and posteriorly along the deep surface of the cartilage to the junction with maxillary and nasal bones and tend to reach the skin at this level passing between the cartilages and bones (Fig. 3.8).

In our experience, these cases are less favorable both for the potential invasion of bone (which is vascularized and notoriously much less resistant than cartilage to tumor infiltration) and for the posterior spread along the internal lining beyond the plane of the pyriform aperture, which makes interstitial interventional radiotherapy more difficult (see Chaps. 1, 5, and 13).

In any case, skin involvement of the ala or of the tip of the nose is almost constant for all the primary locations (Figs. 3.5, 3.6, 3.7, and 3.8) in the lateral wall of the vestibule.

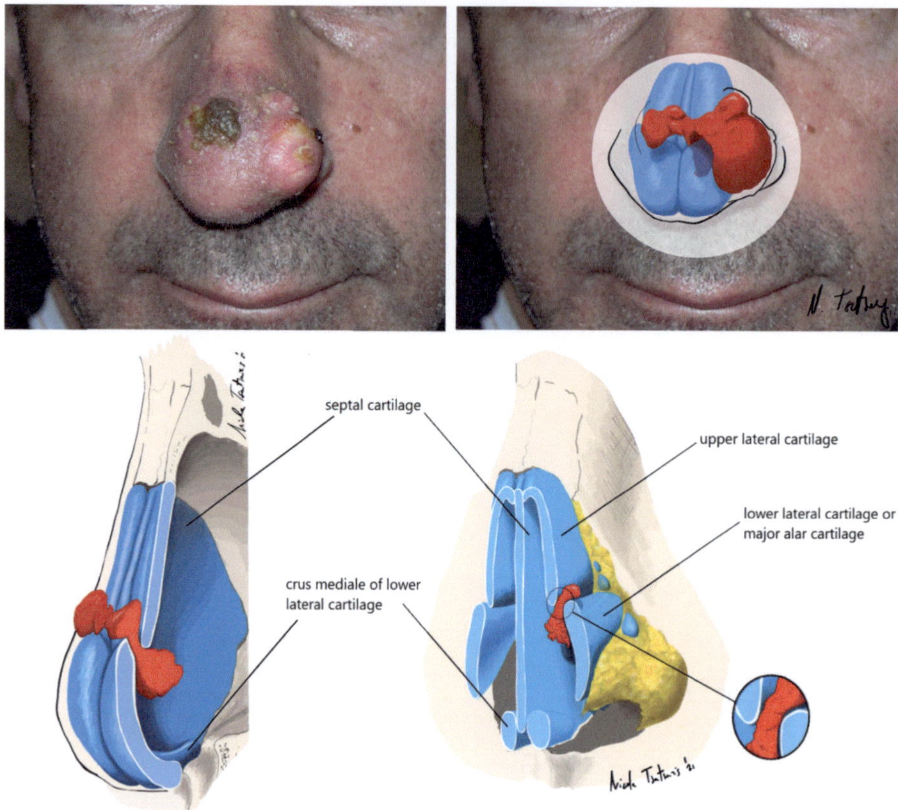

Fig. 3.7 Typical pattern of spread between alar and lateral cartilages

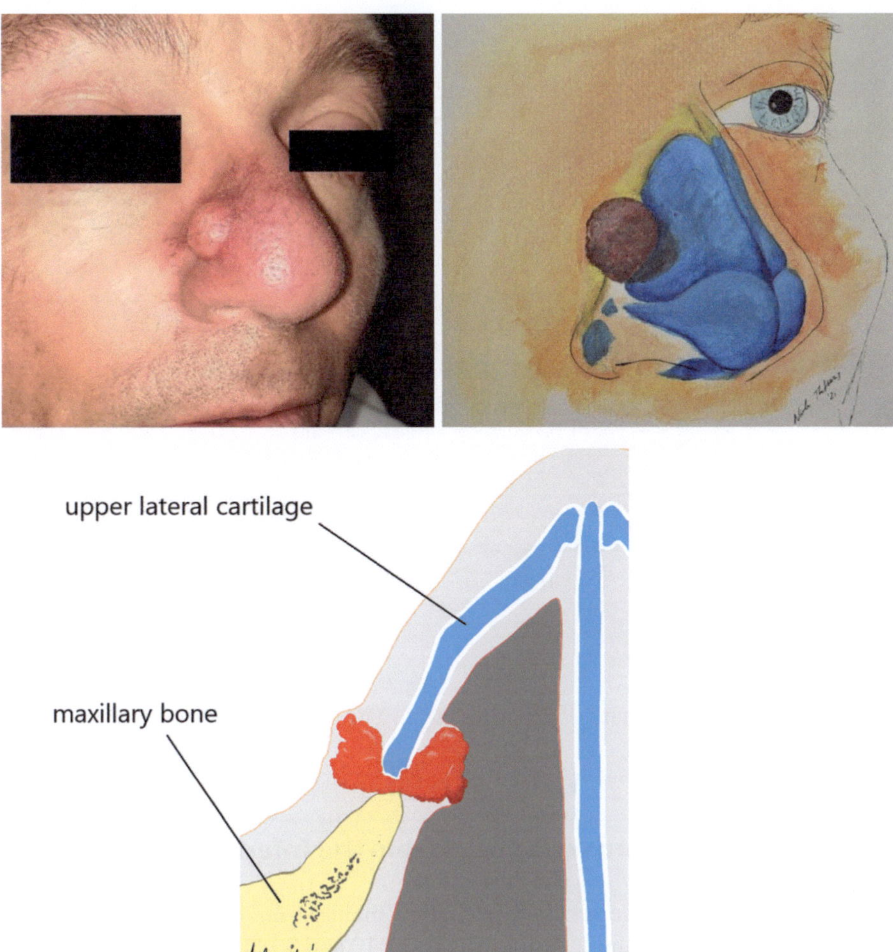

Fig. 3.8 A less frequent case: the visible lesion on the skin arises from the internal surface of the lateral alar cartilage, and from here it comes to invade the skin

3.4 Typical Patterns of Spread from the Medial Wall

When a primary lesion of the medial wall of the vestibule spreads posteriorly, it typically runs along the septal cartilage (Fig. 3.9). For the above cited cartilage resistance, septal perforation is rare except in very bulky primaries or as a consequence of extensive tissue sampling during a diagnostic biopsy. Such posterior spread is not an issue until it remains within the anatomical limits of the nose vestibule (anterior to the coronal plane of pyriform aperture) (Fig. 3.9). Septal/columellar primaries can also share the inferior pattern of spread of inferior wall primaries.

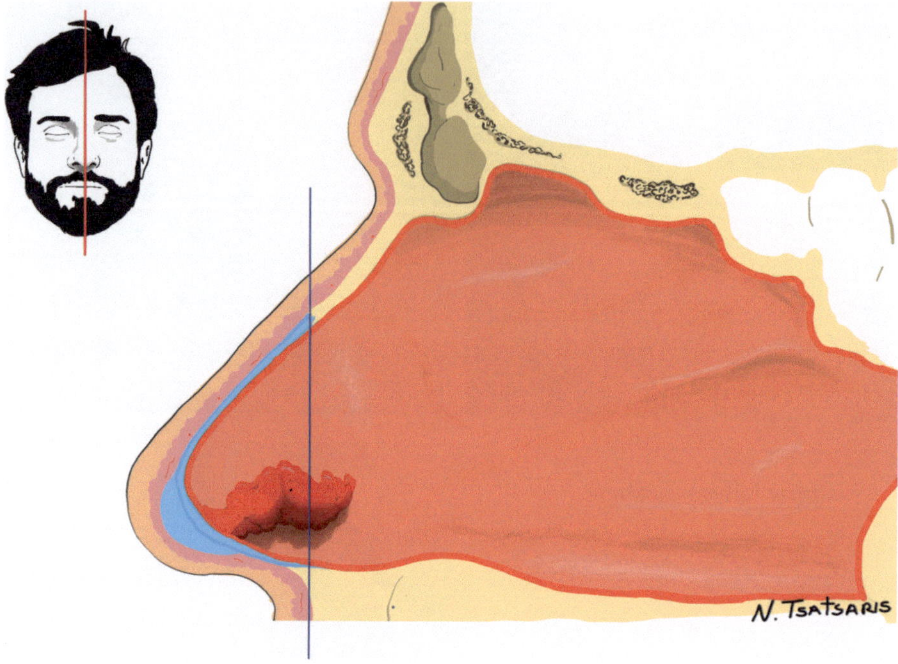

Fig. 3.9 Posterior spread from the septum leading to a cT3 lesion according to our newly proposed T classification

3.5 Typical Patterns of Spread from the Inferior Wall

The inferior spread of nose vestibule primaries (mainly from the inferior and medial walls) typically involves the superior lip (Figs. 3.10 and 3.11). It is therefore another typical route for skin invasion in nose vestibule malignancies.

Primaries of the inferior wall can also spread posteriorly; in this case, as the anteroposterior dimension of the inferior wall is minimal (see Fig. 3.2), it is associated to two orders of issues:

- invasion of the nasal spine and/or of the hard palate with bone involvement (Fig. 3.12), which determines an upstaging according to Wang classification and to our newly proposed T classification [10–12], and most probably a prognostic impairment;
- overcoming of the plane of the pyriform opening, the newly proposed posterior limit of the nose vestibule (Fig. 3.9), which in our opinion should determine an upstaging of the lesion as well (see Chap. 5) as it determines clear issues for treatment by exclusive interstitial brachytherapy (see Chap. 12), which is being demonstrated to be a valuable option in this group of malignancies [10–12].

Fig. 3.10 A typical route of invasion involving the upper lip

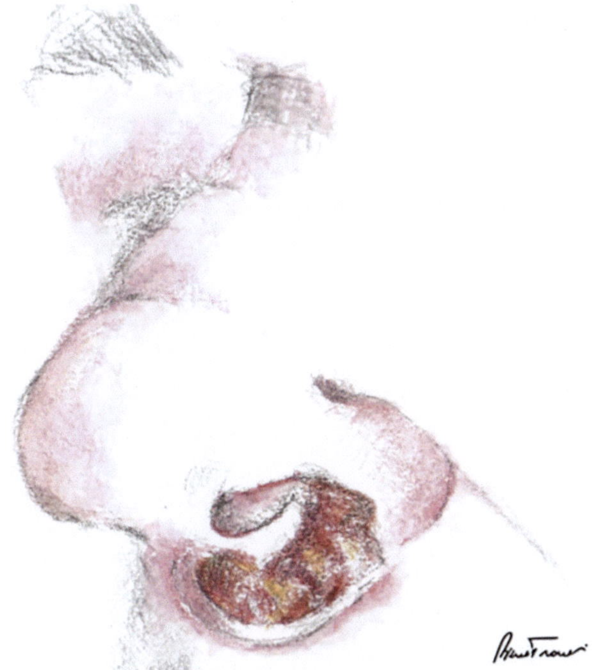

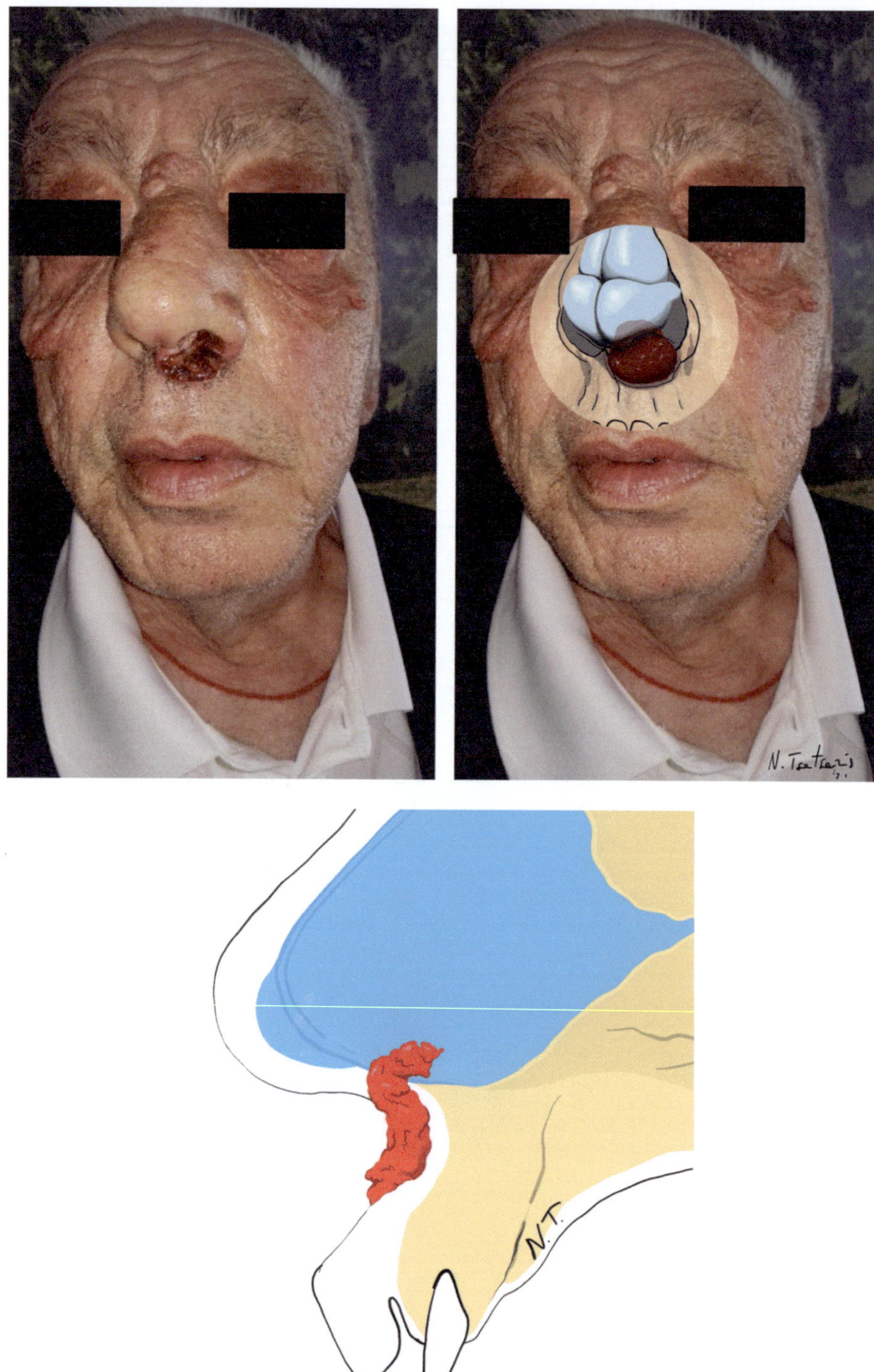

Fig. 3.11 The tumor invades the filter and runs to the upper lip

Fig. 3.12 Inferior spread: invasion of the nasal spine and/or hard palate

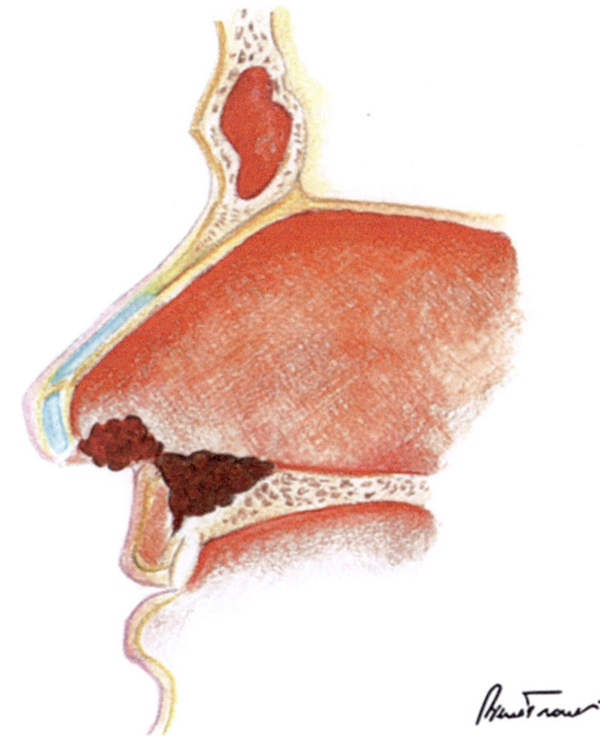

References

1. Jeannon J-P, Riddle PJ, Irish J, O'sullivan B, Brown DH, Gullane P. Prognostic indicators in carcinoma of the nasal vestibule. Clin Otolaryngol. 2007;32:19–23.
2. Bussu F, Tagliaferri L, Mattiucci G, et al. Comparison of interstitial brachytherapy and surgery as primary treatments for nasal vestibule carcinomas. Laryngoscope. 2016;126:367–71.
3. Mor N, Blitzer A. Functional anatomy and oncologic barriers of the larynx. Otolaryngol Clin North Am. 2015;48:533–45.
4. Sandell LJ. Novel functions for type II procollagen. Connect Tissue Res. 2014;55:20–5.
5. Caccialanza M, Piccinno R, Percivalle S, Rozza M. Radiotherapy of carcinomas of the skin overlying the cartilage of the nose: our experience in 671 lesions. J Eur Acad Dermatol Venereol. 2009;23:1044–9.
6. Caccialanza M, Piccinno R, Moretti D, Rozza M. Radiotherapy of carcinomas of the skin overlying the cartilage of the nose: results in 405 lesions. Eur J Dermatol. 2003;13:462–5.
7. Caccialanza M, Piccinno R, Gaiani F, Contini D. Relevance of dermatologic radiotherapy in the therapeutic strategy of skin epithelial neoplasms: excellent results in the treatment of lesions localized on eyelids and skin overlying the cartilage of the nose. G Ital Dermatol Venereol. 2013;148:83–8.
8. Caccialanza M, Bertani E, Piccinno R, Rozza M, Brambilla R, Percivalle S. Radiotherapy of T4 squamous cell carcinoma of the skin of nasal pyramid. J Eur Acad Dermatol Venereol. 2006;0:060606032107062.
9. Bussu F, Tagliaferri L, De Corso E, et al. Functional results of exclusive interventional radiotherapy (brachytherapy) in the treatment of nasal vestibule carcinomas. Brachytherapy. 2021;20:178–84.

10. Bussu F, Tagliaferri L, Piras A, Rizzo D, Tsatsaris N, De Corso E, Parrilla C, Paludetti G. Multidisciplinary approach to nose vestibule malignancies: setting new standards approccio multidisciplinare ai tumori maligni del vestibolo del naso: verso la definizione di nuovi standard. Acta Otorhinolaryngol Ital. 2021;41(1):S158–S165. https://doi.org/10.14639/0392-100X-suppl.1-41-2021-16.
11. Bussu F. New standards for the management of nose vestibule malignancies. Acta Oto-Laryngologica. 2023;143(3):215–22. https://doi.org/10.1080/00016489.2023.2179662.
12. Scheurleer WFJ, Tagliaferri L, Rijken JA, Crescio C, Rizzo D, Mattiucci GC, Pameijer FA, de Bree R, Fionda B, de Ridder M, Bussu F. Evaluation of staging systems for cancer of the nasal vestibule. Cancers. 2023;15(11):3028. https://doi.org/10.3390/cancers15113028.

Current Staging Systems for Nose Vestibule Malignancies

4

Antonio Piras, Davide Rizzo, Emilia Degni, Claudia Crescio, Alessia Re, Giovanni Maria Fadda, Giancarlo Mattiucci, and Antonio Pazzola

4.1 Introduction

4.1.1 Principles of TNM Classification

In the management of cancer, an accurate and reliable staging of the tumor holds the key to successful treatment strategies, to the prediction of clinical outcomes, and to international communication.

The tumor-node-metastasis (TNM) staging system describes the anatomic extent of the primary tumor (T) as well as the involvement of the regional lymph nodes (N) and distant metastasis (M). It should be based on a thorough knowledge of the natural history of tumors at various sites and subsites and on a clear definition of

A. Piras · D. Rizzo (✉)
Otolaryngology Division, Sassari University Hospital, Sassari, Italy

Department of Medicine, Surgery and Pharmacy, University of Sassari, Sassari, Italy
e-mail: davide.rizzo@aouss.it; drizzo@uniss.it

E. Degni · C. Crescio
Otolaryngology Division, Sassari University Hospital, Sassari, Italy
e-mail: emilia.degni@aouss.it; claudia.crescio@aouss.it

A. Re
Radiation Oncology Unit, Mater Olbia Hospital, Olbia, Italy

G. M. Fadda · A. Pazzola
Medical Oncology Division, Sassari University Hospital, Sassari, Italy
e-mail: giovanni.fadda@aouss.it; antonio.pazzola@aouss.it

G. Mattiucci
Radiation Oncology Unit, Mater Olbia Hospital, Olbia, Italy

Università Cattolica del Sacro Cuore, Istituto di Radiologia, Rome, Italy
e-mail: giancarlo.mattiucci@unicatt.it

© Springer Nature Switzerland AG 2023
F. Bussu (ed.), *Malignancies of the Nasal Vestibule*,
https://doi.org/10.1007/978-3-031-32850-3_4

prognostic parameters, as it is expected, first of all, to properly stratify prognosis and hence to guide therapeutic decision.

TNM was developed and is periodically updated by the Union for International Cancer Control (UICC). It is also used by the American Joint Committee on Cancer (AJCC) and by the International Federation of Gynecology and Obstetrics (FIGO). In 1987, the UICC and AJCC staging systems were unified into a single TNM staging system. The generation of scientific evidence leads to continuous updates in the TNM system for all the malignancies.

4.1.2 Current UICC/AJCC TNM Classification for Nose and Paranasal Sinuses Malignancies

Like many other cancers, a fully satisfying stratification of nose/paranasal malignancies has been challenging, mainly because of the numerous anatomic sites and subsites from which tumors can arise and because of the heterogeneity of histologic types that show different clinical behavior and outcomes.

T classification of nose and paranasal sinuses follows two different orders of criteria for maxillary sinus primaries on the one hand and nasal cavities/ethmoid primaries on the other (Tables 4.1 and 4.2).

Many histotypes exist and are also acknowledged as key factors when determining the prognosis. Melanoma, lymphoma, and sarcoma are not included in the UICC/AJCC staging of nose/paranasal sinuses primaries.

The nasoethmoidal complex is divided into two subsites: the nasal cavity and the ethmoid sinuses. The ethmoids are further subdivided into two subsites: left and right, separated by the nasal septum (perpendicular plate of ethmoid). The nasal

Table 4.1 UICC/AJCC 2017, Eighth Edition. Classification of Primary Tumor (T): Maxillary Sinus

T category	T criteria
TX	Primary tumor cannot be assessed
Tis	Carcinoma in situ
T1	Tumor limited to maxillary sinus mucosa with no erosion or destruction of bone
T2	Tumor causing bone erosion or destruction including extension into the hard palate and/or middle nasal meatus, except extension to posterior wall of maxillary sinus and pterygoid plates
T3	Tumor invades any of the following: bone of the posterior wall of the maxillary sinus, subcutaneous tissues, floor or medial wall of orbit, pterygoid fossa, ethmoid sinuses
T4	Moderately advanced or very advanced local disease
• T4a	Moderately advanced local disease Tumor invades anterior orbital contents, skin of cheek, pterygoid plates, infratemporal fossa, cribriform plate, sphenoid or frontal sinuses
• T4b	Very advances local disease Tumor invades any of the following: orbital apex, dura, brain, middle cranial fossa, cranial nerves other than maxillary division of trigeminal nerve (V2), nasopharynx or clivus

Table 4.2 UICC/AJCC 2017, Eighth Edition. Classification of Primary Tumor (T): Nasal cavity and ethmoid sinus

T category	T criteria
TX	Primary tumor cannot be assessed
Tis	Carcinoma in situ
T1	Tumor restricted to any one subsite, with or without bony invasion
T2	Tumor invading two subsites in a single region or extending to involve an adjacent region within the nasoethmoidal complex, with or without bony invasion
T3	Tumor extends to invade the medial wall or floor of the orbit, maxillary sinus, palate, or cribriform plate
T4	Moderately advanced or very advanced local disease
• T4a	Moderately advanced local disease Tumor invades any of the following: anterior orbital contents, skin of the nose or cheek, minimal extension to anterior cranial fossa, pterygoid plates, sphenoid or frontal sinuses
• T4b	Very advanced local disease Tumor invades any of the following: orbital apex, dura, brain, middle cranial fossa, cranial nerves other than maxillary division of trigeminal nerve (V2), nasopharynx or clivus

cavity is divided into four subsites: the septum, the floor, the lateral wall, and the edge of the naris to the mucocutaneous junction, but without any differences in the definition of c- and/or p-T between such different subsites, which are all included in the same topographic code C30.0 (Tables 4.5 and 4.6).

4.1.3 Evolution of UICC/AJCC TNM of Nose and Paranasal Sinus

The current complete 8th UICC/AJCC staging system (2017) for maxillary sinus and nasoethmoid lesions is therefore shown in Tables 4.1, 4.2, 4.3, and 4.4 [1].

The T category (Tables 4.1 and 4.2) is identical to the UICC/AJCC Cancer Staging Manual 7th edition (2009) [2], according to the changes introduced in the 6th edition (2002) concerning the classification of the nasal cavity and paranasal malignancies [3]. Here a new site, the nasal cavity (C30.0), was added for inclusion into the staging system of nose malignancies. In the 6th UICC/AJCC edition, in addition to maxillary sinus, the nasal cavity was merged with the ethmoid in the same T classification, forming the nasoethmoid complex, divided into two regions: the nasal cavity (four subsites: septum, floor, lateral wall, and vestibule) and the ethmoid sinuses (two subsites: right and left).

The sites in this classification are listed by code numbers of the International Classification of Diseases for oncology (Chapter 2 of the 2019 edition of the ICD-10-CM, World Health Organization) [4] (Tables 4.5 and 4.6).

As shown, the nasal vestibule (NV) is included in C30.0 code, the same "billable" ICD code used to specify a diagnosis of malignant neoplasm everywhere in the nasal cavity, considering NV only an unspecified subsite of the nasal cavity [5, 6].

Table 4.3 Definition of regional lymph node (N): Clinical N (cN)

N category	N criteria
NX	Regional lymph nodes cannot be assessed
N0	No regional lymph node metastasis
N1	Metastasis in a single ipsilateral lymph node, 3 cm or smaller in greatest dimension and ENE (−)
N2	Metastasis in a single ipsilateral node larger than 3 cm but no larger than 6 cm in greatest dimension and ENE (−); or metastasis in multiple ipsilateral lymph node, none larger than 6 cm in greatest dimension and ENE (−); or in bilateral or contralateral lymph nodes, none larger than 6 cm in greatest dimension and ENE (−)
• N2a	Metastasis in a single ipsilateral node larger than 3 cm but no larger than 6 cm in greatest dimension and ENE (−)
• N2b	Metastasis in multiple ipsilateral lymph node, none larger than 6 cm in greatest dimension and ENE (−)
• N2c	Metastasis in bilateral or contralateral lymph nodes, none larger than 6 cm in greatest dimension and ENE (−)
N3	Metastasis in a lymph node larger than 6 cm in greatest dimension and ENE (−); or metastasis in any node(s) with clinically overt ENE (+)
• N3a	Metastasis in a lymph node larger than 6 cm in greatest dimension and ENE (−)
• N3b	Metastasis in any node(s) with clinically overt ENE (+)

ENE extranodal extension

Table 4.4 Definition of regional lymph node (N): Pathological N (pN)

N category	N criteria
NX	Regional lymph nodes cannot be assessed
N0	No regional lymph node metastasis
N1	Metastasis in a single ipsilateral lymph node, 3 cm or smaller in greatest dimension and ENE (−)
N2	Metastasis in a single ipsilateral node, 3 cm or smaller in greatest dimension and ENE (+); or larger than 3 cm but no larger than 6 cm in greatest dimension and ENE (−); or metastasis in multiple ipsilateral lymph node, none larger than 6 cm in greatest dimension and ENE (−); or in bilateral or contralateral lymph nodes, none larger than 6 cm in greatest dimension and ENE (−)
• N2a	Metastasis in single ipsilateral or contralateral node 3 cm or less in greatest dimensión and ENE(+); or a single ipsilateral node larger than 3 cm but not larger than 6 cm in greatest dimensión and E N E (−)
• N2b	Metastasis in multiple ipsilateral lymph node, none larger than 6 cm in greatest dimension and ENE (−)
• N2c	Metastasis in bilateral or contralateral lymph nodes, none larger than 6 cm in greatest dimension and ENE (−)
N3	Metastasis in a lymph node larger than 6 cm in greatest dimension and ENE (−); or in a single ipsilateral node larger than 3 cm in greatest dimension and ENE (+); or multiple ipsilateral, contralateral or bilateral node, any with ENE (+)
• N3a	Metastasis in a lymph node larger than 6 cm in greatest dimension and ENE (−)
• N3b	Metastasis in a single ipsilateral node larger than 3 cm in greatest dimension and ENE (+); or multiple ipsilateral, contralateral or bilateral nodes, ant with ENE (+)

Table 4.5 Anatomical sites and subsites

Site	ICD code number	Subsite
Nasal cavity	(C30.0)	Septum Floor Lateral Wall Vestibule
Maxillary sinus	(C31.0)	
Ethmoid sinus	(C31.1)	Left Right

Table 4.6 Coding notes for C30.0

Inclusion terms:
– *Malignant Neoplasm Of Cartilagine Of Nose*
– *Malignant Neoplasm Of Nasal Concha*
– *Malignant Neoplasm Of Internal Nose*
– *Malignant Neoplasm Of Septum Of Nose*
– *Malignant Neoplasm Of Vestibule Of Nose*
Code Type-1 excluded
– *Malignant Neoplasm Of Nasal Bone (Instead, Use Code C41.0)*
– *Malignant Neoplasm Of Nose Nos (Instead, Use Code C76.0)*
– *Malignant Neoplasm Of Olfactory Bulb (Instead, Use Code C72.2)*
– *Malignant Neoplasm Of Posterior Margin Of Nasal Septum And Choana (Instead, Use Code C11.3)*
– *Malignant Neoplasm Of Skin Of Nose (Instead, Use Code C43.31)*
– *Malignant Neoplasm Of Turbinates (Instead, Use Code C41.0)*
– *Other And Unspecified Malignant Neoplasm Of Skin Of Nose 44.301, C44.311, C44.321, C44.391 (Instead, Use Code C44.301)*

In the eighth edition of UICC/AJCC Cancer Staging Manual, as in other head and neck sites, the N category for nasal and parasinuses malignancies was expanded to incorporate extranodal extension (ENE) (Tables 4.3 and 4.4); no changes were made for T classification.

4.1.4 Alternative Staging Systems for Nose Vestibule Malignancies

The nasal vestibule represents a subsite of the nose, defined as that part of the anterior nasal cavity lined by squamous epithelium up to the limen nasi, which corresponds to the junction of the lower and upper lateral cartilages, as well as to the mucocutaneous transition [7]. As a result of this anatomic location, nasal vestibule

Table 4.7 UICC/AJCC 1997, Fifth Edition, Non-melanoma skin cancer classification. Definition of primary tumor (T)

T category	T criteria
T1	Primary tumour 2 cm or less in maximum diameter
T2	Greater than 2 cm but no more than 5 cm in maximum diameter
T3	Greater than 5 cm in maximum diameter
T4	Invasion of cartilagine, bone or nerves
• T4 favourable	Less than 4 cm with no bone invasion
• T4 unfavourable	$\geq$ 4 cm with invasion of the premaxilla or the bone septum

Table 4.8 Staging of the primary lesions of the nose vestibule according to Wang

T1	The lesion is limited to the nasal vestibule, relatively superficial, involving one or more sites within
T2	The lesion has extended from the nasal vestibule to its adjacent structures, such as the upper nasal septum, upper lip, philtrum, skin of the nose and/or nasolabial fold, but not fixed to the underlying bone
T3	The lesion has become massive with extension to the hard palate, buccogingival sulcus, large portion of the upper lip, upper nasal septum, turbinate and/or adjacent paranasal sinuses, fixed with deep muscle and bone involvement

malignancies show distinct histological and, most of all, clinical features (see Chap. 3).

Such peculiarities lead many oncologists, who deal with nose vestibule malignancies, to use different classifications, such as the UICC/AJCC classification for non-melanoma skin cancers (Table 4.7) [8–10]. We do not deem it acceptable as the nose vestibule is part of the nasal cavity and not of the cutaneous surfaces.

Nevertheless, the T classification proposed by Wang [11] back in 1976 specifically for nose vestibule carcinomas was reported in different series to predict survival better than the UICC/AJCC classification itself (Table 4.8) [9, 10, 12–20]. For

Table 4.9 The comparison of different T classification in the three named staging systems

	UICC/AJCC staging for tumors of nasal cavity and ethmoid (2017, eighth edition)	UICC/AJCC staging for non melanoma skin cancer (1997, fifth edition)	T nose vestibule Wang' s classification
T1	Tumor restricted to any one subsite, with or without bony invasion	Primary tumour 2 cm or less in maximum diameter	The lesion is limited to the nasal vestibule, relatively superficial, involving one or more sites within
T2	Tumor invading two subsites in a single region or extending to involve an adjacent region within the nasoethmoidal complex, with or without bony invasion	Greater than 2 cm but no more than 5 cm in maximum diameter	The lesion has extended from the nasal vestibule to its adjacent structures, such as the upper nasal septum, upper lip, philtrum, skin of the nose and/or nasolabial fold, but not fixed to the underlying bone
T3	Tumor extends to invade the medial wall or floor of the orbit, maxillary sinus, palate, or cribriform plate	Greater than 5 cm in maximum diameter	The lesion has become massive with extension to the hard palate, buccogingival sulcus, large portion of the upper lip, upper nasal septum, turbinate and/or adjacent paranasal sinuses, fixed with deep muscle and bone involvement
T4	• **T4a** moderately advanced local disease Tumor invades anterior orbital contents, skin of cheek, pterygoid plates, infratemporal fossa, cribriform plate, sphenoid or frontal sinuses	Invasion of cartilagine, bone or nerves • Less than 4 cm with no bone invasion	–
	• **T4b** very advances local disease. Tumor invades any of the following: Orbital apex, dura, brain, middle cranial fossa, cranial nerves other than maxillary division of trigeminal nerve (V2), nasopharynx or clivus	• ≥4 cm with invasion of the premaxilla or the bone septum	

this reason, nowadays, many head and neck clinicians use UICC/AJCC classification for N and M and resort to Wang criteria for T classification.

The comparison of different T classification in the three named staging systems is shown in Table 4.9.

References

1. Institute NC, National Cancer Institute. AJCC Cancer Staging Manual. Definitions. 8th ed; 2020. https://doi.org/10.32388/b30ldk.
2. Cancer AJC on American Joint Committee on Cancer. AJCC Cancer Staging Manual. 2010. https://doi.org/10.1007/978-0-387-88441-7.
3. Edge SB. AJCC cancer staging handbook: from the AJCC cancer staging manual. 6th ed. Berlin: Springer; 2002. p. 469.
4. WHO. International Statistical Classification of Diseases and Related Health Problems. 2019. https://icd.who.int/browse10/2019/en.
5. Bussu F, Tagliaferri L, Piras A, et al. Multidisciplinary approach to nose vestibule malignancies: setting new standards Approccio multidisciplinare ai tumori maligni del vestibolo del naso: verso la definizione di nuovi standard. Acta Otorhinolaryngologica Italica. 2021; 41(Suppl. 1):S158–S165. https://doi.org/10.14639/0392-100X-suppl.1-41-2021-16.
6. Bussu F et al. New standards for the management of nose vestibule malignancies. Acta Oto-Laryngologica. 2023;143(3):215–22. https://doi.org/10.1080/00016489.2023.2179662.
7. Gray H, Gray H, Clemente CD. Anatomy of the human body. Philadelphia, PA: Lippincott Williams & Wilkins; 1985.
8. Vital D, Morand G, Huber GF, Studer G, Holzmann D. Outcome in squamous cell carcinoma of the nasal vestibule: a single center experience. Head Neck. 2015;37:46–51.
9. Mendenhall WM, Stringer SP, Cassisi NJ, Mendenhall NP. Squamous cell carcinoma of the nasal vestibule. Head Neck. 1999;21:385–93.
10. Poulsen M, Turner S. Radiation therapy for squamous cell carcinoma of the nasal vestibule. Int J Radiat Oncol Biol Phys. 1993;27:267–72.
11. Wang CC. Treatment of carcinoma of the nasal vestibule by irradiation. Cancer. 1976;38:100–6.
12. Jeannon J-P, Riddle PJ, Irish J, O'sullivan B, Brown DH, Gullane P. Prognostic indicators in carcinoma of the nasal vestibule. Clin Otolaryngol. 2007;32:19–23.
13. Kummer E, Rasch CRN, Keus RB, Bing Tan I, Balm AJM. T stage as prognostic factor in irradiated localized squamous cell carcinoma of the nasal vestibule. Head Neck. 2002;24:268–73.
14. Agger A, von Buchwald C, Madsen AR, et al. Squamous cell carcinoma of the nasal vestibule 1993-2002: a nationwide retrospective study from DAHANCA. Head Neck. 2009;31:1593–9.
15. Bussu F, Tagliaferri L, De Corso E, et al. Functional results of exclusive interventional radiotherapy (brachytherapy) in the treatment of nasal vestibule carcinomas. Brachytherapy. 2021;20:178–84.
16. Bussu F, Tagliaferri L, Mattiucci G, et al. Comparison of interstitial brachytherapy and surgery as primary treatments for nasal vestibule carcinomas. Laryngoscope. 2016;126:367–71.
17. Bussu F, Tagliaferri L, Mattiucci G, et al. HDR interventional radiotherapy (brachytherapy) in the treatment of primary and recurrent head and neck malignancies. Head Neck. 2019;41:1667–75.
18. Tagliaferri L, Fionda B, Bussu F, et al. Interventional radiotherapy (brachytherapy) for squamous cell carcinoma of the nasal vestibule: a multidisciplinary systematic review. Eur J Dermatol. 2019;29:417–21.
19. Dowley A, Hoskison E, Allibone R, Jones NS. Squamous cell carcinoma of the nasal vestibule: a 20-year case series and literature review. J Laryngol Otol. 2008;122:1019–23.
20. Chabrillac E, Talawdekar A, Garikipati S, Varley I, Sionis S, Beasley N, Jackson R. A single centre's experience of 23 cases of total rhinectomy for the treatment of squamous cell carcinoma involving the nasal vestibule. Eur Arch Otorhinolaryngol. 2021;279:2069. https://doi.org/10.1007/s00405-021-06972-6.

A Proposal for a Consistent Classification of Nasal Vestibule Carcinomas

5

Francesco Bussu, Roberto Gallus, Davide Rizzo, Pierangela Tramaloni, Nicola Tsatsaris, Luca Tagliaferri, Jacopo Galli, and Piero Nicolai

F. Bussu . D. Rizzo (✉)
Otolaryngology Division, Sassari University Hospital, Sassari, Italy

Department of Medicine, Surgery and Pharmacy, University of Sassari, Sassari, Italy
e-mail: fbussu@uniss.it; drizzo@uniss.it

R. Gallus
Otolaryngology Division, Mater Olbia Hospital, Olbia, Italy
e-mail: roberto.gallus@materolbia.com

P. Tramaloni
Otolaryngology Division, Sassari University Hospital, Sassari, Italy
e-mail: pierangela.tramaloni@aouss.it

N. Tsatsaris
Neurosurgery Residency Program, University of Verona, Verona, Italy

L. Tagliaferri
Radiotherapy Division, Fondazione Policlinico Universitario Agostino Gemelli, Rome, Italy
e-mail: luca.tagliaferri@policlinicogemelli.it

J. Galli
Istituto di Otorinolaringoiatria, Universitá Cattolica del Sacro Cuore, Rome, Italy
e-mail: Jacopo.Galli@unicatt.it

P. Nicolai
Department of Neurosciences, University of Padua, Padua, Italy
e-mail: piero.nicolai@unipd.it

© Springer Nature Switzerland AG 2023
F. Bussu (ed.), *Malignancies of the Nasal Vestibule*,
https://doi.org/10.1007/978-3-031-32850-3_5

5.1   Definition of the Nose Vestibule

The nose vestibule (NV) has been defined as that part of the anterior nasal cavity lined by squamous epithelium up to the limen nasi, which is the muco-cutaneous junction [1, 2]. We propose to change the anatomical borders of the nose vestibule, switching to radiological landmarks (so that the posterior limit of NV would be the tangential plane to the pyriform opening, see Chap. 1) (Fig. 5.1) [3].

SCC of the NV is currently considered a relatively rare condition, which is commonly considered to account for about 1% of all head and neck malignancies. A Danish group recently estimated, as a rounded down approximation, an annual incidence of squamous cell of the nasal vestibule of 0.41 per 100.000 inhabitants [4]. According to the AJCC/UICC staging system [5], primary epithelial malignancies of the nasal vestibule, in particular SCCs, are classified together and assigned to the same WHO topography code (C30.0) with those of the rest of the nasal cavity (nasal cavity proper) (see Chap. 4). However, such absence of a specific topography code for nose vestibule malignancies in the WHO ICD-O classification contributes to an underestimation of their incidence, as most often they cannot be discriminated from all the other nasal cavity primaries in the databases extracted from the cancer registries and clinical records [3].

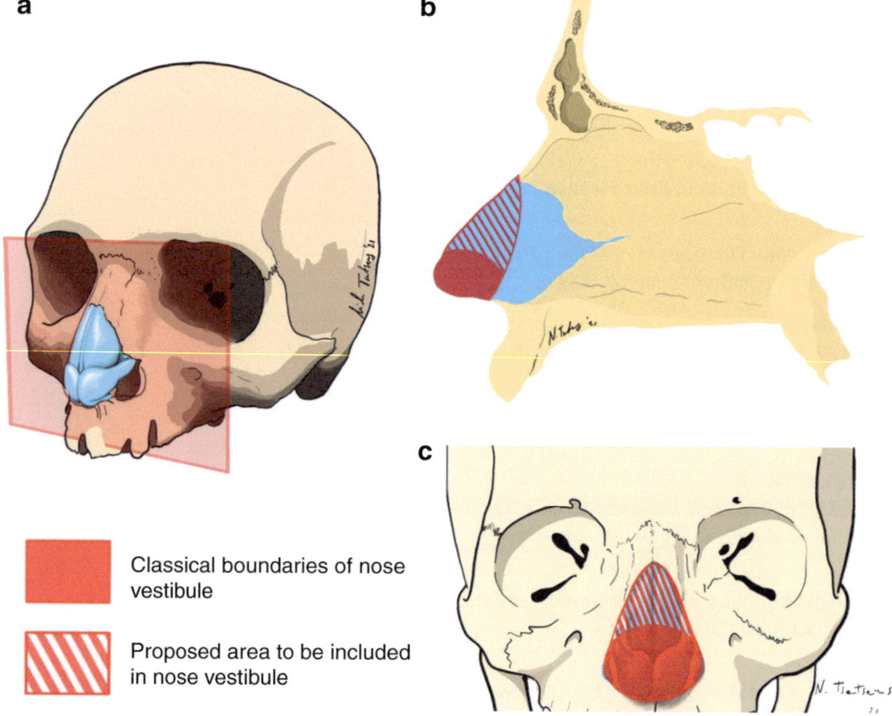

Fig. 5.1 Tridimensional (**a**), sagittal (**b**), and frontal (**c**) view of the new proposed definition of nose vestibule subsite

5.2   Misdiagnosis for Skin Primary

Another factor contributing to such underestimation is for sure the frequent misdiagnosis and misclassification of these lesions as cutaneous neoplasms. This is favored by the typical and early pattern of spread from the lateral wall of the vestibule, through the junctions between alar and lateral cartilages and between lateral cartilages and nasal bones, directly to the skin (see Chap. 3) (Fig. 5.2) [3, 6], so that nose vestibule primaries are usually first assessed by dermatologists or plastic surgeons. We recommend that every lesion of the nose skin be always evaluated also by an otolaryngologist to exclude a vestibular primary and differentiate it from a skin primary [3]. This has a clear deep impact on staging and most of all on treatment strategy. In fact, in case of a vestibule primary involving the skin, the resection most often shall involve all the layers of the nasal walls including hard framework (cartilages and/or bones) and mucosal lining, with clear reconstructive needs and issues, and cosmetic consequences (see Chaps. 7 and 8). On the other hand, the exclusive focus on the skin component of the malignancy with a complete miss of the mucosal origin, as in our experience can often happen, will induce to treat the lesion as a skin cancer thus leaving gross tumor in the primary site (R2) and certainty of local

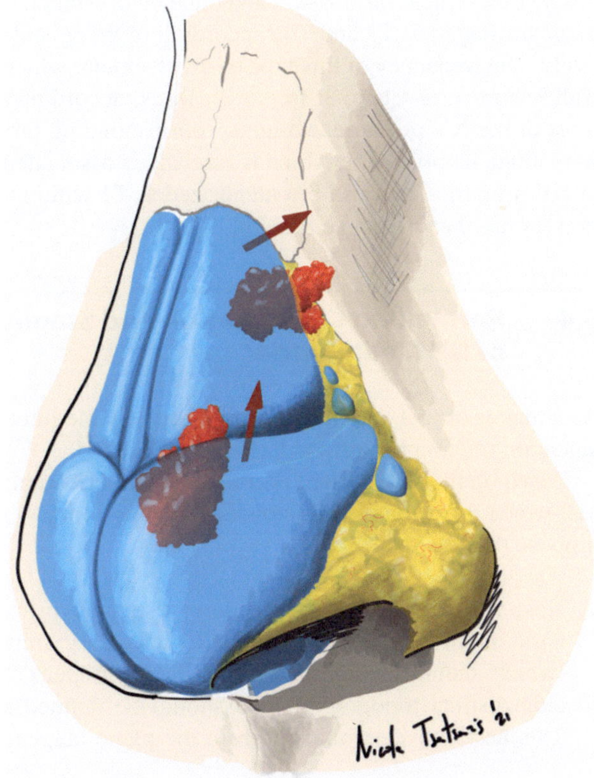

Fig. 5.2 Patterns of cutaneous spread of carcinomas from the lateral wall of nose vestibule

recurrence with obvious prognostic impairment. Therefore, the lack of cooperation with an otolaryngologist in managing nose cancers often leads—in our experience— to gross mistakes, as a skin invasion by a NV primary treated as a skin primary will most probably lead to oncological and cosmetic disasters [3].

5.3 General Issues in TNM Staging

In regard to the TNM staging system, some authors, also recently, have used the AJCC classification for non-melanoma skin cancers [7–9], which is not anatomically justified, as the primary site is completely different, and such an approach may increase the rate of misdiagnosis of NV lesions as skin primaries.

On the other hand, the staging criteria for the primary lesion (T) arising from the NV, sticking to the AJCC TNM, are the same as nasal cavity proper and ethmoid, but anatomical features and peculiar pattern of spread make such criteria clearly inadequate for NV (see Chap. 3). In fact, while the recent AJCC staging system is generally accepted for nodal disease (N), when it comes to primary lesion (T), Wang classification [11] has been reported to predict prognosis much better and remains the most used for nose vestibule malignancies [2, 8–10, 12–18].

The critical key parameters, whose weight is clearly different in Wang versus AJCC T classification, are skin and bone involvement. NV lesions with skin involvement are staged as T2 and T4a according to Wang and AJCC classification, respectively. The frequency of this type of involvement, which is almost constant in lateral wall lesions (see Chap. 3, Fig. 5.2), leads, according to AJCC, to classify as cT4 most of the NV primaries without a corresponding prognostic impact. On the contrary, bone involvement, which is rare and is associated with an ominous prognosis in NV primaries, can still be categorized as T1 within the AJCC/UICC T classification for nasal cavity and ethmoid [19].

5.4 Rethinking Classification and Staging of NV Malignancies

As a matter of fact, a shared, specific and reliable international standard for T classification of NV primaries is lacking and needed.

Based on the above listed peculiarities (described in detail in Chap. 3) and on the real-world diffusion and acknowledged superiority of the Wang classification, we propose that [3, 6]:

1. Nose vestibule should be considered a separate primary subsite of nose and paranasal malignancies, in addition to maxillary sinus and ethmoid/nasal cavity (which should include only nasal cavity proper/posterior nasal cavity). A specific distinct topography code should be defined in the ICD-O classification. This new subsite would go from the plane tangential to the pyriform aperture

posteriorly, to the external skin of the nose, cheek, superior lip anteriorly (see Chap. 1, see Fig. 5.1). This will allow better defining the incidence, more properly considering the most relevant features, and better assessing prognosis of malignancies of the NV.

2. The T classification criteria for this new subsite should be modified, mostly borrowing them from Wang's classification.

However, Wang's classification, although more specific to the nasal vestibule, cannot be grafted as it is in the AJCC staging system for the following reasons:

- only 3 T classes are provided, and not 4 as in all head and neck malignancies,
- cartilages, which always have a close yet variable relationship with NV primaries, are not even mentioned (not in AJCC for nose/paranasal nor in Wang classification),
- objective anatomical and dimensional boundaries are not provided. For example, upper lip or nasal septum can be involved in T2, a massive involvement of any of them leads to stage the lesion as T3, but the definition of "massive" is subjective and no objective criteria allowing to distinguish a T2 from a T3 are provided in the Wang classification.

Therefore, we propose to keep the "weight" attributed by Wang's classification respectively to skin involvement (compatible with a T2 class) and bone involvement (always determining a T4 stage) but to introduce clearer criteria and cutoffs to discriminate different stages, at the same time defining 4 (from T1 to T4), instead of 3 (as in the original Wang classification), T classes (Table 5.1). Among the additional criteria, there is cartilage destruction, which usually occurs only in larger primaries, when blood supply through perichondrium has been disrupted, and has a clear

Table 5.1 A preliminary proposal for redefinition of T classification in nose vestibule malignancies

T1	The lesion is limited to the nasal vestibule internal surface (skin and/or mucosa) (Fig. 5.3)
T2a	The lesion invades superficial structures outside the nasal cavity (skin and subcutaneous planes) and in particular upper lip, philtrum, skin of the nose and/or nasolabial fold, but does not destroy cartilage, nor invades bony structures, nor structures beyond the plane of the pyriform aperture (septum, lateral wall, turbinates, etc.) (Fig. 5.4)
T2b	Disruption of cartilages is evident, without invasion of bony structures, nor of structures beyond the plane of the pyriform aperture (septum, lateral wall, turbinates, etc.) (Fig. 5.5)
T3	The lesion extends beyond the pyriform aperture (septum, lateral wall, turbinates, etc.) (Fig. 5.6)
T4a	The lesion invades bony structures as hard palate, nasal bones, frontal process of the maxilla, ethmoid, and the orbit (Fig. 5.7)
T4b	Tumor invades any of the following: orbital apex, dura, brain, anterior and middle cranial fossa, cranial nerves other than (V2), nasopharynx, or clivus (Fig. 5.8)

impact on cosmetic results also when primary treatment is not surgical. The radiological boundary for nose vestibule (the tangential plane to piriform aperture) is another important parameter as lesions spreading posteriorly are more difficult to access and, most of all, cannot be covered by fully interstitial brachytherapy implants (see Chap. 13), invasion beyond this level would upstage the lesion to T3. For T4a, the main criterion is bone infiltration, while criteria for T4b are similar to those already set by AJCC T classification. This novel staging system has been recently preliminarily evaluated with very promising results [19]

Some examples of the changes in T classification deriving from the new proposal are shown in Figs. 5.3, 5.4, 5.5, 5.6, and 5.7.

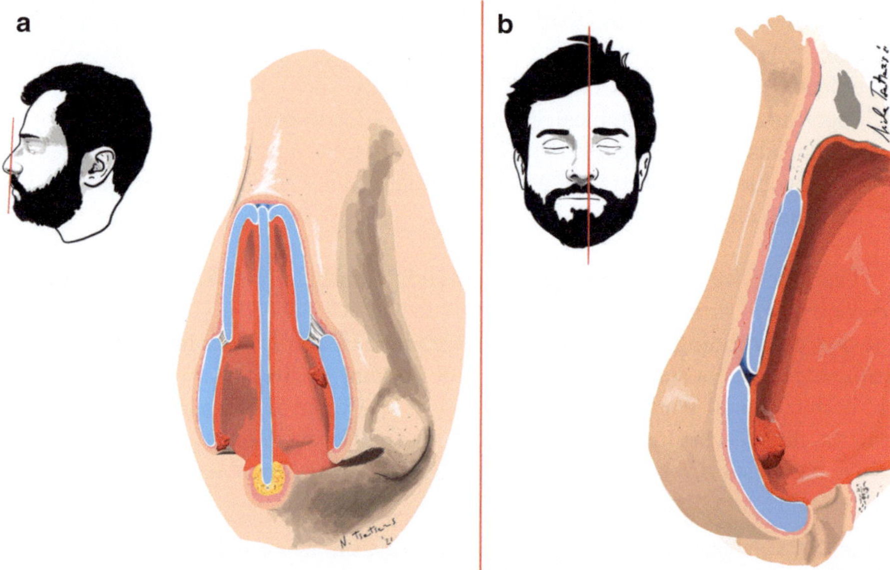

Fig. 5.3 The lesion is limited to the nasal vestibule internal surface (skin, transitional area, and/or mucosa) (examples in coronal, **a**, and sagittal, **b**, plane). In this case, the lesion is a cT1 in any staging system. (Current proposal, Wang, and AJCC classification)

Fig. 5.4 Nose vestibule SCC extends to the skin passing between the alar and lateral cartilage. According to the current proposal, this would be classified as a cT2a; in Wang's classification, it is a T2; in AJCC classification, it is a cT4a

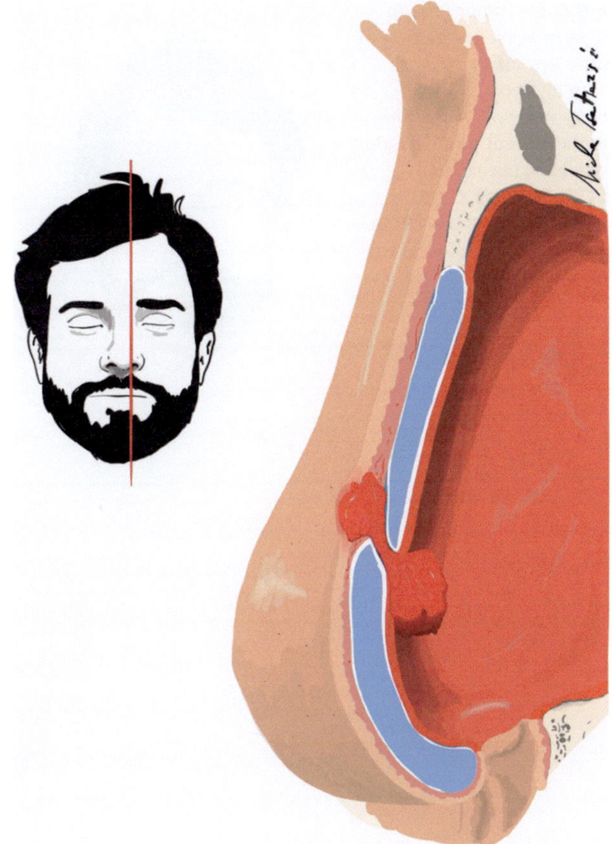

Fig. 5.5 Tumor growth determines a destruction of nose tip cartilages, with skin invasion, without bony invasion. According to the current proposal, this would be classified as a cT2b; in Wang's classification it is a T2; in AJCC classification, it is a cT4a

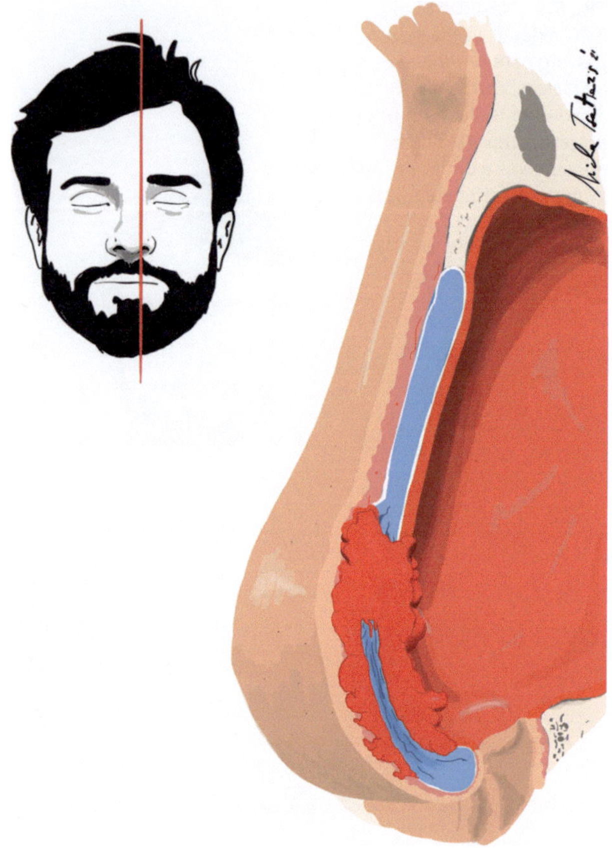

Fig. 5.6 The lesion extends beyond the pyriform aperture along the nasal septum. According to the current proposal, this would be classified as a cT3, in Wang and AJCC classification, it is a T1

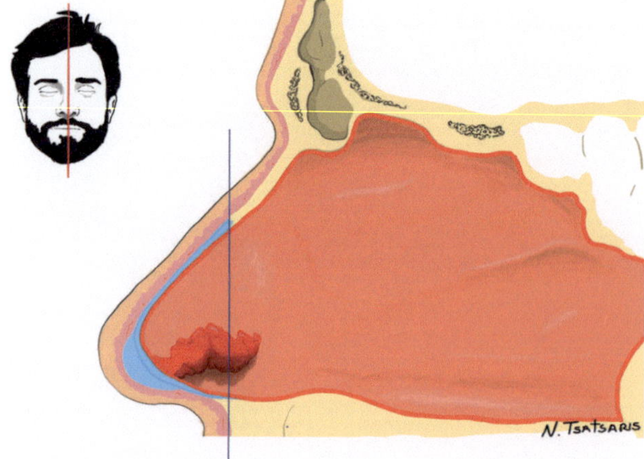

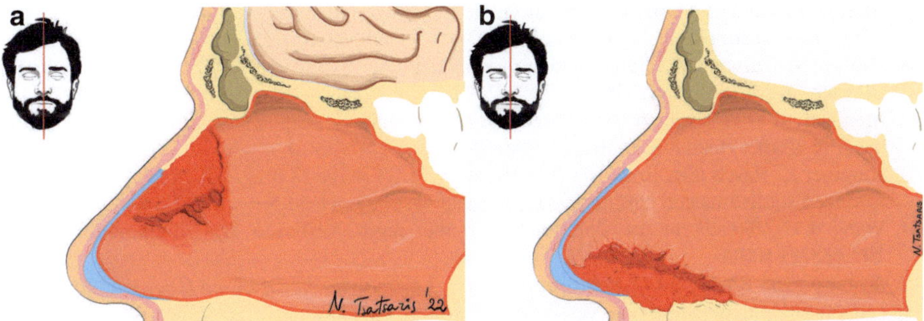

Fig. 5.7 The lesion invades bony structures as nasal bones (**a**) or hard palate (**b**). According to the current proposal, these would be classified as a cT4a, in Wang classification as T3, in AJCC as <u>cT1</u> (**a**) or cT3 (**b**)

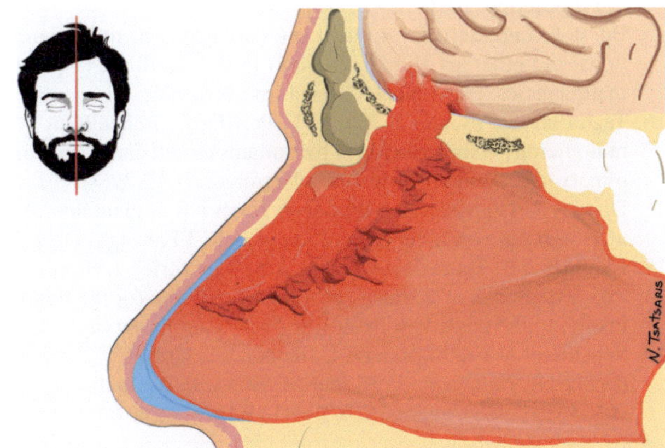

Fig. 5.8 The lesion sliding along the deep surface of nasal bones invades the intracranial space. In this case, the lesion is a cT4b according to both the current proposal and AJCC classification and T3 according to Wang classification

References

1. Gray H. Anatomy of the human body. Philadelphia: Lea & Febiger.
2. Jeannon JP, Riddle PJ, Irish J, O'Sullivan B, Brown DH, Gullane P. Prognostic indicators in carcinoma of the nasal vestibule. Clin Otolaryngol. 2007;32(1):19–23.
3. Bussu et al. New standards for the management of nose vestibule malignancies Acta Oto-Laryngologica. 2023;143(3):215–22. https://doi.org/10.1080/00016489.2023.2179662.
4. Horsmans JD, Godballe C, Jorgensen KE, Bastholt L, Lontoft E. Squamous cell carcinoma of the nasal vestibule. Rhinology. 1999;37(3):117–21.
5. Amin MB. AJCC cancer staging manual, vol. 17. 8th ed. Berlin: Springer International; 2017. p. 1032.
6. Bussu F, Tagliaferri L, Piras A, Rizzo D, Tsatsaris N, De Corso E et al. Multidisciplinary approach to nose vestibule malignancies: setting new standards Approccio multidisciplinare ai tumori maligni del vestibolo del naso: verso la definizione di nuovi standard Acta Otorhinolaryngologica Italica. 2021;41(Suppl. 1):S158–S165 https://doi.org/10.14639/0392-100X-suppl.1-41-2021-16.

7. Vital D, Morand G, Huber GF, Studer G, Holzmann D. Outcome in squamous cell carcinoma of the nasal vestibule: a single center experience. Head Neck. 2015;37(1):46–51.

8. Poulsen M, Turner S. Radiation therapy for squamous cell carcinoma of the nasal vestibule. Int J Radiat Oncol Biol Phys. 1993;27(2):267–72.

9. Mendenhall WM, Stringer SP, Cassisi NJ, Mendenhall NP. Squamous cell carcinoma of the nasal vestibule. Head Neck. 1999;21(5):385–93.

10. Kummer E, Rasch CR, Keus RB, Tan IB, Balm AJ. T stage as prognostic factor in irradiated localized squamous cell carcinoma of the nasal vestibule. Head Neck. 2002;24(3):268–73.

11. Wang CC. Treatment of carcinoma of the nasal vestibule by irradiation. Cancer. 1976;38(1):100–6.

12. Agger A, von Buchwald C, Madsen AR, Yde J, Lesnikova I, Christensen CB, et al. Squamous cell carcinoma of the nasal vestibule 1993-2002: a nationwide retrospective study from DAHANCA. Head Neck. 2009;31(12):1593–9.

13. Bussu F, Tagliaferri L, De Corso E, Passali GC, Lancellotta V, Mattiucci GC, et al. Functional results of exclusive interventional radiotherapy (brachytherapy) in the treatment of nasal vestibule carcinomas. Brachytherapy. 2020;20:178.

14. Bussu F, Tagliaferri L, Mattiucci G, Parrilla C, Dinapoli N, Micciche F, et al. Comparison of interstitial brachytherapy and surgery as primary treatments for nasal vestibule carcinomas. Laryngoscope. 2016;126(2):367–71.

15. Bussu F, Tagliaferri L, Mattiucci G, Parrilla C, Rizzo D, Gambacorta MA, et al. HDR interventional radiotherapy (brachytherapy) in the treatment of primary and recurrent head and neck malignancies. Head Neck. 2019;41(6):1667–75.

16. Tagliaferri L, Fionda B, Bussu F, Parrilla C, Lancellotta V, Deodato F, et al. Interventional radiotherapy (brachytherapy) for squamous cell carcinoma of the nasal vestibule: a multidisciplinary systematic review. Eur J Dermatol. 2019;29(4):417–21.

17. Dowley A, Hoskison E, Allibone R, Jones NS. Squamous cell carcinoma of the nasal vestibule: a 20-year case series and literature review. J Laryngol Otol. 2008;122(10):1019–23.

18. Chabrillac E, Talawdekar A, Garikipati S, Varley I, Sionis S, Beasley N, et al. A single centre's experience of 23 cases of total rhinectomy for the treatment of squamous cell carcinoma involving the nasal vestibule. Eur Arch Otorhinolaryngol. 2022;279:2069.

19. Scheurleer WFJ, Tagliaferri L, Rijken JA, Crescio C, Rizzo D, Mattiucci GC, Pameijer FA, de Bree R, Fionda B, de Ridder M, Bussu F. Evaluation of Staging Systems for Cancer of the Nasal Vestibule Cancers. 2023;15(11):3028. https://doi.org/10.3390/cancers15113028.

Acknowledged Therapeutic Options in Nose Vestibule Malignancies

6

Tropiano Paolo, Fois Paolo, Melis Andrea, Laura Maria De Luca, Francesco Miccichè, Di Mario Dalila, Andrea D'Aviero, Giovanni Maria Fadda, Luca Tagliaferri, and Davide Rizzo

6.1 Introduction

SCC is the most frequent malignancy of the nose vestibule, it is considered to account for <1% of head and neck malignant lesions [1], but its prevalence is probably underestimated (see Chaps. 3 and 16) [2, 3]. As early symptoms are lacking and mostly analog to infectious/inflammatory processes (vestibulitis) or traumatic lesions, diagnosis is often delayed. This leads to a sure, even if difficult to quantify,

T. Paolo · F. Paolo · M. Andrea · L. M. De Luca (✉)
Otolaryngology Division, Azienda Ospedaliero Universitaria Sassari, Sassari, Italy
e-mail: andrea.melis@aouss.it

F. Miccichè · A. D'Aviero · L. Tagliaferri
Radiotherapy Division, Fondazione Policlinico Universitario Agostino Gemelli, Rome, Italy
e-mail: luca.tagliaferri@policlinicogemelli.it

D. M. Dalila
Radiation Oncology Division, Sassari University Hospital, Sassari, Italy

G. M. Fadda
Medical Oncology Division, Sassari University Hospital, Sassari, Italy
e-mail: giovanni.fadda@aouss.it

D. Rizzo
Otolaryngology Division, Azienda Ospedaliero Universitaria Sassari, Sassari, Italy

Department of Medicine, Surgery and Pharmacy, University of Sassari, Sassari, Italy
e-mail: drizzo@uniss.it

© Springer Nature Switzerland AG 2023
F. Bussu (ed.), *Malignancies of the Nasal Vestibule*,
https://doi.org/10.1007/978-3-031-32850-3_6

impact on survival [4] and viable therapeutic options because of almost constant tumoral extension to adjacent structures (e.g., skin, nasal cavities and paranasal sinuses, superior lip, nasal septum or bones) at diagnosis [5].

Due to the relative rarity of this malignancy and to the frequent misdiagnosis (see Chaps. 3, 5, and 16), there are no univocal recommendations for treatment choice. Both surgery and radiotherapy (RT) are generally accepted modalities for first-line treatment of primary tumor (T) and regional metastasis (N). However, in the literature most of the described series are small and involve patients primarily treated with only one modality with just few works describing larger series and/or comparing different treatment modalities (e.g., surgical versus non-surgical).

Comparison of different studies is further complicated by the absence of consensus concerning the staging system, and also among the works cited in the following paragraphs, T classification has been non-consistently alternatively defined using AJCC or Wang classification (and in some cases, even NMSC AJCC classification) [6].

In Table 6.1, a summary of the literature evidence concerning the different treatment modalities for primary NVSCC is reported.

Table 6.1 Main literature series of nasal vestibule, with a summary of populations described and treatment strategies

Author	Year	Histology	No of patients	Primary surgery	Primary EB RT	Primary IRT	No curative treatment/ BSC/lost	Adjuvant/complementary EBRT
DesPrez [42]	1967	Mixed histologies	6	6 (100%)	0	0	0	0
Haynes [26]	1974	SCC	22	0(0%)	9 (40%)	13 (60%)	0	0
Goepfert [7]	1974	SCC	26	10 (38%)	16 (62%)	0	0	0
Wang [18]	1976	SCC	36	0	NP	NP	5	NP
Mak [19]	1980	BCC and SCC	47	3 (6%)	41 (88%)	2 (4%)	1	2 (4%)
Kagan [8]	1981	SCC	42	28 (67%)	14 (33%)	0	0	13 (31%)
De Jong [20]	1981	SCC	22	9 (40%)	13 (60%)	0	0	0
Johansen [22]	1984	SCC	66	7 (11%)	56 (85%)	0	3	NP
Mendenhall [43]	1984	SCC	13	0	6 (46%)	7 (54%)	0	3 (23%)
Baris [23]	1985	SCC	22	0	0	22 (100%)	0	3 (14%)
Wong [24]	1986	SCC	56	0	56 (100%)	0	0	0
Mendenhall [44]	1987	SCC	27	0	8	14	5	8
Chobe [27]	1988	SCC	32	0	21(66%)	11 (34%)	0	0
Mazeron [45]	1989	BCC and SCC	1668[a]	0	914 (55%)	762 (45%)	0	0
Levendag [28]	1990	SCC	63	0	18 (29%)	45 (71%)	0	8 (13%)
Patel [10]	1992	SCC	30	10 (33%)	0	20 (67%)	0	23 (77%)
Poulsen [30]	1993	SCC	29	7 (24%)	22 (76%)	0	0	7 (24%)
McCollough [46]	1993	SCC	39	0	12 (31%)	27 (69%)	0	18 (46%)

(continued)

Table 6.1 (continued)

Author	Year	Histology	No of patients	Primary surgery	Primary EB RT	Primary IRT	No curative treatment/ BSC/lost	Adjuvant/complementary EBRT
Pantelakos [11]	1994	SCC	25	21 (84%)	4 (16%)	0	0	11 (44%)
Turner [31]	1995	SCC	21	0	21 (100%)	0	0	0
Evensen [32]	1996	SCC	23	4 (17%)	0	19 (83%)	0	7 (30%)
Mendenhall [33]	1999	SCC	60	0	16 (27%)	44 (73%)	0	31 (52%)
Fornelli [12]	2000	SCC	32	23 (72%)	9 (28%)	0	0	8 (25%)
Langendijk [35]	2004	SCC	56[h]	0	56 (100%)	0	0	47 (84%)
Levendag [29]	2006	BCC and SCC	64[i]	14 (22%)	0	50 (78%)	0	14 (22%)
Jeannon [25]	2007	SCC	84	17 (20%)	65 (77%)	0	2 (3%)	10 (12%
Wallace [47]	2007	SCC	79	0	24 (30%)	55 (70%)	0	42 (53%)
Dowley [4]	2008	SCC	26	12 (46%)	14 (54%)	0	0	2 (8%)
Agger [13]	2009	SCC	174	50 (29%)	120 (69%)	0	4 (2%)	28 (16%)
Ladderose [14]	2013	SCC	10	10 (100%)	0	0	0	2 (20%)
Koopmann [48]	2014	SCC	30	30 (100%)	0	0	2 (7%)	7 (23.3%)
Lipman [36]	2014	SCC	83	11 (13%)	9 (11%)	60 (72%)	1 (1.2%)	14 (17%)
Vital [1]	2014	SCC	30	21 (70%)	9 (30%)	0	2 (7%)	6 (20%)
Wray [34]	2015	SCC	99	13 (13%)	39 (39%)	15 (15%)	1 (1%)	52 (52%)
Bussu [39]	2016	SCC	12	6 (50%)	0	6 (50%)	0	0
Taxy	2016	SCC	5	5 (100%)	0	0	0	3 (60%)
Vanneste [38]	2016	SCC	81	0	38 (47%)	41 (51%)	0	2 (2%)

Czerwinski [37]	2018	SCC	141	0	0	102 (72%)	0	0
Zaoui [5]	2018	SCC	26	26 (100%)	0	0	0	2 (8%)
Federspril [15]	2020	SCC	16	16 (100%)	0	3 (19%)	0	0
Tagliaferri [40]	2020	SCC	14	0	0	14 (100%)	0	0
Lambertoni [16]	2021	SCC	45	45 (100%)	0	0	0	0
Chabrillac [17]	2021	SCC	23	23 (100%)	0	0	0	17 (73.9%)
Czerwinski [41]	2022	SCC	225	0	65 (29%)	153 (68%)	0	7 (3%)

Primary	Recurrences	Wang T classification	AJCC T classification	N classification	Primary management of N0	OS	DSS	RFS
6 (100%)	0	NP	NP	NP	Observation	83% (2 yrs)	100% (2 yrs)	100% (2 yrs)
22 (100%)	0	NP	NP	NP	Observation	NP	86% (2 yrs)	73% (2 yrs)
20 (77%)	6 (23%)	NP	NP	AJCC	Observation	78% (5 yrs)	NP	77% (2 yrs)
36 (100%)	0	Yes	NP	AJCC	Observation	NP	NP	74%
45 (96%)	2 (4%)	NP	NP	NP	Observation	NP	NP	67%
42 (100%)	0	NP	NP	NP	NP	64%	74%	64%

(continued)

Table 6.1 (continued)

Primary	Recurrences	Wang T classification	AJCC T classification	N classification	Primary management of N0	OS	DSS	RFS
22 (100%)	0	Yes	NP	NP	Observation	NP	NP	50%
NP	NP	Yes	NP	AJCC	Observation	61.4%	79%	59%
8 (62%)	5 (38%)	NP	AJCC skin	AJCC	ENI	71% (5 yrs)	100% (5 yrs)	77% (3 yrs)
19 (84%)	3 (14%)	NP	NP	NP	ENI	92%	95%	95%
56 (100%)	0	NP	NP	NP	Observation	64% (5 yrs)	87% (5 yrs)	80% (5 yrs)
15 (68%)	7 (32%)	NP	AJCC skin	AJCC	ENI	77% (2 yrs)	91% (2 yrs)	NP
32(100%)	0	NP	NP	NP	ENI	NP	NP	87.5%
1356 (81%)	312 (19%)	NP	NP	NP	NP	NP	NP	93%[b]
63 (100%)	0	Yes	NP	AJCC	NP	65% (5 yrs)	90%	80% (5 yrs)
30 (100%)	0	Yes	NP	AJCC	NP	NP	~80%[c] (5 yrs)	NP
29 (100%)	0	NP	AJCC skin	AJCC	Observation	64% (5 yrs)	NP	61%
29 (74%)	10 (26%)	NP	AJCC skin	AJCC	Mixed	75%	~90%[d]	54%[e]
25 (100%)	0	NP	NP	NP	Observation	NP	8	52%
21 (100%)	0	NP	NP	NP	Observation	57% (3 yrs)	86% (3 yrs)	81% (3 yrs)
23 (100%)	0	NP	AJCC skin	AJCC	Observation	78%	96%	87%

49 (82%)	11 (18%)	NP	AJCC skin	AJCC	Mixed	74%[f]	91%[g]	NP
32 (100%)	0	NP	NP	NP	Mixed	50% (5 yrs)	66%	42% (5 yrs)
56 (100%)	0	Yes	NP	NP	Observation	66%	87%	NP
64 (100%)	0	Yes	NP	NP	Observation	59% (5 yrs)	NP	92% (5 yrs)
84 (100%)	0	Yes	AJCC skin	NP	Observation	58%	NP	52%
67 (85%)	12 (15%)	NP	AJCC skin	AJCC	Mixed	76% (5 yrs)	90% (2 yrs)	NP
26 (100%)	0	Yes	AJCC nose	AJCC	Observation	68%	77%	NP
NP	NP	Yes	AJCC nose	AJCC	Observation	50% (5 yrs)	74% (2 yrs)	NP
10 (100%)	NP	Yes	NP	AJCC	Observation	NP	NP	NP
30 (100%)	NP	Yes	AJCC nose	AJCC	NP	92%	92%	NP
NP	NP	Yes	NP	AJCC	NP	70%	95%	92%
NP	NP	NP	AJCC skin	AJCC	Observation	92% (1 yr)	96% (1 yr)	70% (5 yrs)
NP	NP	NP	AJCC skin	AJCC	ENI	75% (5 yrs)	91% (5 yrs)	NP
12 (100%)	NP	Yes	NP	AJCC	Mixed	NP	83%[j]	83%
5 (100%)	NP	NP	NP	NP	NP	NP	NP	40%
81 (100%)	NP	Yes	NP	NP	NP	59%	NP	57%
0	NP	Yes	NP	NP	NP	72%	94%	NP

(continued)

Table 6.1 (continued)

Primary	Recurrences	Wang T classification	AJCC T classification	N classification	Primary management of N0	OS	DSS	RFS
26 (100%)	NP	NP	AJCC skin	AJCC	Observation	92% (3 yrs)	96%	86.7% (5 yrs)
0	NP	Yes	AJCC nose	AJCC	Observation	NP	NP	78% (5 yrs)
14 (100%)	NP	Yes	NP	NP	NP	67.3% (3 yrs)	92.3% (3 yrs)	NP
45 (100%)	NP	Yes	AJCC skin	NP	NP	81.9% (5 yrs)	92% (3 yrs)	61.9% (5 yrs)
17 (73.9%)	6 (26.1%)	Yes	AJCC nose	NP	NP	67.5% (5 yrs)	80.7% (5 yrs)	66.3% (5 yrs)
NP	NP	Yes	NP	AJCC	ENI	82% (3 yrs)	94% (3 yrs)	NP

NP not provided, *yr or yrs* year or years

[a] Cancers of the nasal skin are included together with nasal vestibule primaries without distinction

[b] Only local relapse free survival

[c] 100% N0, 38% N+

[d] 93% stage I–II; 83% stage III–IV

[e] In T4 group

[f] For 56 patients treated with RT alone

[g] For 56 patients treated with RT alone

[h] All T1/2 N0 (T3/N+ were excluded)

[i] All T1/2 N0 (T3/N+ were excluded)

[j] 83% in RT group; 80% in surgical group

6.2   Surgery

As an advocate of surgery, in 1974, Goepfert et al. published a series of ten patients treated with surgery at University of Texas, MD Anderson. After 2 years of follow up, they reported a local control rate of 90% and an ultimate local control rate after salvage of 100%, reaching the conclusion that in small cancers, if a surgical resection followed by immediate repair is possible, surgical option has equal effectiveness than radiotherapy with the advantage of no local radiotherapy side effect and optimal cosmetic result [7].

Between 1960 and 1977, Kagan and colleagues collected 38 early NVSSC and 4 advanced tumors. Fourteen patients underwent surgery alone with a local control (LC) rate of 93%, seven patients were treated with RT alone with LC rate of 71%, and 17 underwent RT and surgery with LC rate of 47%. They reported considerable sequelae due to irradiation as dryness, even if without cartilage destruction, so they proposed surgery as an adequate alternative to irradiation for early lesion or for RT recurrences, as well as irradiation for primary surgery recurrences [8].

In 1988, Weimberger published a small series of five patients who underwent surgery for early (4) or locally advanced (1) NVSSC with a locoregional control in 100% [9]. In 1992, Patel et al. described a bigger group of 30 patients treated at Free University Hospital in Amsterdam. Five of them had Wang T1 NVSSC treated by RT, with 1 local recurrence salvaged with surgery; 22 had Wang T2 disease, 15 of whom were primarily treated by RT (60% later underwent surgery for local recurrence), 7 were primarily treated by surgery (1 case with the addition of adjuvant RT); 3 T3 cases underwent surgery (2 with additional postoperative RT). The 5-year DSS was 100% for T1, 76% for T2, with a local control rate for T1/T2 treated with RT of 50% and an ultimate local control rate after salvage surgery of 90% and only 1/7 recurrence in the surgery group. Based on their results, Patel advocated for surgery because of better cosmetic results in T1 and better local control in rT2 lesions and proposed surgery and postoperative RT in T3 [10].

Between 1975 and 1991, at North Carolina Baptist Hospital and at the Bowman Gray School of Medicine (Winston-Salem), 25 patients with NVSSC underwent surgery (10), EBRT (4), or combined treatment (11) in one of the few comparative studies present in the literature. Three out of four subjects who were treated with EBRT recurred and two died from the disease. Seven out of ten patients of the surgery group had a local recurrence and underwent RT with an ultimate local control rate of 80%. Larger lesions, treated with a combination of surgery and EBRT, recurred in two out of 11 subjects with ultimate local control in ten of them. Authors concluded that an aggressive initial surgical resection, eventually followed by RT, can obtain better control than surgery or RT alone [11].

In 2000, Fornelli et al. published a dual institution experience (University Hospital Morgantown, West Virginia and Hershey, Pennsylvania) in which 32 patients with de novo N0 NVSCC were treated with surgery (15), EBRT (9), or surgery and postoperative EBRT (8). No elective neck dissection was performed, while elective neck irradiation was performed in 19% of subjects. They described a 2-year OS of 69% and a 5-year RFS and OS of 42% and 50%, respectively. Surgery group presented 2 local and 4 regional recurrences (9 out of 15 free to relapse), EBRT group showed 2 local and 6 regional recurrences (1 out of 9 free to relapse) while group treated with combination of surgery and RT showed 4 out of 8 recurrences, 1 local and 3 regional. Finally, Fornelli advocated for surgery that showed the best overall cure rate and a locoregional control rate better than EBRT alone, suggesting elective neck irradiation (ENI) only for selected patients [12].

Dowley et al. presented in 2008 a 20-year experience in which 26 patients were treated with RT alone or surgery. In the first group, 6/13 presented a local recurrence and 4/13 a regional recurrence, while in the surgery group, only 1 out of 10 subjects had a local recurrence, and regional control rate was 90%. The OS observed was 68%. The author described that Wang T2/T3 tumor treated with RT recurred in four cases of five, while 100% of subjects treated with surgery alone or with combined RT were disease-free. So, if a radical surgical resection and a high-quality reconstruction, potentially followed by RT, are possible, patients would obtain a better survival rate with an adequate quality of life [4].

In 2009, Agger et al. published the results of the DAHANCA forum that pooled data from five Danish H&N cancer centers from 1993 to 2002. They collected 174 patients: 120 were treated with EBRT, 22 underwent surgery, 28 were given surgery plus postoperative RT, and 4 received palliative or no treatment. Local control rate and locoregional control rate were 80% and 67%, respectively, while 5-year DSS and OS were 74% and 50%. Locoregional control rate was better in the surgery group, followed by group treated with a combination of the two treatments, while EBRT was associated with a worst locoregional control rate. So, the authors suggested minimal surgery or hypofractionated RT for Wang T1, while in Wang T2/T3, combined treatments (surgery + radiotherapy) or intensified RT was proposed [13].

Between 2008 and 2010, at Ludwig-Maximilians-University Munich ENT Department, ten Wang (and UICC) T1/T2 NVSCCs were treated with endonasal surgical en bloc resection of lesion supplemented by a circular resection to a safe margin. Only two adjuvant RTs were performed for close margin or N+. Local and locoregional control rates observed were 100%, while functional results were satisfactory, with some external retraction and internal nasal scarring and only one monolateral obstruction that did not require surgical revision. Basing upon such good cosmetic results, negligible morbidity, and optimal local control, the authors suggested endonasal approach for carefully selected patients [14].

Vital et al. presented in 2015 a series of 30 patients observed between 1995 and 2012 at University Hospital, Zurich: 21 treated with surgical resection, followed by reconstruction with transposition flap in 2 cases, composite graft in 4, paramedian forehead flap in 3; 5 resections did not require reconstruction, and 7 total rhinectomies were reconstructed by epithesis. In six cases, postoperative intensity-modulated RT was performed. Nine lesions were treated with IMRT alone. The authors observed an RFS at 1–5 years of 81% and 70%, respectively, and a DSS at 1 year of 96%, with equal control in early NVSCC treated with surgery or RT. They also observed a high risk of locoregional recurrence in case of insufficient margin in surgery resection, even in case of postoperative RT, so they advocated an aggressive surgical treatment to obtain safe margins in spite of cosmetic disadvantages [1].

In 2018, Zaoui et colleagues presented a series of 26 patients treated between 2005 and 2013 at the Department of Oncology, Head and Neck Surgery at the University Hospital Heidelberg, with surgical external approach: 7 lateral rhinotomies, 6 partial rhinectomies, and 13 total rhinectomies. Reconstruction was performed in 14 cases with nasal prosthesis, in 5 patients with forehead flap, in 7 with anterior-based septal mucoperichondrial flap and cartilage grafts. Nine patients underwent concomitant neck dissection for cN+, but only in one case pathological exam confirmed a pN1. Adjuvant radiation was performed in 8% of patients. Outcomes described by the authors (RFS at 1 year 96.2%, 4 years 92.1%, 5 years 86.7%; 5-year DSS 96.2%, 5-year OS 91.8%), in particular the absence of local recurrence after primary surgical treatment of advanced stage, made them advocate for surgery for early and advanced SCCNV [5]. In an update of the previous series, authors evaluated 16 patients who underwent skin-preserving excision of the tumor as a primary procedure via lateral rhinotomy with a 1–2 week delayed reconstruction. They proposed a septal rotation and free auricular cartilage grafts for the framework reconstruction, combined with an anteriorly pedicled septal mucoperichondrial flap for the inner lining. Five-year local control and ultimate local control rate were 83%, and 100%, respectively, and progression-free survival was 78% after 5 years. Partial necrosis of the mucoperichondrial flap occurred in 6.25% of cases without further surgical intervention needed, skin breakdown in one patient, nasal breathing was normal or near normal in 75% of patients, nasal deviation occurred in 6.25% of patients, and alar retraction in 6.25% of patients. According to these results, the authors advocated for lateral rhinotomy for primary malignant not involving skin lesions, thanks to highly satisfactory aesthetical and functional outcomes [15].

Between October 2010 and December 2018, at University of Insubria, Varese, Italy, 45 patients underwent a surgical excision for NVSCC: a combined endoscopic-assisted/transfacial approach or open rhinoplasty approach, with a reconstructive procedure in 38 cases: local flaps for defects involving only the skin, a cartilaginous graft covered by forehead flap in case of partial involvement of nasal structures, a cartilaginous graft with mucoperichondrium flap or an endonasal composite chondromucosal septal flap for skeleton/mucosa defects, and a medial femoral condyle free flap for reconstruction of the framework, a septal mucoperichondrium flap for inner lining, and interpolated forehead flap to cover in case of defect of nasal dorsum or sidewalls. The authors observed that 5-year OS, DSS, and DFS were 81.9%, 87.4%, and 61.9%, respectively, while overall locoregional control rate was 66% at 5 years. So they advocated for surgical resection as a reliable treatment in the management of selected cases of nasal and pyramid SCC and suggested an algorithm for reconstruction strategy based on layers removed and related to defect characteristics and site [16].

In the United Kingdom, at Sheffield Teaching Hospital, Chabrillac et colleagues revised their series of 23 NV SCC treated with total rhinectomy (TR) between September 2003 and February 2021, in 73.9% as a primary treatment and in 26.1% as a salvage treatment after radiotherapy or partial rhinectomy. Five patients underwent reoperation due to positive excisional margins, while 17 patients required adjuvant treatment (radiotherapy or chemoradiotherapy). Almost all of the patients (91.3%) were rehabilitated with prosthesis. Five-year OS was 67.5%, DFS was 66.3% while DSS was 80.7%. According to their observations, the authors concluded that TR can be chosen as the reference treatment option [17].

6.3 Radiotherapy

A larger number of series about RT treatment for NVSCC is available in the literature. Year by year, the technical improvements made RT a more and more suitable option for these tumors. Most studies put attention on oncological and functional outcomes to evaluate the gold standard treatment not only between surgery and radiotherapy but also between the different techniques for irradiation, mainly external beam radiotherapy (EBRT) and interventional radiotherapy (IRT, brachytherapy, administered with different modalities and in particular endocavitary, interstitial, through molds).

Between 1960 and 1974, at the Department of Radiation Medicine, Massachusetts General Hospital, 31 of 36 patients with NVSCC were treated with RT. The authors observed a RFS at 3 years of 74%, a regional control rate in 26 N0 patients of 81% at 3 years, and no clinically significant complications. So, they advocated for EBRT and IRT in T1/T2 tumors and surgery +/− preoperative RT in T3 lesions, and no indication for ENI or elective ND was given [18].

In 1980, Mark et al. presented a series with 47 patients, 32 of them irradiated with the same modality, at Rotterdamsch Radio-Therapeutisch Instituut, The Netherlands, in 1968–1978, with a total dose of 43–60 Gy and daily fractions of 2.5–3 Gy given by electron-beam RT. Local control rate was 72% for early tumors (tumours ≤1.5 cm) and 50% for locally advanced lesions (tumours >1.5 cm), reaching the conclusion that electron-beam radiotherapy can be a useful option for the primary lesion [19].

The next year, De Jong published a series of 22 patients observed at University of Leiden, The Netherlands, between 1960 and 1978, for SCC of nasal vestibule: 13 underwent RT and 9 patients were treated with surgery, obtaining local control in 8 out of 9 cases in surgery group and in 7 out of 13 cases in irradiated patients (4 of these local recurrence were outfield). The conclusion of the paper was that adequate treatment of the primary tumor can be achieved either by surgery or by RT, and from a cosmetic point of view, RT is the treatment of choice [20].

In an editorial in 1984, Chassagne presented 27 T1/T2 primary NVSCC treated with BRT alone with afterloading techniques employing continuous iridium wire sources at Institut Gustave Roussy, Villejuif, France, which reached a local control rate of 100% in T1 tumor and 93% in T2, without major compliances, proposing brachytherapy as an adequate technique for the oncological outcomes, the adaptability to local anatomy and tissue tolerance [21].

In the same year, Johansen reported a series of 63 patients treated at the Department of Oncology and Radiotherapy, Radiumstationen between 1956 and

1982. In total, 56 underwent EBRT while seven cancers were surgically resected. Local control rate was 65%, with an RFS of 59% and an ultimate RFS of 78%. The regional recurrence rate was 19%, while 13 patients died of disease. The authors advocated for RT for small and medium lesions due to mild side effects and good cosmetic results, while, in locally advanced tumors, higher recurrence rate in RT group led to consider surgery a better option despite aesthetic mutilation. Moreover, they suggested prophylactic neck dissection in case of local recurrence [22].

Between 1981 and 1984, 22 patients were treated with IRT, in three cases in association with EBRT, at Rotterdam RadioTherapeutic Institute. Only one patient had a recurrence and underwent total rhinectomy, the 2-year survival was 92%, and no major complications were described. The authors proposed IRT with iridium alone as standard treatment for early and superficial tumor and a combination of IRT and EBRT for invasive tumors, while surgery should be reserved only for recurrence [23].

Wong et al. presented in 1986 a series of 56 patients treated between 1958 and 1986 with EBRT at Princess Margaret Hospital, Toronto, which showed a 5-year local control rate and a DSS respectively of 80% and 87%. In particular, they analyzed tumors with bone or cartilage invasion and observed an initial and ultimate local control rate of 57% and 79%. They observed a rate of clinically relevant complications of 7%, in particular two cases of maxillary osteonecrosis, epistaxis requiring hospitalization, nasal obstruction that needed a surgical procedure [24].

In an update of 84 cases observed in 1979–2000, 65 patients were treated with primary radical EBRT, 10 patients underwent surgery and postoperative EBRT, 7 lesions were treated exclusively with surgery, and 2 patients were treated with EBRT for palliative intention. Seventeen patients were saved with surgery after primary treatment. Observed OS and DFS were respectively 58% and 52%, and no significant differences were found among different primary treatments. So, the authors advocated for radical radiotherapy as primary treatment [25].

At MD Anderson Hospital, Houston, Texas, 22 N0 patients with less than 3 cm diameter cancer were collected between 1953 and 1969. Nine were treated with IRT, nine with EBRT, and four with intracavitary molds. Local control rate and ultimate local control rate after salvage surgery were 86% and 91%, with only one significant complication. Initial and ultimate regional control rates were 77% and 95%, respectively [26]. In an update from 1967 to 1984, in the same institution, 32 patients were treated primarily with irradiation, in 18 patients only on the primary lesion, and in the other 14 with an ENI. Local control rate was 97% with only 3% of major complications (osteonecrosis of maxilla). The authors advocated for IRT in case of early lesion thanks to excellent cosmetic results and a locoregional control that is similar to surgical excision, while irradiation of the neck was proposed only for large and undifferentiated tumors [27].

Levendag and colleagues in 1990 published a series of 63 patients treated in 1978–1988 at Dr. Daniel den Hoed Cancer Center (Rotterdam, the Netherlands). Eighteen patients were irradiated with EBRT alone, 37 patients were implanted for brachytherapy, and in 8 cases, a combination of the two modalities had been chosen.

Local control rate in T1 according to Wang or less than 2 cm lesions was respectively 89% and 97%, while in T2 according to Wang or bigger than 2 cm tumors was respectively 64% and 57%, with an overall survival in the whole series of 65% and an RFS of 80% [28]. In a more recent series, collected between 1991 and 2005 in the same institution, 64 Wang T1/T2 N0 cancers were treated with HDR-IRT: in 50 patients primarily, in 14 cases after an extensive excision biopsy. 5-year LRFS and OS observed were 89% and 58% in T1 tumor and 100% and 78% in T2 lesion, respectively. One-hundred percent of patients reported a maximum score in cosmetic and functional outcome evaluation for IRT while the patients with previous extensive excision biopsy presented worse cosmetic outcomes. Based on these results and on the relatively low cost of IRT, the authors advocated for this technique [29].

In 1993, Poulsen presented a series of 29 patients treated between 1960 and 1989 at Queensland Radium Institute South Brisbane, in 22 cases with primary EBRT, in the other 7 with surgery and postoperative EBRT. They observed a 5-year OS and RFS of 64% and 61% in the whole series, in RT alone group 67% and 63% and in the combined therapy group 57% and 57%, respectively. Patients treated with surgery and RT presented a local and regional control rate of 66% and 57%. In RT alone group, initial and ultimate local control rates were 59% and 63%, while initial and ultimate regional control rates were 86% and 90%. Only minor complications were described: two cases of septal necrosis and one nasoalveolar fistula in irradiated patients. As no advantages were observed in surgery plus radiotherapy combined treatments versus irradiated group, the authors advocated for RT alone [30].

Between 1986 and 1994, at Mount Vernon Hospital, Northwood, 21 patients underwent continuous hyperfractionated accelerated radiotherapy (CHART), 3 daily fractions over 12 consecutive days for a total dose of 54 Gy, on primary lesion. No ENI was performed. Overall recurrence-free survival and local control rate were 81% and 86%. One major complication was described (a bilateral blindness due to optic nerves and chiasma damage), while no late skin alterations were observed. Due to survival outcome comparable to surgery or other radiotherapy technique, optimal tolerance even in elderly patients, excellent aesthetic results, and adaptability to small as well as extensive lesions, CHART was presented as a possible schedule for RT, the treatment of choice of NVSCC [31].

At Norwegian Radium Hospital between 1985 and 1994, 23 NVSCC were treated. Four patients underwent surgery and postoperative brachytherapy, obtaining a locoregional control rate of 100%. In the group of seven patients treated with EBRT and brachytherapy, the authors described a local recurrence and a regional recurrence, with an ultimate locoregional control of 100%. The other 12 patients underwent brachytherapy, presenting a local control in 11/12 cases and an ultimate local control and regional control of 100%. In the whole series, they observed soft tissue necrosis in four patients and two cartilage necrosis. The authors advocated BRT for UICC T1/T2 SCC due to high rate of local control and good cosmetic results shown in the series, while in UICC T3/T4 suitable for implantation, they suggested that EBRT should precede brachytherapy. Finally in no implantable locally advanced lesions, EBRT alone was recommended [32].

In 1999, Mendenhall published a series of 60 patients treated at University of Florida in 1970–1995. In total, 56 lesions were primary irradiated, and 4 T4 cancers underwent high dose preoperative irradiation followed by surgical resection. Sixteen patients were treated with EBRT, 13 patients implanted with IRT, 31 patients received a combination of the two modalities. Local control rate after radiotherapy alone was 85%: 94% in UICC T1/T2 cancer, 83% in T4 without bone invasion, 0/3 in case of bone invasion. Initial and ultimate regional control rate was 88% in N0 with primary site controlled and no ENI. Five-year OS observed in case of RT alone was 74%. No severe complications were described in RT alone group, only minimal or moderate soft tissue necrosis in 21% of patients, while significant sequelae-like bone exposure, wound breakdown, or surgery for suspected but not real recurrence was observed in three out of four patients who underwent surgery after RT [33]. In 2016, Wray et al. presented an update of the series to 99 patients: 13 patients underwent RT and surgery while 86 patients were treated with RT alone, 39 patients with EBRT, 15 patients with brachytherapy, and 45 with a combination of the two modalities. ENI was performed in 25 N0 advanced tumors (T4 or poorly differentiated lesions). Five-year initial and ultimate local control rates were 88% and 94% in the whole series, 88% and 93% in RT alone group. Five-year initial and ultimate N0 regional control rates were 87% and 97%, while OS and DSS were 75% and 91% in all patients and 77% and 94% in RT alone group. The authors observed an overall local control of 100% in patients treated with brachytherapy: a local control rate of 88% in T1/T2 tumors and 75% in T3/T4 cancer treated with combination of EBRT and brachytherapy, and a local control rate of 86% in T1/T2 tumors and 77% in T3/T4 tumors irradiated with EBRT alone. So, Wray and colleagues concluded that primary RT is recommended for tumors smaller than 4 cm, while for bigger lesions they suggested a combination of surgery and RT. ENI was recommended only in T3/T4 tumors or in case of recurrence [34].

At VU University Medical Center, Amsterdam, 56 Wang T1/T2 NVSCCs were primarily irradiated between 1980 and 2000: before 1997, 32 patients were treated with EBRT and IDR brachytherapy boost; after 1997, 9 patients underwent EBRT alone, and 15 lesions were treated with EBRT and HDR Brachytherapy boost. Two-year initial local control rate was 79% in whole series; in particular, in EBRT + IDR group was 75%, in EBRT group 88%, and in EBRT + HDR group 86%. Two-year initial and ultimate regional control rates were 87% and 97%. At 5-year follow-up, the authors observed ultimate local control rate of 95%, OS of 66%, and DSS of 87%. In conclusion, the authors advocated for radiotherapy in T1/T2 tumors, choosing the technique depending on the extension of primary lesion and on radiation oncologists' training [35].

In 2015, Lipman et al. presented a series of 60 Wang T1/T2 NVSCCs treated with high-dose Iridium[192] exclusive brachytherapy at Department of Radiation Oncology of Radboud University Nijmegen Medical Centre between 1992 and 2010: 38 patients with interstitial catheters and 22 with a mold technique. Three-year initial and ultimate local control rates were 91% and 96%, while initial and ultimate regional control rates were 93% and 96% [36]. In an update of this series, 42 new patients were treated in 2010–2014 for a total of 102 Wang T1/T2 patients.

Authors observed that 5-year initial and ultimate local control rates were 95% and 98% (100% in patients treated after 2010) and an initial and ultimate regional control rates of 91% and 96%, 88% in the group enrolled after 2010. After 5 years of follow-up, OS and DSS were 72% and 94% in the whole series, 83% and 97% in the new patients enlisted group. Toxicity due to radiation was considered acceptable, patients reported good functional and cosmetic outcomes. The authors advocated for brachytherapy for Wang T1 and T2 and even in well-selected larger lesions, while ENI was not recommended [37].

Between 1977 and 2012, at Netherlands Cancer Institute-Antoni Leeuwenhoek Hospital, 81 patients were irradiated for NVSCC, 38 with HDR HBRT, 41 with Iridium[192] IRT, and 2 cases with EBRT and Iridium[192]. No ENI was performed. The authors described a 5-year local control rate of 97% in 48 Wang T1 tumors, 68% in 26 T2 lesions, and 53% in 7 T3 cancers; OS was 59% and progression-free survival 57%. The authors concluded that IRT is a successful option for Wang T1/T2 tumor, invasion of lip is not an absolute contraindication for IRT, while EBRT is not recommended as a single treatment for T3 cancer but only in combination with IRT [38].

In the same year, Bussu et al. presented a series of 12 patients treated in 2009–2013 at Università Cattolica del Sacro Cuore, Rome. Six patients underwent surgery, and other six patients were treated with IRT. Elective neck dissection was performed in cT3 lesion. The authors described a DSS of 80% in the surgery group, 83% in brachytherapy, and a RFS of 83% in both groups. Functional and cosmetic outcomes were evaluated in both groups, showing a significantly higher value in the IRT group. Authors advocated for IRT as primary treatment and EBRT in case of recurrence or positive nodes with adverse features at pathological report [39]. In an update that analyzed 14 patients treated with exclusive IRT between 2012 and 2019, authors observed two local recurrences with a 3-year LC of 85.7%, and two regional recurrences with a 3-year RC of 81.2%, who underwent neck dissection and adjuvant EBRT. At 3-year follow-up, DFS was 67.3%, OS 69.2%, and DSS 92.3%. Cosmetic results were very good, confirming that IRT provides excellent tumor control and high patient's aesthetic satisfaction and could be considered as a definitive treatment in nasal vestibule cancer [40].

In 2021, Czerwinski published a six Nederland oncological hospital multicenter cohort study in which comparison between IRT and EBRT for Wang T1-T2 NV cancers in terms of oncological outcomes, nose preservation rate, and late toxicity was performed. At 3-year follow-up, regional control rate of the 225 patients treated between 2010 and 2016 was 89% (ultimate 95%), while OS and DSS were 82% and 94%, with no significant difference between the two treatment modalities for each statistical parameter. Three-year LC rate was 87%, with an ultimate 3-year LC rate of 96%, and a statistic significant difference between the IRT (95%) and the EBRT (71%) groups. Also, the percentage of survival with nose preservation was different according to the irradiation technique, being higher in the IRT-treated patients (82%) than in the EBRT group (61%), so that at multivariate analysis EBRT resulted to decrease survival with preserved nose besides being the sole significant risk factor for local relapse. On the contrary, radiation toxicity-free survival at 5 years was

71%, resulted to be worse in the IRT subgroup in which ulcers occurred significantly more often than in EBRT-treated patients, without however impacting patient satisfaction in a major way. According to this multicenter study results, the author suggested that IRT can be recommended as first-line treatment for Wang T1-T2 (and Bussu up to T3) NV cancers [2, 3, 41].

References

1. Vital D, Morand G, Huber GF, Studer G, Holzmann D. Outcome in squamous cell carcinoma of the nasal vestibule: a single center experience. Head Neck. 2015;37:46–51.
2. Bussu F, et al. New standards for the management of nose vestibule malignancies Acta Oto-Laryngologica. 2023;143(3):215–22. https://doi.org/10.1080/00016489.2023.2179662.
3. Bussu F, Tagliaferri L, Piras A, Rizzo D, Tsatsaris N, De Corso E et al. Multidisciplinary approach to nose vestibule malignancies: setting new standards Approccio multidisciplinare ai tumori maligni del vestibolo del naso: verso la definizione di nuovi standard Acta Otorhinolaryngologica Italica. 2021;41(Suppl. 1):S158–S165. https://doi.org/10.14639/0392-100X-suppl.1-41-2021-16.
4. Dowley A, Hoskison E, Allibone R, Jones NS. Squamous cell carcinoma of the nasal vestibule: a 20-year case series and literature review. J Laryngol Otol. 2008;122:1019–23.
5. Zaoui K, Plinkert PK, Federspil PA. Primary surgical treatment of nasal vestibule cancer—therapeutic outcome and reconstructive strategies. Rhinology. 2018;56:393–9.
6. Evaluation of Staging Systems for Cancer of the Nasal Vestibule Cancers. 2023;15(11):3028. https://doi.org/10.3390/cancers15113028.
7. Goepfert H, Guillamondegui OM, Jesse RH, Lindberg RD. Squamous cell carcinoma of nasal vestibule. Arch Otolaryngol. 1974;100:8–10.
8. Kagan AR, Nussbaum H, Rao A, Chan P, Gilbert H, Hintz B, Ryoo M, Miles J, Rice D. The management of carcinoma of the nasal vestibule. Head Neck Surg. 1981;4:125–8.
9. Weinberger JM, Briant TD, Cummings BJ, Wong CS. The role of surgery in the treatment of squamous cell carcinoma of the nasal vestibule. J Otolaryngol. 1988;17:372–5.
10. Patel P, Tiwari R, Karim AB, Nauta JJ, Snow GB. Squamous cell carcinoma of the nasal vestibule. J Laryngol Otol. 1992;106:332–6.
11. Pantelakos ST, McGuirt WF, Nussear DW. Squamous cell carcinoma of the nasal vestibule and anterior nasal passages. Am J Otolaryngol. 1994;15:33–6.
12. Fornelli RA, Fedok FG, Wilson EP, Rodman SM. Squamous cell carcinoma of the anterior nasal cavity: a dual institution review. Otolaryngol Head Neck Surg. 2000;123:207–10.
13. Agger A, von Buchwald C, Madsen AR, et al. Squamous cell carcinoma of the nasal vestibule 1993-2002: a nationwide retrospective study from DAHANCA. Head Neck. 2009;31:1593–9.
14. Ledderose GJ, Reu S, Englhard AS, Krause E. Endonasal resection of early stage squamous cell carcinoma of the nasal vestibule. Eur Arch Otorhinolaryngol. 2014;271:1051–5.
15. Federspil PA, Plinkert PK, Zaoui K. Early nasal reconstruction after skin-preserving excision of squamous cell carcinoma of the nasal vestibule. J Plast Reconstr Aesthet Surg. 2020;73:1683–91.
16. Lambertoni A, Cherubino M, Battaglia P, et al. Squamous cell carcinoma of nasal vestibule and pyramid: outcomes and reconstructive strategies. Laryngoscope. 2021;131:E1198–208.
17. Chabrillac E, Talawdekar A, Garikipati S, Varley I, Sionis S, Beasley N, Jackson R. A single centre's experience of 23 cases of total rhinectomy for the treatment of squamous cell carcinoma involving the nasal vestibule. Eur Arch Otorhinolaryngol. 2021;279:2069. https://doi.org/10.1007/s00405-021-06972-6.
18. Wang CC. Treatment of carcinoma of the nasal vestibule by irradiation. Cancer. 1976;38:100–6.

19. Mak ACA, van Andel JG, Van Woerkom-Eijkenboom WMH. Radiation therapy of carcinoma of the nasal vestibule. Eur J Cancer. 1980;16:81–5.
20. Jong JMA, Schalekamp W, Hordijk GJ. Squamous carcinoma of the nasal vestibule. Clin Otolaryngol. 1981;6:205–8.
21. Chassagne D, Wilson JF. Brachytherapy of carcinomas of the nasal vestibule. Int J Radiat Oncol Biol Phys. 1984;10:761.
22. Johansen LV, Hjelm-Hansen M, Andersen AP. Squamous cell carcinoma of the nasal vestibule. Treatment results. Acta Radiol Oncol. 1984;23:189–92.
23. Baris G, Visser AG, van Andel JG. The treatment of squamous cell carcinoma of the nasal vestibule with interstitial iridium implantation. Radiother Oncol. 1985;4:121–5.
24. Wong CS, Cummings BJ, Elhakim T, Briant TD. External irradiation for squamous cell carcinoma of the nasal vestibule. Int J Radiat Oncol Biol Phys. 1986;12:1943–6.
25. Jeannon J-P, Riddle PJ, Irish J, O'sullivan B, Brown DH, Gullane P. Prognostic indicators in carcinoma of the nasal vestibule. Clin Otolaryngol. 2007;32:19–23.
26. Haynes WD, Ducote Haynes W, Tapley ND. Radiation treatment of carcinoma of the nasal vestibule. Am J Roentgenol. 1974;120:595–602.
27. Chobe R, McNeese M, Weber R, Fletcher GH. Radiation therapy for carcinoma of the nasal vestibule. Otolaryngol Head Neck Surg. 1988;98:67–71.
28. Levendag PC, Pomp J. Radiation therapy of squamous cell carcinoma of the nasal vestibule. Int J Radiat Oncol Biol Phys. 1990;19:1363–7.
29. Levendag PC, Nijdam WM, van Moolenburgh SE, Tan L, Noever I, van Rooy P, Mureau MAM, Jansen PP, Munte K, Hofer SOP. Interstitial radiation therapy for early-stage nasal vestibule cancer: a continuing quest for optimal tumor control and cosmesis. Int J Radiat Oncol Biol Phys. 2006;66:160–9.
30. Poulsen M, Turner S. Radiation therapy for squamous cell carcinoma of the nasal vestibule. Int J Radiat Oncol Biol Phys. 1993;27:267–72.
31. Turner SL, Lochrin CA, Dische S, Saunders MI, Maher EJ. Continuous hyperfractionated accelerated radiotherapy in the treatment of carcinoma of the columella and vestibule of the nose. Eur J Cancer B Oral Oncol. 1995;31B:368–72.
32. Evensen JF, Jacobsen AB, Tausjø JE. Brachytherapy of squamous cell carcinoma of the nasal vestibule. Acta Oncol. 1996;35(Suppl 8):87–92.
33. Mendenhall WM, Stringer SP, Cassisi NJ, Mendenhall NP. Squamous cell carcinoma of the nasal vestibule. Head Neck. 1999;21:385–93.
34. Wray J, Morris CG, Kirwan JM, Amdur RJ, Werning JW, Dziegielewski PT, Mendenhall WM. Radiation therapy for nasal vestibule squamous cell carcinoma: a 40-year experience. Eur Arch Otorhinolaryngol. 2016;273:661–9.
35. Langendijk JA, Poorter R, Leemans CR, de Bree R, Doornaert P, Slotman BJ. Radiotherapy of squamous cell carcinoma of the nasal vestibule. Int J Radiat Oncol Biol Phys. 2004;59:1319–25.
36. Lipman D, Verhoef LC, Takes RP, Kaanders JH, Janssens GO. Outcome and toxicity profile after brachytherapy for squamous cell carcinoma of the nasal vestibule. Head Neck. 2015;37:1297–303.
37. Czerwinski MD, van Leeuwen RGH, Kaanders JHAM, Zwijnenburg EM, Lipman D, Takes RP, Verhoef CG. Image guided brachytherapy for cancer of the nasal vestibule: local control and cosmesis. Int J Radiat Oncol Biol Phys. 2019;103:913–21.
38. Vanneste BGL, Lopez-Yurda M, Tan IB, Balm AJM, Borst GR, Rasch CR. Irradiation of localized squamous cell carcinoma of the nasal vestibule. Head Neck. 2016;38(Suppl 1):E1870–5.
39. Bussu F, Tagliaferri L, Mattiucci G, et al. Comparison of interstitial brachytherapy and surgery as primary treatments for nasal vestibule carcinomas. Laryngoscope. 2016;126:367–71.
40. Tagliaferri L, Carra N, Lancellotta V, et al. Interventional radiotherapy as exclusive treatment for primary nasal vestibule cancer: single-institution experience. J Contemp Brachytherapy. 2020;12:413–9.
41. Czerwinski MD, Jansen PP, Zwijnenburg EM, Al-Mamgani A, Vergeer MR, Langendijk JA, Wesseling FWR, Kaanders JHAM, Verhoef CG. Radiotherapy as nose preservation treat-

ment strategy for cancer of the nasal vestibule: the Dutch experience. Radiother Oncol. 2021;164:20–6.

42. DesPrez JD, Kiehn CL. Carcinoma of the nasal vestibule. Am J Surg. 1967;114:587–91.

43. Mendenhall NP, Parsons JT, Cassisi NJ, Million RR. Carcinoma of the nasal vestibule. Int J Radiat Oncol Biol Phys. 1984;10:627–37.

44. Mendenhall NP, Parsons JT, Cassisi NJ, Million RR. Carcinoma of the nasal vestibule treated with radiation therapy. Laryngoscope. 1987;97:626–32.

45. Mazeron JJ, Chassagne D, Crook J, Bachelot F, Brochet F, Brune D, Brunin F, Bunescu U, Daly N, Danczak S. Radiation therapy of carcinomas of the skin of nose and nasal vestibule: a report of 1676 cases by the Groupe Europeen de Curiethérapie. Radiother Oncol. 1988;13:165–73.

46. McCollough WM, Mendenhall NP, Parsons JT, Mendenhall WM, Stringer SP, Cassisi NJ, Million RR. Radiotherapy alone for squamous cell carcinoma of the nasal vestibule: management of the primary site and regional lymphatics. Int J Radiat Oncol Biol Phys. 1993;26:73–9.

47. Wallace A, Morris CG, Kirwan J, Amdur RJ, Werning JW, Mendenhall WM. Radiotherapy for squamous cell carcinoma of the nasal vestibule. Am J Clin Oncol. 2007;30:612–6.

48. Koopmann M, Weiss D, Savvas E, Rudack C, Stenner M. Clinicopathological and immunohistochemical characteristics of surgically treated primary carcinoma of the nasal vestibule—an evaluation of 30 cases. Clin Otolaryngol. 2015;40:240–7.

Surgery in Nose Vestibule Malignancies: The Ablative Phase

7

Tito Poli, Davide Lanfranco, Davide Rizzo, Eleonora Longoni, Antonio Tullio, Francesco Bussu, Jacopo Galli, and Enrico Sesenna

7.1 Introduction

Cancers of the nasal vestibule are considered rare and reported to account for less than 1% of all tumors of the head and neck [1] but their prevalence is probably largely underestimated [2, 3]. The nasal vestibule is separated anatomically from the nasal cavity, classically by the limen nasi (even if the plane tangential to the pyriform opening has been proposed as more reliable boundary, see Chap. 1). Cancers originating from the nasal vestibule behave differently from squamous cell

T. Poli · D. Lanfranco · E. Sesenna
Maxillo-Facial Surgery Division, Head and Neck Department, University Hospital of Parma, Parma, Italy
e-mail: tito.poli@unipr.it; enrico.sesenna@unipr.it

E. Longoni (✉)
Otolaryngology Division, Azienda Ospedaliera Universitaria, Sassari, Italy

A. Tullio
Maxillo-Facial Surgery Division, Department of Medicine and Surgery, University of Perugia, Perugia, Italy

Maxillo-Facial Surgery Unit, Santa Maria Della Misericordia Hospital, San Sisto, Perugia, Italy
e-mail: antonio.tullio@unipg.it

D. Rizzo · F. Bussu
Otolaryngology Division, Azienda Ospedaliera Universitaria, Sassari, Italy

Department of Medicine, Surgery and Pharmacy, University of Sassari, Sassari, Italy
e-mail: drizzo@uniss.it; fbussu@uniss.it

J. Galli
Otolaryngology Division, Fondazione Policlinico Universitario Agostino Gemelli IRCCS, Rome, Italy

Department of Head-Neck and Sensory Organs, Università Cattolica del Sacro Cuore, Rome, Italy

© Springer Nature Switzerland AG 2023
F. Bussu (ed.), *Malignancies of the Nasal Vestibule*,
https://doi.org/10.1007/978-3-031-32850-3_7

carcinomas of the skin and are distinct histological and clinical entities from those arising from the nasal cavity proper (see Chaps. 1, 3, 5). Thus, these tumors must be considered separately also when the surgical approach is concerned.

The goal of therapy is to achieve the best oncologic outcome with the least morbidity in terms of both cosmesis and nasal function. There are no large clinical trials that have established the optimal treatment for these patients; treatment modalities are currently based upon institutional specific expertise and attitudes or are decided individually on the basis of a multidisciplinary discussion (see Chap. 6).

7.2 Surgery

Surgery is probably the most used treatment modality for nose vestibule malignancies worldwide. It is made up of an ablative phase (resection) and of a reconstructive phase. The approach, including surgery, to the neck will be discussed in a separate chapter, and in general is similar for all midface malignancies, including vestibule, but also superior lip and labial commissure/cheek primaries. On the other hand, the ablative surgery of the primary lesion in malignancies of the nose vestibule presents typical issues. It is usually relatively easy, yet positive margins at pathology and local recurrences are not infrequent. The reason for that is most often the attitude of the surgeon to preserve as much as possible of the osteo-cartilaginous framework of the nose tip in order to avoid cosmetic deformity or anyway facilitate the much more difficult following phase, that is reconstruction. This can turn out to be a tragic mistake, as positive margins strongly affect survival as recently reported in a total rhinectomy series [4]. As a matter of fact, local recurrences are always difficult to manage and often result in regional metastasis, oncological failure, and death, while in every oncological surgery, the main aim must always be eradication of the disease. So, our advice, in surgically treated nose vestibule malignancies, is to complete the resection of primary lesion with the objective of the wider and safer margins as possible, keeping the ablative phase completely separated from the reconstructive one (see Chap. 8), whose issues must not affect in any case the extent of the resection.

7.3 Resection

The approach to the tumor is most often external or combined (external + endoscopic). Endoscopic approach or midfacial degloving have a limited role, also because the "external" skin is most often involved (see Chap. 3).

Depending on the extent of the cancer and on the attitude of the surgeon, resection may range from a wide demolition, including a maxillectomy, to Mohs micrographic surgery. We do believe that, with very few exceptions, this last option is generally unsafe. In nose vestibule primary SCCs the most notable difference from primary skin cancers in terms of surgical approach is that a radical surgical resection requires most often a through resection including all the nasal wall from the skin to mucosa. In fact, most skin cancers arising on the nose tip can be safely and radically resected while sparing the cartilage, dissecting when needed under the perichondral plane. On the other hand, in case of primaries of the nasal vestibule, with the goal of complete tumor removal with microscopically tumor-free margins, deep structures, such as the upper and lower nasal cartilages, septal cartilage, and nasal and maxillary bones, most often need to be resected. Such resection must be planned with details in advance basing upon radiological, clinical, and endoscopic data; in our opinion, relying upon intraoperative findings and frozen section reports is far too unsafe in nose vestibule malignancies, where the complex tridimensional anatomy of internal and external surfaces and cartilaginous planes makes in our opinion the intraoperative sampling totally unreliable. For these reasons, the surgical sample must be single, delivered en-bloc, and well oriented, possibly with an early discussion with the histopathologist concerning the cutting and sampling of the specimen itself. In case of positive margins, a surgical widening of the resection is recommended and therefore is of utmost importance that histological margins are as reliable as possible. In case of need, in particular for unexpectedly positive margins in the final histopathology report, the reresection will be far simpler in case of delayed reconstruction or resort to an epithesis (Fig. 7.1).

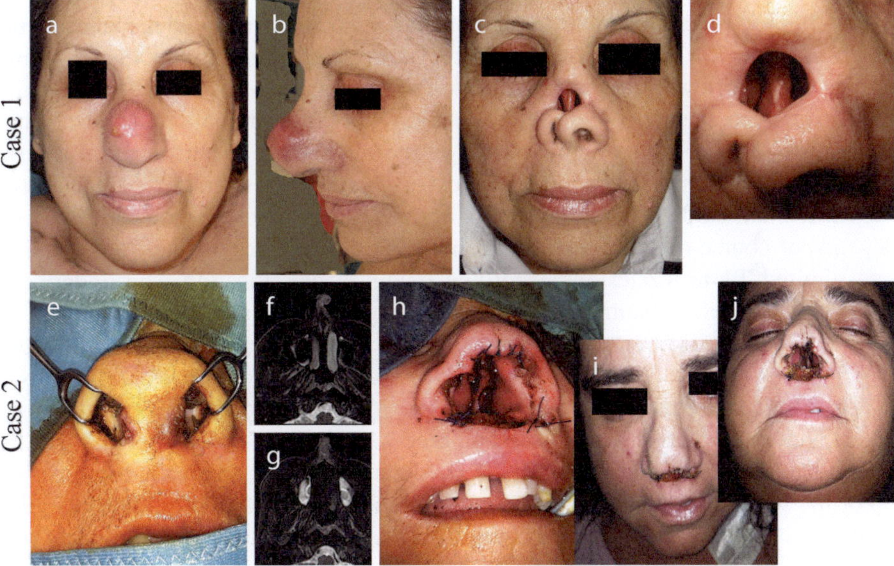

Fig. 7.1 Preoperative findings (**a, b, e, f, g**) and postoperative results (**c, d, h, i, j**) in two patients treated by primary surgery are shown. Case 1 came to our observation with a primary SCC arising from the limen nasi and spreading to the tip and the alar skin without clear cartilagineous destruction (**a, b**) (T2 stage according to Wang, T2a according to Bussu, T4a according to AJCC/UICC [2, 3, 5]). R0 resection was performed, with the preservation of nostril rims, but the aesthetic result without a prosthesis 12 months after surgery is not satisfactory at all (**c, d**). Case 2 displayed at physical exam (**e**) and at MR imaging (**f, g**), an SCC of the columella spreading toward the superior lip (T2 stage according to Wang, T2a according to Bussu, T4a according to AJCC/UICC [2, 3, 5]). Six weeks after the R0 resection, the results of the primary closure are objectively better (**h, i, j**) but still not fully satisfactory for the patient

Table 7.1 Classification of the resection for nose vestibule malignancies

Type of resection	Structures involved	Preferred rehabilitation/reconstruction
Minimal muco-cutaneous resection	Internal lining (skin and mucosa) ± alar/lateral cartilage *No external skin included*	Secondary healing
Lateral through defect	Internal lining (skin and mucosa), alar/lateral cartilage, external skin	Local flaps
Medial-inferior through defect	Internal lining (skin and mucosa), alar/lateral cartilage, external skin + superior lip and/or columella septum	Local flaps/Prostetic rehabilitation
Total rhinectomy	Total subtotal defect of cartilaginous framework and overlying skin ± (part of) nasal bones ± nasal process of the maxilla	Prosthetic rehabilitation/free flaps/forehead flap
Enlargement to the maxillary bones	Level I: Premaxilla/nasal floor Level II: Maxillary face/premaxilla/nasal floor Level III: Medial maxillectomy Level IV: Subtotal maxillectomy Level V: Anterior craniofacial	Prosthetic rehabilitation/free flaps

We do believe that the best way to define, and therefore classify, the resection of a primary nose vestibule malignancy is to list the structures included in the resection itself. In Table 7.1, we stratify the ablative surgery according to the level of complexity of the following reconstruction. As, by definition, nose vestibule malignancies arise from the muco-cutaneous junction [6], the minimal resection always includes an area of mucosa and/or skin in the most anterior part of nasal cavity. Unluckily, such minimal resection is almost never sufficient to eradicate the disease, even if a small study reports the results of such an approach, whose effectiveness depends of course on the correct indications [7]. Such series included ten patients with limited T1 to T2 lesions according to AJCC classification who underwent endonasal resection resulting in 100% local control with a median follow-up of 37 months [7], two patients underwent adjuvant RT for a close margin and positive lymph nodes.

The surgical resection in nose vestibule carcinoma most often leads to a through defect including internal lining (skin and mucosa), cartilage, and "external" skin. It can be lateral, for lesions arising in the ala/dorsum, include an area in the superior lip or the septum for lesions arising in the inferior aspect of the vestibule or in the columella, or become a total rhinectomy defect for total/subtotal resection of the cartilaginous framework of the nose often including part of the bony framework [8–10]. Rhinectomy can extend to various degrees to maxillary bones, as defined by Dias [8] (Table 7.1).

Anyway, there is no doubt that ablative surgery in nose vestibule carcinomas can usually obtain tumor-free margins, issues arise in the perspective of the successive reconstruction (Fig. 7.1). In fact, surgically treated patients have usually very good locoregional control rates [11] if the above listed principles are followed.

This is confirmed by literature series, even if surgical series purely composed of nose vestibule carcinomas are small and a thorough and definite analysis of outcomes and predictors is not possible [12, 13]. The most recent of these series, composed of 23 patients treated with total rhinectomy (in 73.9% as a primary treatment), reports a 67.5% overall survival and a 80.7% disease-specific survival, confirming excision margins as one of the most important predictive factors for tumor recurrence after total rhinectomy [4].

References

1. Patel P, Tiwari R, Karim AB, Nauta JJ, Snow GB. Squamous cell carcinoma of the nasal vestibule. J Laryngol Otol. 1992;106:332–6.
2. Bussu et al. New standards for the management of nose vestibule malignancies Acta Oto-Laryngologica. 2023;143(3):215–22. https://doi.org/10.1080/00016489.2023.2179662.
3. Bussu F, Tagliaferri L, Piras A, Rizzo D, Tsatsaris N, De Corso E et al. Multidisciplinary approach to nose vestibule malignancies: setting new standards Approccio multidisciplinare ai tumori maligni del vestibolo del naso: verso la definizione di nuovi standard Acta Otorhinolaryngologica Italica. 2021;41(Suppl. 1):S158–S165. https://doi.org/10.14639/0392-100X-suppl.1-41-2021-16.
4. Chabrillac E, Talawdekar A, Garikipati S, Varley I, Sionis S, Beasley N, Jackson R. A single centre's experience of 23 cases of total rhinectomy for the treatment of squamous cell carcinoma involving the nasal vestibule. Eur Arch Otorhinolaryngol. 2021;279:2069. https://doi.org/10.1007/s00405-021-06972-6.
5. Scheurleer WFJ, Tagliaferri L, Rijken JA, Crescio C, Rizzo D, Mattiucci GC, Pameijer FA, de Bree R, Fionda B, de Ridder M, Bussu F. Evaluation of Staging Systems for Cancer of the Nasal Vestibule Cancers. 2023;15(11):3028. https://doi.org/10.3390/cancers15113028.
6. Jeannon J-P, Riddle PJ, Irish J, O'sullivan B, Brown DH, Gullane P. Prognostic indicators in carcinoma of the nasal vestibule. Clin Otolaryngol. 2007;32:19–23.
7. Ledderose GJ, Reu S, Englhard AS, Krause E. Endonasal resection of early stage squamous cell carcinoma of the nasal vestibule. Eur Arch Otorhinolaryngol. 2014;271:1051–5.
8. Dias FL. Rhinectomy. In: Ferris RL, Myers EN, editors. Master techniques in otolaryngology-head and neck surgery: larynx, hypopharynx, oropharynx, oral cavity and neck. Philadelphia, PA: Lippincott Williams & Wilkins; 2013. p. 183–90.
9. Teichgraeber JF, Goepfert H. Rhinectomy: timing and reconstruction. Otolaryngol Head Neck Surg. 1990;102:362–9.
10. Stanley RJ, Olsen KD. Rhinectomy for malignant disease: a 20-year experience. Arch Otolaryngol Head Neck Surg. 1988;114:1307–11.
11. Bussu F, Tagliaferri L, Mattiucci G, et al. Comparison of interstitial brachytherapy and surgery as primary treatments for nasal vestibule carcinomas. Laryngoscope. 2016;126:367–71.
12. Weinberger JM, Briant TD, Cummings BJ, Wong CS. The role of surgery in the treatment of squamous cell carcinoma of the nasal vestibule. J Otolaryngol. 1988;17:372–5.
13. Dowley A, Hoskison E, Allibone R, Jones NS. Squamous cell carcinoma of the nasal vestibule: a 20-year case series and literature review. J Laryngol Otol. 2008;122:1019–23.

Surgery in Nose Vestibule Malignancies: The Reconstructive Phase

8

Luca Salvatore Calabrese, Davide Rizzo, Luigi Angelo Vaira, Francesco Giuseppe Riu, Corrado Rubino, and Giacomo De Riu

8.1 Introduction

NV is the anterior part of the nasal cavity classically consisting of the internal lining of the lateral crus and alar soft tissue, the medial crus of the lower lateral cartilage, the nasal floor, and the dome. The medial part of the NV includes the columella, the medial alar cartilage, and the medial membranous nasal septum. It has been

L. S. Calabrese
Otolaryngology Division, Regional Hospital of Bolzano, Bolzano, Italy

D. Rizzo (✉)
Otolaryngology Division, Sassari University Hospital, Sassari, Italy

Department of Medicine Pharmacy and Surgery, University of Sassari, Sassari, Italy
e-mail: davide.rizzo@aouss.it, drizzo@uniss.it

L. A. Vaira
Department of Medicine Pharmacy and Surgery, University of Sassari, Sassari, Italy

Maxillofacial Surgery Division, Sassari University Hospital, Sassari, Italy
e-mail: lavaira@uniss.it

F. G. Riu
Otolaryngology Division, Sassari University Hospital, Sassari, Italy
e-mail: francesco.riu@aouss.it

C. Rubino
Department of Medicine Pharmacy and Surgery, University of Sassari, Sassari, Italy

Plastic Surgery Division, Sassari University Hospital, Sassari, Italy
e-mail: corubino@uniss.it

G. De Riu
Department of Clinical, Surgical and Experimental Medicine, University of Sassari, Sassari, Italy

Maxillofacial Surgery Division, Sassari University Hospital, Sassari, Italy
e-mail: gderiu@uniss.it

© Springer Nature Switzerland AG 2023
F. Bussu (ed.), *Malignancies of the Nasal Vestibule*,
https://doi.org/10.1007/978-3-031-32850-3_8

classically considered to extend from the nostrils approximately 1.5 cm upward to limen nasi, which marks the "classical" ill-defined boundary between the NV and the nasal cavity [1, 2], even if in the present monograph we propose an extension as well as more objective/radiological definition of the anatomical boundaries (see Chap. 1).

Treatment of tumors of NV is a debated issue in the literature.

The ablative surgery has been discussed in a specific section of this text. However, before talking about reconstruction, it is necessary to remark on some relevant issues. Tumors of NV can show submucosal and subcutaneous pattern of spread; along the above cited cartilages (see Chap. 3) [3, 4]; consequently, the authors recommend to consider delaying the reconstructive phase after ablative step. Indeed, even if guided by frozen sections, in a limited space and anatomically complex region, it is not possible to have certainty about free margins until and sometimes even after the definitive histologic examination.

8.2 Principles of Reconstruction

Planning reconstruction after resection of tumors of NV requires to keep in mind several issues:

1. NV is composed of different layer of tissues (mucosa, skin, cartilaginous layer) that make architecture of this site very complex.
2. Tumors of NV are often diagnosed in advanced stages, when adjacent subsites are involved (due to the differential diagnosis with inflammatory diseases), especially in AJCC/UICC classification, for which the early almost constant skin involvement already makes up for a T4a [5].
3. Surgery is usually the treatment of choice in very early or advanced-stage tumors. While small defects do not require intricate reconstruction, complexity of NV makes surgical reconstruction for mild and large-size defects demanding.

As a general rule, we need to imagine the NV as a tetrahedral space: the base is extended from the anterior nares to the limen nasi, a mucosal fold formed by the upper margin of the alar cartilage and the lower margin of the upper lateral cartilage; the medial wall is built of the nasal septum, columella, and medial section of the alar cartilage; the lateral wall is mainly composed of the alar cartilage and superiorly, of the triangular cartilage. These intersecting structures are difficult to reconstruct with a satisfactory cosmetic result because, differently from cutaneous tumors of nasal pyramid, the cartilaginous layer is often involved, and resection must be extended to the latter, thus removing support and symmetrical spatial projection to the vestibule.

Burget and Menick analyzed the nose as a facial unit with subunits based on the skin quality, border outline, and three-dimentional contour of each region [6]. The so-called aesthetic units of the nose include: dorsum, pair sidewalls, tip lobule, pair alae, pair soft triangles, and columella. The NV includes the four latter. According to Baker, when a portion of the nose is missing, the ideal surgical approach is to repair it with an equal amount of similar tissue, neither underfilling, nor overfilling the defect, with a covering flap of the proper thinness and with appropriate midlayer

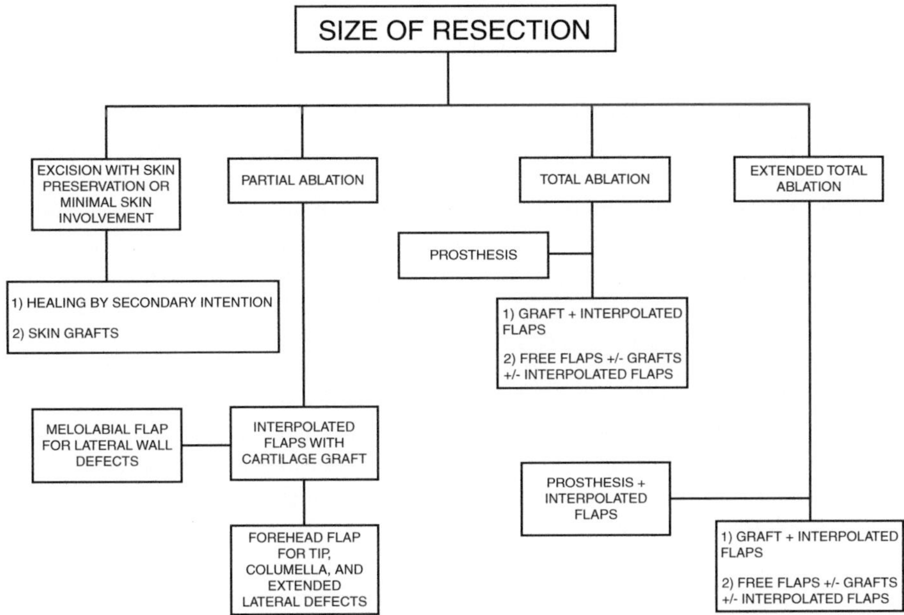

Fig. 8.1 A decisional algorithm for the reconstruction techniques based on the size/site of the defect

framework to support shape and brace the repair. If resection encompasses more than 50% of the subunit, it is better to excise normal tissue and reconstruct the entire unit.

In Fig. 8.1 is represented our algorithm of reconstruction techniques based on the size of the defect of NV.

8.3 Limited-Size Defects with Skin Preservation or Minimal Skin Involvement

8.3.1 Healing by Secondary Intention

There is still a role for healing by second intention, especially for small, superficial defects. In addition, patients may choose this option to avoid further procedures or if they have significant medical comorbidities that preclude additional surgery [7].

8.3.2 Skin Grafts

Skin grafts are considered a good option for internal lining when a limited resection is required. Indeed, although for full-thickness defects are preferred folded flaps or combination of intranasal and extranasal flap, a skin graft is useful to help healing of surgical site, preventing retracting scar [8].

Skin grafts can be harvested in several different forms. Regardless of the type of graft, graft viability depends on several factors: blood supply to the recipient site, microcirculation on the surface of the recipient site, vascularity of donor graft tissue, contact between graft and recipient site, and systemic illnesses. Contact between the skin graft and recipient site is essential: a bolster dressing is helpful to prevent fluid collection beneath the graft postoperatively. Bolsters also prevent shearing forces from disrupting fibrous connections between the graft and wound bed. Recipient site conditions that are not favorable to graft survival include irradiated tissue; excessive fibrosis; exposed bone, or cartilage; and a bleeding wound. Grafts placed over avascular defects smaller than 1 cm [9] may survive through nutritional support via wound edges; however, grafting over avascular wounds larger than this is unlikely to succeed [10]. A number of donor sites for skin grafts are available in most individuals, depending on the location and size of the nasal vestibule defect. Preauricular or supraclavicular skin can be used for the upper part of the nose. Repair of the tip or ala with skin grafts must be avoided because of the thickness and texture of these units. The only exception, according to Menick, is forehead full thickness skin graft [11].

8.4 Reconstruction in Partial Ablation

The most common resection for tumors of the NV is the full thickness. As a general principle, we can divide the defect according to nasal units mostly involved: lateral defect (ala), medial defect (tip and columella), and composite defect (from lateral to medial). Moreover, the resection could be variable extended to other structures such as nasal septum, upper lip, and cheek.

Full-thickness nasal defects require three-layered reconstruction in order to provide restoration of the internal lining, skeletal support, and cutaneous cover.

8.4.1 Internal Lining

The internal lining can be restored with different available sources. For pure alar defects, a folded interpolated flap represents a valuable option because it avoids additional procedure on nasal cavities, shortening surgical time. Other options include septal flaps and inferior turbinate flap [12]. One of the most common flaps utilized for lining reconstruction is the septal hinge flap [13]. Septal hinge flap is based on the anterior septal artery and is useful for defects of the ala, tip, and sidewall. A superiorly based septal flap can also be created [14], based on the dorsal septum and raised with the distal portion of the flap along the floor of the nose. The width of the flap depends on the size of the defect. This septal flap can be delivered through a small defect created below the most dorsal aspect of the nasal septum. Septal flaps can also incorporate the septal cartilage. The de Quervain flap is created following elevation of a contralateral septal flap in such a way that the vertically oriented septal flap and attached cartilage are rotated into the contralateral defect so that the septal cartilage provides structure for the nasal sidewall.

The inferior turbinate flap, as described by Murakami et al. [15], is a versatile and valuable option. It can be used as a primary lining flap or in conjunction with other techniques. Baker recommends the turbinate flap for defects of limited size and a lateral location [14].

8.4.2 Skeletal Support

One of the most important tenets in NV reconstruction is to establish and maintain support of the soft tissues to minimize functional sequelae such as nasal obstruction, as well as to diminish the risk of contraction of the reconstructed segments. Cartilage grafts are used liberally in nasal reconstruction because they help prevent contraction of the overlying soft tissues, reduce nasal obstruction, and serve as a rigid framework to prevent movement of subunit structures. In these circumstances, the grafts are sutured to the underlying lining tissues to minimize dead space that might occur. The best example is the placement of cartilage grafts in the alar region, restoring the shape of the alar subunit while preventing alar collapse and alar retraction [12]. Most nasal defects can be reconstructed with septal and/or conchal cartilage. In particular, conchal cartilage optimizes reconstruction of alar defects because of the curvature of the graft. Using the opposite ear for alar reconstruction has been observed to provide better contour for the alar subunit [12] (Fig. 8.2). The skeletal

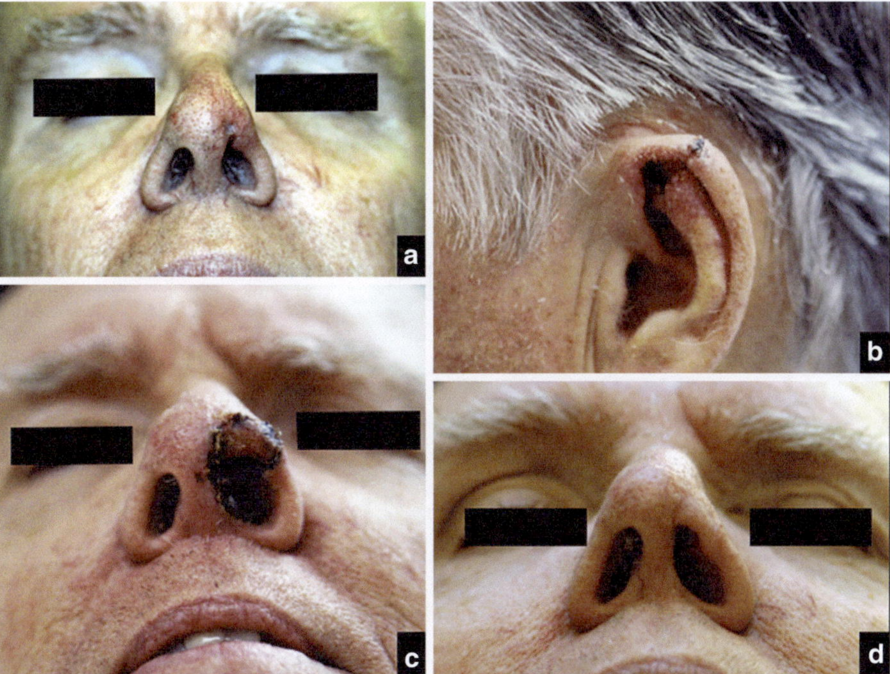

Fig. 8.2 (**a**) Columellar SCC involving the lateral wall. (**b**) Skin and cartilage grafts donor site. (**c**) Seven days and (**d**) 2 -month follow-up after reconstruction with helix graft

support to the tip of the nose can be obtained with a double graft of conchal cartilage, when the defect is almost symmetrical. More complex reconstruction of the tip can be obtaining with costal cartilage or calvarial bone grafts; however, these grafts are usually bounded to near total nasal reconstruction and will be discussed in the dedicated section.

Porous polyethiene implants (Medpore) are widely used for aesthetic rhinoplasty. Their application in reconstructive surgery as cartilagineous support increased over the last years. Implants area already shaped to replace small cartilage defects: columella strut, tip, nasal valve. Some authors describe their use also as scaffold in prelaminated flaps for total nasal reconstruction. The great advantage in their use is to avoid donor site morbidity. The cost is considered affordable, and the rate of infection (3–4%) can be estimated to be low [16–18].

8.4.3 Cutaneous Reconstruction

8.4.3.1 Melolabial Flap

The melolabial flap continues to be ideal for reconstruction of the ala nasi. Ala nasi can be constructed using either an island pedicle flap or a superiorly based pedicle flap [19, 20] (Figs. 8.3 and 8.4). The melolabial flap can be utilized for cutaneous defects of the ala in which cartilage grafts provide contour and support, both with an internal lining flap, or folding the melolabial flap itself. Drisco and Baker [21] have pointed out that this flap is best utilized for defects less than 4 cm. Generally,

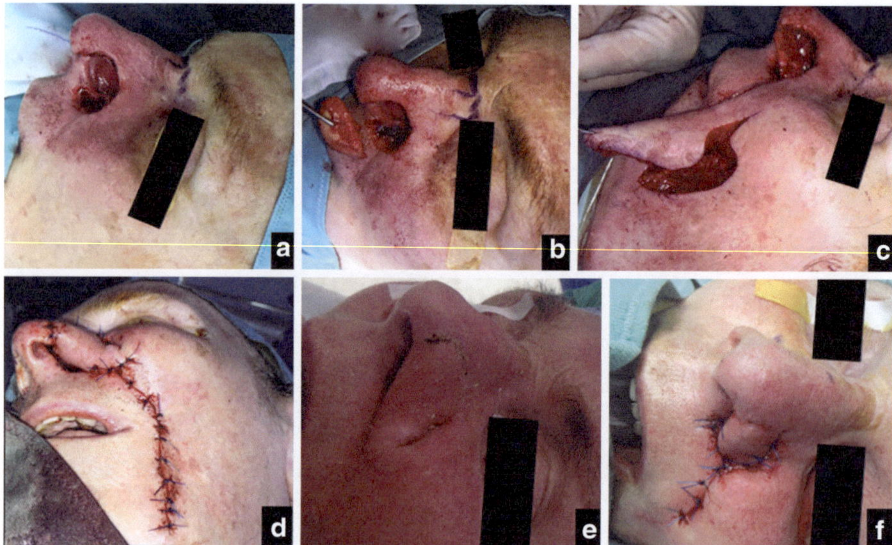

Fig. 8.3 (**a**) Alar SCC ablation defect with delayed reconstruction. (**b**) Cartilage graft from septum. (**c**) Melolabial flap preparation. (**d**) Immediate result after alar reconstruction with cartilage grafts as internal lining. (**e**) Two -month follow-up. (**f**) Flap remodeling

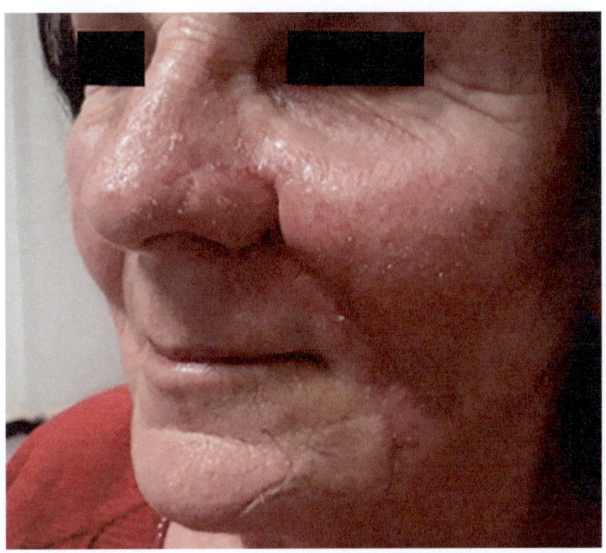

Fig. 8.4 Final result for melolabial flap

two surgical steps are sufficient to have a satisfactory aesthetic result. Although primarily used for alar defects, it can provide predictable results for alar defects with modest extensions onto the tip and nasal sidewall.

Surgical technique: The interpolated melolabial flap can be harvested as a peninsular flap with a linear axis based on a cutaneous pedicle that connects the flap to the cheek, or as an island flap, which does not have a cutaneous pedicle and is connected to the cheek by subcutaneous tissue. Whether a peninsular or island flap, the pedicle is developed at the superior aspect of the donor site. In both cases, the design should be based on a template of the defect.

The peninsular flap depends on the dermal and subdermal vascular plexus of the cutaneous pedicle to provide vascularity to the distal flap. The cutaneous pedicle must be of sufficient width and depth to ensure this vascularity. The peninsular flap is elevated in a subcutaneous tissue plane, maintaining 3 mm of fat on the undersurface of the cutaneous pedicle.

The island design has greater freedom to pivot on its pedicle and may have a better blood supply by incorporating within the pedicle of the flap a greater number of perforating vessels arising from the angular artery. The pedicle of the island flap does not require tailoring and inset following division of the pedicle. The subcutaneous tissue pedicle is simply excised, and the skin edges surrounding the pedicle are freshened and closed primarily. However, harvesting the island flap is technically more difficult than harvesting the peninsular flap because the plane of dissection is considerably deeper, placing the branches of the facial nerve supplying the zygomatic major and minor muscles at greater risk of injury. Both the flaps pivot 90° toward the midline and are sutured to the nose in a similar fashion. Care is taken not to kink the pedicle upon transferring the flap.

Interpolated melolabial flap may be thinned as necessary to replicate the thickness of the recipient site. The proximal portion of the flap bridging between cheek and nose is not thinned to ensure an ample vascular supply. According to Baker [20], the flap remains attached to the cheek for 3 weeks to enable the establishment of collateral vascularity. The pedicle is divided at a second stage, and the proximal portion of the pedicle is inset in the cheek by opening the superior portion of the donor site scar for 1–2 cm. The wound edges are spread widely, creating a space to accommodate the proximal pedicle. The skin adjacent to the opened wound is undermined for 2 cm. This allows the cheek skin to contract, assisting with enlarging nostril margin [20].

8.4.3.2 Forehead Flap

The paramedian forehead flap remains the primary workhorse for any significant NV defect for many reasons: potential for abundant skin and tissue, axial pattern blood supply, and ability to be shaped and thinned. Moreover, it has an abundant blood supply, providing for revascularization of cartilage and bone grafts covered by the flap.

The midline forehead flap is a modification that places the donor site scar in the midline of the forehead to facilitate the closure of donor site, However, according to Baker, the paramedian forehead flap based on a single supratrochlear artery has replaced the median forehead flap for nasal reconstruction because it has a more axial design, narrower base, and more effective length [20].

Surgical technique: The design of the flap should be based on a template of the defect. The base of the pedicle is centered over the supratrochlear artery. The vertical axis of the supratrochlear artery is 2 cm lateral to the midline, which corresponds to the medial border of the eyebrow. Therefore, the base of the flap is centered over the medial border of the brow. The base width is 1.5 cm wide and is not flared as this restricts the pivotal movement of the flap. Giving the flap angular rather than curvilinear borders reduces the propensity for developing trap-door deformity. If the defect occupies more than 50% of the surface area of the tip or alar aesthetic unit, the border of the unit is marked for removal of the remaining skin. To limit and adapt the size of the forehead flap according to the defect minimizes the deformity of the forehead. In the literature, the use of forehead flap for nasal reconstruction is widely discussed, and many tricks are suggested to obtain the best functional and cosmetic results. According to Baker, in most instances, freeing the flap from the frontalis muscle and most of its subcutaneous fat is essential when using the forehead for tip, columella, and alar defects [20]. Proper thinning of the flap will ensure that the shape and contour of the underlying nasal framework are manifested. The supratrochlear artery runs in the subdermal plan from 1 cm above the level of the eyebrow, and that enables flap thinning without concern for compromising vasculature [20].

As the melolabial flap, forehead flap can be folded. Folded forehead flaps for internal lining are thicker than hinge or contralateral septal grafts, but they have the significant advantage of axial rather than random-pattern blood supply, and they can be designed into just about any shape or size needed for internal lining reconstruction. They do require debulking, and they move the hair to the inside of the nose. All in all, they provide many advantages for a variety of reconstructive scenarios, and their disadvantages are easily managed. Regarding surgical steps, a recent study by Menick [22] highlights the major principles and key concepts in the contemporary use of the paramedian forehead flap. This study also covers the indications for a two-staged versus three-staged forehead flap. Indeed, an elevation of the flap during an intermediate operation allows the vascularity to be significantly greater than when it was transferred and much greater than that of a "thinned" two-stage flap at its initial transfer. However, it is important to underlie, as mentioned above, that the reconstruction in tumors of the NV must usually be delayed after resection, and therefore, the balance of a further surgical step under general anesthesia should be considered.

8.4.4 Additional Face Units' Defects

It is not infrequent, when dealing with tumors of NV, the need to extend the resection to other units of the face. Indeed, tumors of low NV (columella, floor of vestibule) can easily extend to the upper lip, while tumors involving the ala nasi may extend to the cheek. Whatever the addiction defect, it is important to reconstruct adjacent facial unit independently of the nasal reconstruction. In particular, for extensive defects involving the upper lip and cheek, it is recommended that these areas be reconstructed prior to nasal reconstruction in order to provide a solid and stable foundation for the nose [12].

8.4.5 Reconstruction in Total and Extended Total Ablation

Total nasal reconstruction represents an extremely challenging procedure and requires a great surgical experience to produce an acceptable functional and aesthetic result. According to the literature, three options are in the surgical armamentarium: prosthesis, grafts with interpolated flaps, and free flaps with or without grafts, and with or without interpolated flaps. The decision to perform reconstruction or prosthesis rests with the patient at the counsel of the surgeon. Depending on the patients' overall health and desire to avoid a prosthesis, they may or may not be motivated to undergo further procedures involved with reconstructing the nose.

8.4.5.1 Prosthesis

In specific indications, midfacial defects can be addressed to prosthetic rehabilitation, that can give a superior aesthetic outcome, combined with a less intensive surgical strain on the patient (see Chap. 9) [23]. Modern prostheses are made of specialized silicones and are flexible and adaptable; their thin and transparent edges merge almost perfectly with surrounding skin. An expert anaplastologist can master the prosthesis with modern coloring technique and tattooing skin features. The success of implant placement depends on planning for placing in the desired position and angle of the supports. An in-depth discussion on this topic will be done in the next chapter.

8.4.5.2 Surgical Reconstruction

Internal Lining and Skeletal Support in Total Nasal Reconstruction

Important differences with partial nose ablation must be taken into account in internal lining and skeletal support in total nasal reconstruction. Indeed, despite their obvious convenience, septal flaps may not provide adequate tissue in the total nasal defect; they are thin and fragile, thus more easy to devascularize, and frequently more difficult to harvest. Moreover, usually bilateral conchal cartilage is not sufficient for support extended tip defects.

In the last decades, several options have been described as alternatives for lining and supporting nasal reconstruction. A variety of regional turn-in, rotational, and transposition flaps have been described in reconstruction of the nasal lining. In fact, paramedian forehead flap, melolabial flap, and random turn-in flap can be used also for it in combination with other local interpolated or free flaps [24]. The major disadvantages of these flaps are the limited availability of tissue and the transfer of dry skin; however, they may be used in concert with other techniques. Given the principle role of the forehead flap in reconstructing the envelope, most surgeons reserve its use for this layer.

According to Cannady et al., another solution is the facial artery musculomucosal flap (FAMM) [24]. It is an axial pattern flap first described by Pribaz et al. based on the facial artery that can be transposed into the nasal cavity to provide mucosal lining that is both moist and well vascularized [25]. The major disadvantage of the FAMM flap is its bulk, which often will require subsequent thinning for nasal lining. In addition, the FAMM flap may not provide enough nasal lining to fill the total nasal defect even when harvested bilaterally and thus may be used in combination with other local flaps.

Lastly, one option is the microvascular free flaps. Forearm flap is the workhorse for internal lining reconstruction in total nasal defect. The flap is wrapped around skeletal support in order to create a tridimensional structure that will be used as framework for the following surgical steps. Several authors explored free tissue transfer for this defect to provide adequate volume of vascularized tissue for single-stage reconstructions of the total nasal defect, but the choice of a prelaminated single stage forearm flap must be reserved in selected cases with poor chance of reconstruction.

Regarding skeletal support, it is obviously fundamental to provide an acceptable functional and aesthetic result. This result is accomplished by providing central structure to allow for tip projection and prevent midvault collapse and by contouring of the lateral subunits and alae to recreate distinct nasal features. Although graft material is available from the calvarium, septal cartilage and bone, rib, and auricular cartilage, the best combination of choices is case-dependent. According to Cannady et al., as a general rule, monocortical calvarial bone or rib cartilage can provide the central support, while conchal cartilages the lateral reconstruction [24]. The calvarial bone or the rib cartilage should be fashioned into an L-strut to the remaining nasal bones superiorly and the floor of the nose inferiorly and affixed with miniplates, thus creating central stability and the basis of a structural tripod. The conchal cartilage is then used to reconstitute the lateral sidewalls of the nose with conchal bowl curvature used to the advantage of the surgeon, completing the tripod.

Gaggl [26] and Cherubino [27] promoted the use of medial femoral condyle free flap to solve most of the requirements needed for internal and skeletal nasal reconstruction, reducing surgical steps. Indeed, the pliable cortical bone of medial femoral condyle offers stable and long-lasting skeletal support, while periosteum will ultimately mucosalize, providing the internal lining. The flap is designed and harvested as a rectangle. The cortical bony aspect of the flap is trimmed, and the flap is folded into an acute-angle vault to reproduce a tent-like shape. The periosteal surface of the flap is turned into internal lining part and sutured to remaining nasal mucosa, while the bone is stabilized with plates or mesh. The arterial and venous anastomoses are performed end-to-end to angular or facial vessels. According to the authors, any dysfunction of the knee after the operation is not reported by the patient.

Cutaneous Reconstruction

The last layer in the reconstruction is the cutaneous covering to the support grafts, and internal lining is the envelope or external skin. Again, multiple options exist. Transposition flaps that reconstruct part, but not all, of the total nasal defect tend to cross subunits and leave unsightly, noticeable scarring; options include melolabial flaps and cheek advancement flaps. Thus, the paramedian forehead flap, the oldest and most well-described nasal reconstructive technique, remains the best local flap for total nasal reconstruction. It can be created with ample length to reconstruct defects down to the columella or even parts of the internal nasal lining via infolding. We already described in another section of the chapter the surgical technique for flap harvesting.

Finally, free flap reconstruction of the envelope has also been employed. Some argue that the skin match with free tissue transfer is less ideal than a forehead flap; however, free flaps remain a viable option in some situations.

Helix free flap is becoming a popular option for alar reconstruction . The flap was firstly described by Pribax and Falco in 1993. It is based on the branches of superficial temporal vessels. Li in 2005 described its use also as reverse flap based on the terminal upper branches of the temporalis vessels. The purpose was lengthening the pedicle. The flap is easy to harvest, donor site morbidity at the ear is considered acceptable, and color match to the nose quite good. Anastomosis on facial vessels at the nasolabial fold is sometimes tedious. The great advantage of this flap is the very low rate of deformation due to its unique shape. Even if the first indication was alar reconstruction, the flap can be adopted also for more extended reconstruction of the sidewalls and tip with satisfactory results [28, 29].

Specific Considerations in Total and Extended Total Nasal Reconstruction

According to Burget and Walton, use of free flaps alone for reconstructing the nose frequently falls short of achieving an aesthetic result. Indeed, it is difficult to estimate correctly the deep tissue volume of the defect and meet the lining requirements for alae, columella, and adjacent facial units [30]: so the authors suggested always the combination of free flaps, in particular the radial forearm, for internal lining and forehead flap for external covering, with an ideal case-dependent skeletal support. The authors stated to consider the nose and adjacent face in layers, from posterior to anterior, from the bottom of the defect, up.

The deepest layer is the one that fills the deep recesses of the defect. This first establishes the base for the second posterior-to-anterior layer. This second layer is the facial plane of the cheek and upper lip, floor of the nasal airway, and the platform on which the new nose will rest. Although this plane is usually reconstructed with a single, large, free microvascular flap, two separate paddles are sometimes necessary. In some cases, the free microvascular flap that forms the facial plane of the cheek and upper lip has been allowed to flow over into the nasal cavity to line the floor of the nose. The plane of the cheeks, upper lip, nasal floor, and nasal platform should be well established before the new nose is reconstructed on it.

Installed in a separated surgical step, the third layer of reconstruction is the lining flap for the nasal vestibule and columella. The fourth and fifth layers of the central face are the framework of cartilage grafts or calvarial bones, and a paramedian forehead flap designed to fit over this framework [30].

An alternative two-stage approach to reconstruction after total rhinectomy, based exclusively on local flaps and rib grafts, with very satisfying cosmetic results is shown in Figs. 8.5 and 8.6 [31].

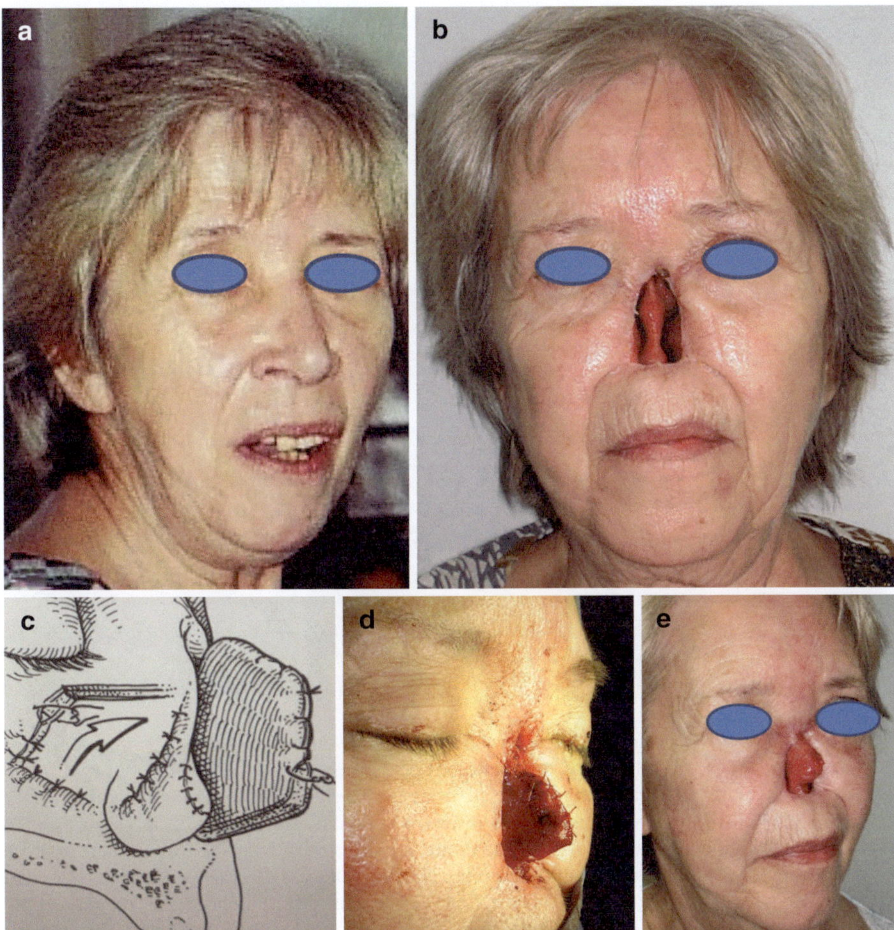

Fig. 8.5 (**a**) 73 y.o. female, Caucasian patient, SCC of the nasal vestibule, extended bilaterally and on the vault of the nose. (**b**) About a year after the rhinectomy. (**c**) First surgical step: a lower pedicle septal flap is rotated anteriorly and fixed superiorly to the radix of the nose. (**d**) The flap in place will provide, in the second phase of the reconstruction, a support for the dorsum and lining mucosa for the nasal vault. (**e**) The septal flap is stable at 8 weeks

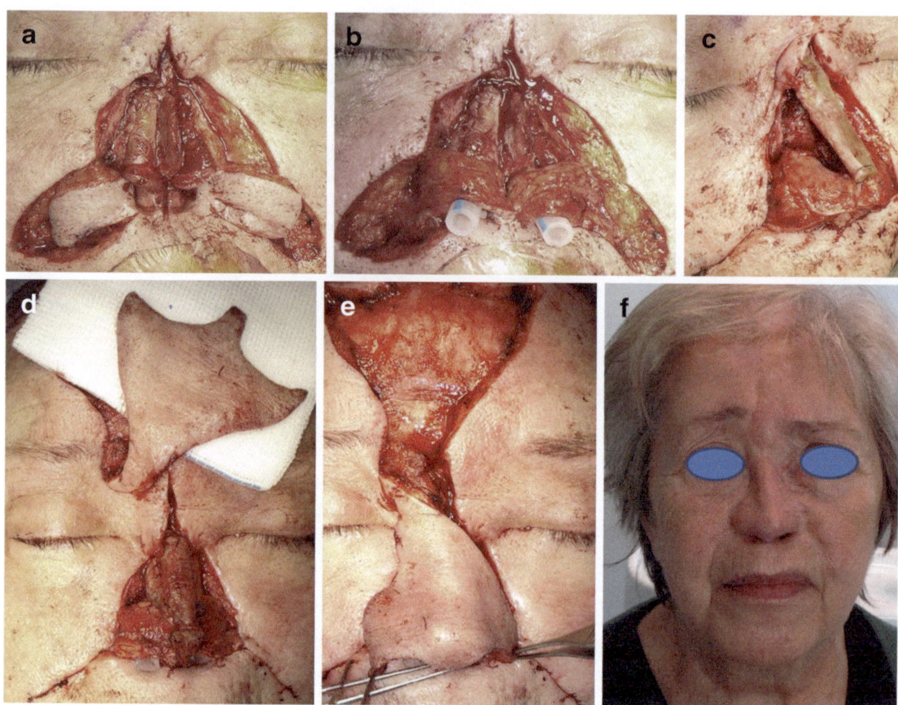

Fig. 8.6 (**a**) Second reconstructive step for the same case of the previous Fig. 8.5: the mucosa of the septal flap is elevated bilaterally, then reflected posteriorly and sutured to lateral nasal lining tissues, to provide the internal lining for the rib grafts that will form the cartilaginous framework of the nose. (**b**) Two melolabial flaps, rotated inside the nose and sutured to the nasal spine, provide the inner lining of the vestibule. Two silicone drains are inserted into the nostrils and left in place for about 2 months to prevent collapse and retraction. (**c**) The nasal framework is reconstructed with cartilaginous grafts harvested from the right eighth rib. (**d–e**) Forehead flap rotated on the cartilage framework, providing color matching skin cover. (**f**) Two-year follow-up, after some outpatient operations to dissect the pedicle and reduce the subcutaneous fat

References

1. Jeannon J-P, Riddle PJ, Irish J, O'sullivan B, Brown DH, Gullane P. Prognostic indicators in carcinoma of the nasal vestibule. Clin Otolaryngol. 2007;32:19–23.
2. Agger A, von Buchwald C, Madsen AR, et al. Squamous cell carcinoma of the nasal vestibule 1993-2002: a nationwide retrospective study from DAHANCA. Head Neck. 2009;31:1593–9.
3. Francesco B, Tagliaferri L, Piras A, Rizzo D, Tsatsaris N, De Corso E et al. Multidisciplinary approach to nose vestibule malignancies: setting new standards Approccio multidisciplinare ai tumori maligni del vestibolo del naso: verso la definizione di nuovi standard Acta Otorhinolaryngologica Italica. 2021;41(Suppl. 1):S158–S165. https://doi.org/10.14639/0392-100X-suppl.1-41-2021-16.
4. Bussu et al. New standards for the management of nose vestibule malignancies Acta Oto-Laryngologica. 2023;143(3):215–22. https://doi.org/10.1080/00016489.2023.2179662.

5. Scheurleer WFJ, Tagliaferri L, Rijken JA, Crescio C, Rizzo D, Mattiucci GC, Pameijer FA, de Bree R, Fionda B, de Ridder M, Bussu F. Evaluation of staging systems for cancer of the nasal vestibule. Cancers. 2023;15(11):3028. https://doi.org/10.3390/cancers15113028.

6. Burget GC, Menick FJ. The subunit principle in nasal reconstruction. Plast Reconstr Surg. 1985;76:239–47.

7. Zitelli JA. Secondary intention healing: an alternative to surgical repair. Clin Dermatol. 1984;2:92–106.

8. Jewett BS, Baker SR. Skin and composite grafts. In: Principles of nasal reconstruction; 2011. p. 133–61.

9. Goding GS, Hom DB. Skin flap physiology. In: Baker SR, Swanson NA, editors. Local flaps in facial reconstruction. St. Louis: Mosby; 1995.

10. Glogau RG, Haas AF. Skin grafts. In: Baker SR, Swanson NA, editors. Local flaps in facial reconstruction. St. Louis: Mosby; 1995.

11. Menick F. Aesthetic nasal reconstruction: principles and practice. W & E, 2017. ISBN 1619565439, 9781619565432.

12. Austin GK, Shockley WW. Reconstruction of nasal defects: contemporary approaches. Curr Opin Otolaryngol Head Neck Surg. 2016;24:453–60.

13. Burget GC, Menick FJ. Nasal support and lining: the marriage of beauty and blood supply. Plast Reconstr Surg. 1989;84:189–202.

14. Baker SR. Nasal lining flaps in contemporary reconstructive rhinoplasty. Facial Plast Surg. 1998;14:133–44.

15. Murakami CS, Kriet JD, Ierokomos AP. Nasal reconstruction using the inferior turbinate mucosal flap. Arch Facial Plast Surg. 1999;1:97–100.

16. Romo T 3rd, Pearson JM. Nasal implants. Facial Plast Surg Clin North Am. 2008;16:123–32, vi.

17. Romo T 3rd, McLaughlin LA, Levine JM, Sclafani AP. Nasal implants: autogenous, semisynthetic, and synthetic. Facial Plast Surg Clin North Am. 2002;10:155–66.

18. Tsiliboti D, Antonopoulos D, Spyropoulos K, Naxakis S, Goumas P. Total nasal reconstruction using a prelaminated free radial forearm flap and porous polyethylene implants. J Reconstr Microsurg. 2008;24:449–52.

19. Burget GC, Menick FJ. The superiorly based nasolabial flap: technical details. In: Aesthetic reconstruction of the nose, vol. 95. Maryland Heights, MO: Mosby Year Book; 1994. p. 593.

20. Baker SR. Interpolated melolabial flaps: reconstruction of alar and columellar units. In: Principles of nasal reconstruction. Ann Arbor, MI: Springer; 2011.

21. Drisco BP, Baker SR. Reconstruction of nasal alar defects. Arch Facial Plast Surg. 2001;3:91–9.

22. Menick FJ. Forehead flap: master techniques in otolaryngology-head and neck surgery. Facial Plast Surg. 2014;30:131–44.

23. Vander Poorten V, Meulemans J, Delaere P. Midface prosthetic rehabilitation. Curr Opin Otolaryngol Head Neck Surg. 2016;24:98–109.

24. Cannady SB, Cook TA, Wax MK. The total nasal defect and reconstruction. Facial Plast Surg Clin North Am. 2009;17:189–201.

25. Pribaz J, Stephens W, Crespo L, Gifford G. A new intraoral flap: facial artery musculomucosal (FAMM) flap. Plast Reconstr Surg. 1992;90:421–9.

26. Gaggl AJ, Bürger H, Chiari FM. Reconstruction of the nose with a new double flap technique: microvascular osteocutaneous femur and microvascular chondrocutaneous ear flap--first clinical results. Int J Oral Maxillofac Surg. 2012;41:581–6.

27. Cherubino M, Stocco C, Tamborini F, Maggiulli F, Sallam D, Corno M, Bignami M, Battaglia P, Valdatta L. Medial femoral condyle free flap in combination with paramedian forehead flap for total/subtotal nasal reconstruction: level of evidence: IV (therapeutic studies): level of evidence: IV (therapeutic studies). Microsurgery. 2020;40:343–52.

28. Lassus P, Husso A, Vuola J, Lindford AJ. More than just the helix: a series of free flaps from the ear. Microsurgery. 2018;38:611–20.

29. Li S, Cao W, Cheng K, Yin C, Qian Y, Cao Y, Chang T-S. Microvascular reconstruction of nasal ala using a reversed superficial temporal artery auricular flap. J Plast Reconstr Aesthet Surg. 2006;59:1300–4.
30. Burget GC, Walton RL. Optimal use of microvascular free flaps, cartilage grafts, and a Paramedian forehead flap for aesthetic reconstruction of the nose and adjacent facial units. Plast Reconstr Surg. 2007;120:1171–207.
31. Burguet GC, Menick FJ. Aesthetic reconstruction of the nose. Maryland Heights, MO: Mosby Year Book; 1986.

Prostheses for Cosmetic and Functional Restoration After Ablative Surgery for Nose Vestibule Malignancies

9

Gianmarco Saponaro, Roberto Gallus, Sasha Budiman, Paolo Tropiano, Giovanni Giorgetti, Nikolaos Machouchas, and Luca Salvatore Calabrese

9.1   A Brief History, Rationale, and Indications

The face is central to our self-image. Facial damages lead to altered perception and experience of a person's identity and environment. As a result, the correction of facial defects is important not only for functional reasons but also for psychosocial reasons. Such essential need for rehabilitation of physical defects is reflected by the amount of historical artifacts related to prosthetic devices, with evidence of devices dating back as far as ancient Egypt [1] and ancient India 600 B.C. [2]. In the sixteenth century, Ambroise Paré, a French surgeon considered the father of modern surgery, extensively described eyeball, orbital, and auricular prostheses, along with the first nose epitheses from gold, silver, and "papier mâché," retained by a metal brace fitted around the head [3]. As reported by Wilson [4], Tycho Brahe, the great Danish astronomer of the sixteenth century, after losing his nose during a duel, made a new one for himself out of silver and gold. In the 1832 issue of The London Medical Gazette is discussed in great detail the case of a French soldier nicknamed the "Gunner with the Silver Mask' 'in reference to his mask forged in metal and

G. Saponaro
Maxillo-Facial Surgery Unit, IRCSS "A. Gemelli" Foundation - Catholic University of the Sacred Heart, Rome, Italy
e-mail: gianmarco.saponaro@unicatt.it

R. Gallus (✉)
Otolaryngology, Mater Olbia Hospital, Olbia, Italy
e-mail: roberto.gallus@materolbia.com

S. Budiman · G. Giorgetti · L. S. Calabrese
Division of Otorhinolaryngology, "San Maurizio" Hospital, Bolzano, Italy
e-mail: sascha.budiman@sabes.it; giovanni.giorgetti@sabes.it; luca.calabrese@sabes.it

P. Tropiano · N. Machouchas
Otolaryngology Division, Azienda Ospedaliero Universitaria, Sassari, Italy
e-mail: paolo.tropiano@aouss.it; nikolaos.machouchas@aouss.it

© Springer Nature Switzerland AG 2023
F. Bussu (ed.), *Malignancies of the Nasal Vestibule*,
https://doi.org/10.1007/978-3-031-32850-3_9

leather to cover the lower aspect of his face after having been hit by a shrapnel. The entire prosthesis was retained by rubber bands stretched over the head and neck [5]. The first example of external retention by using a pair of glasses and rubber bands comes from Delabarre, who published the technique in 1820 [6]. In 1932, Kazanjian described an early example of anatomical retention by exploiting the undercuts of an orbital defect with reinforcement obtained using a pair of glasses [7]. The development of silicone prosthesis and modern anchorage systems, such as the one based on percutaneous titanium fixtures described by Tjellström, has led to a modernization and wider application of prosthetic solutions [8].

Total rhinectomy and partial rhinectomy leave behind the bone, cartilage, and soft tissue defects located in the central midface, with profound aesthetic and psychosocial impact and therefore require a satisfactory reconstruction [9–12]. Patients with acquired facial disfigurement are usually more impacted than those with congenital defects by psychological problems, self-acceptance, and physical impairment [13, 14]. Head and neck cancer patients are particularly prone to mental health conditions and psychological distress due to the impact of their disease on essential functions [15]. Such effects of demolitive surgery are particularly pronounced when the eye and nose are involved and can provoke posttraumatic stress disorder symptoms and social isolation [10, 16–23]. The nose is an essential landmark of our midface, involved in facial recognition, perception, and attractiveness [9, 11, 24, 25]. The importance of proper reconstruction is crucial, especially because most of these patients have long-term survival rates [26, 27]. It is thereby very important to give them a good reconstruction outcome and keep their reconstructive surgery as unnoticeable as possible [28]. This last point in particular is meant to avoid social stigma, an important social determinant that can lead to treatment dropout, delay in seeking medical help, and psychological problems [21, 29, 30].

The nose is a complex anatomical and functional unit, with a peculiar three-dimensional composite structure made by soft tissues (skin and mucosa) and an osteocartilaginous framework. The surface has a complex shape, characterized by highlights and shadow points, and multiple peculiar features as the dorsum, the tip, alar rims, sidewalls, soft triangles, and columella. The skin has its variability too, with areas of different thicknesses, pliability, and abundance of sebaceous glands. Moreover, the nose has key functional roles such as warming, humidification, and filtration of inhaled air, along with the sense of smell [31]. The main rehabilitative options routinely employed after partial and total rhinectomy are simple nasal dressing, prosthetic rehabilitation, and surgical reconstruction. As stated earlier, proper reconstruction is of utmost importance for the psychological and social well-being of the patient. Surgical reconstruction of the nose after such a demolitive surgery is a technical challenge for the reconstructive surgeon [32]. When satisfactory reconstructive surgery is impossible for technical reasons, refused by the patient or with undesirable expected outcomes, maxillofacial prostheses made of artificial materials are the treatment of choice, able to provide both protection to the exposed structures and aesthetic restoration. Other than functional and aesthetically as close as possible to normal tissues, the ideal prosthesis should be easy to use to clean and maintain, durable and stable over time, comfortable, cheap, and easy to produce [33].

Some of the reasons that may justify the preference for a prosthetic rehabilitation include an easier oncologic follow-up and direct checking of the resected area, especially if the risk of recurrence is high (inspection and biopsies); shorter hospitalization time and shorter surgery times; lack of motivation to undergo a complex multi stage surgical procedure; patient's age; lack of well-vascularized tissue caused by eventual radiotherapy; lack of tissue to grant a complete reconstruction; patients' specific contraindications to sustain a surgical procedure. The ideal timing for surgical reconstruction is unclear, and recommendations range from 1 to 2 years after completion of therapy [26, 34]. Nasal epitheses usually require a single surgical procedure to implant the bone anchoring system, and while still debated, it seems that implant survival is only partially affected by radiotherapy, thus allowing for an earlier intervention and earlier social rehabilitation [23, 33, 35–40]. However, at least one study underlines a societal preference for surgical reconstruction over prosthetic rehabilitation [41]. Despite many advantages, there is still a psychological problem to be considered, which is intrinsic to the removable and non-definitive nature of prosthesis itself. Due to the scope and focus of the present book, we will focus on prosthetic rehabilitation for nasal defects, as other prosthesis on the facial area go under the name of "epitheses."

9.2   Current Standards

Recent years' advancements have covered all aspects from retaining systems to manufacturing of the epitheses and types of material involved. The transformative role of prosthetics for those suffering tissue loss or disfigurement cannot be underestimated. These personalized treatments restore aesthetics and function to missing or malformed tissue using synthetic materials that mimic the characteristics of natural tissue. Since the first attempts with rudimentary materials, the science and art of prosthetics have come a long way. Now the association of advanced manufacturing with sophisticated polymer science promises highly personalized and realistic prosthetics. The impact of the advanced manufacturing revolution is significant; traditional time-consuming approaches involving physical casting and hand-crafting are being replaced by 3D scanning, computer modeling, and multi-material 3D printing [42]. Although digital technology has been used in prosthetics for the past 30 years, it is only the last decade that has seen its rapid development. This change in practice is evidenced by the significant fraction of recent literature describing advances in 3D printed prostheses, including technological advances and clinical reports. Further innovations involving collaborations between clinicians, academics, and industry, promise even greater capabilities.

9.3　Manufacturing

9.3.1　Traditional Manufacturing

The traditional method of manufacturing involves the use of moulages and multiple casts, the usual flowchart includes the following steps: A facial moulage is taken after rhinectomy employing alginate and stonecast materials. A stone gypsum moulage of the facial region with the nasal defect is created as anatomical template. A nose wax model is formed onto the template. At this point, patient's requests regarding the morphology can be taken in consideration in order to obtain best acceptance of the future episthesis. Presurgical photographs, 3d-facial scans, and 3d-models of the nose should be used as a guide to contour the prototype. From the wax plastic thereupon, a casting mold in gypsum is formed; this matrix is used later for the silicone prosthesis molding process [43].

9.3.2　Computer-Aided Manufacturing

The traditional method of manual manufacturing might be facilitated or gradually supplanted by use of Computer-Aided Design and Manufacturing (CAD/CAM) systems, completed by computer supported Rapid Prototyping techniques (RP). Digital Imaging (DICOM) data files obtained via computer tomographic scans or optical 3d-facial scans deliver the basic data of individual anatomy.

9.3.3　Prototypting

Prototype techniques are based on different materials and production methods: many different fast prototyping techniques are commercially available including Stereolithic tomography (Stereolithography-SLA), Layered Object Manufacturing (Laminated Object Manufacturing-LOM), Selective Laser Sintering (Select and Laser Sintering-SLS), Model Generation in Stacking Ergiterek (Fused deposition modeling-FDM), Material Spray Three- Dimensional Modeling (Inkjets, Photopolymer Phase Change Ink jets, 3D Printing), and laser engineered net shaping (LENS).

　　Distinctive steps are required to form prosthetic geometry: computer-aided designing and successive transforming the CAD-model into a production-compatible file format, e.g., a stereolithographic file format. Once obtained a hardware model from the software project, it is necessary to implement the cleaning of the completed model.

9.3.4 Digital Library

A prototype of an epithesis might be produced by use of a prefab computer-designed model obtained from a digital library of prosthetic models. In order to create a digital library, anatomic details and profiles of patients of different gender, age, and physiognomy are collected by use of conventional medical imaging techniques, laser surface scanners, and optical systems. Combining these data via computer-aided designing technologies, a catalog of a broad range of different prosthetics prototypes can be created. The advantage of this method is the redundancy of physical contact to soft tissues avoiding distortion and other imprecisions during acquisition. Furthermore, the digital image acquisition allows the registration of deeper endonasal anatomical regions, which by traditional moulage techniques are hardly accessible. These data allow reproducing a mesostructure, which maintains also functional aspects of the airways in the epithesis.

9.3.5 Materials and Techniques

Digital models are used to form successful prototypes with CAD/CAM and fast prototyping technologies. Even though SLA technology has gained a lot of popularity during the recent years as manufacturing method for facial prostheses because of its advantages, it is limited to produce only resin-based prototypes of the facial epithesis. They cannot be directly turned into silicone and need an intermediate step of molding a wax model, increasing the risk of introducing errors and imprecisions during manufacturing process and prolongation of delivery time. The SLS technology however allows the direct production of a wax prototype, therefore surmounting the limits of the SLA technology. It is expected that in the future, facial prostheses will be prepared by directly freezing the silicone molds [33].

One of the first polymers to be used in prosthetics, polymethyl methacrylate (PMMA), was developed in response to the glass shortages in the World Wars of the twentieth century. This polymer went on to become the most common prosthetic material of the time and still finds use today in artificial eyes and prosthetic substructures. Further innovations in the twentieth century produced many new polymers, such as vinyls, copolymers, plastisols, and of course, silicone. Discovered in the early 1900s by Fredrick Kipping, silicone was first used in prosthetics by George W Barnhart in 1960. This versatile polymer remains a primary prosthetic material today due to its soft tissue–like properties, ease of manipulation, chemical inertness, durability, and excellent biocompatibility. Recent innovations have brought new specialized material blends and cross-linking methods optimized for 3D printing, enabling a large range of mechanical and visual properties. Innovation often comes from the 3D printer manufacturers themselves that develop, produce, and sell materials comprising proprietary blends of polymers suitable for printing only on their machines. Many of these polymers also contain complex blends of methacrylates, urethanes, and other engineered polymers that are subject to biocompatibility testing and regulatory approval that limit their clinical application, although some of these advanced polymers have received ISO-10993, USP Class VI, or other biocompatibility certification. This increases their potential for use in the routine fabrication of soft tissue prosthetics, eventually rendering traditional prosthetic fabrication approaches obsolete [42].

9.3.6 Future Aspects

Computer-aided designing and manufacturing allow the combination and structural conjunction of different materials in order to create endonasal replica mesostructures covered by state-of-the-art silicone surface respecting not only an external morphology but taking into consideration the endonasal functionality as aerodynamic air flow and gaining a reduction of the total weight of the epithesis. In conclusion, with the possibility of starting with a three-dimensional scan of the face and the possibility of repeating or creating a mirror effect, CAD/CAM technology allows any customised prosthesis to be made.

9.3.7 Examples

Case 9.1 Carcinoma of Upper Maxilla, Resection and Reconstruction with Fibula
Anchorage strategy: transcutaneous bone anchorage onto nasal bone using epiplating bridge preserving the fibula from iatrogenic trauma; fixation of the episthesis superiorly by magnets onto the epiplating bridge and inferiorly by anatomical fixation into the defective area tissue (natural clipping effect) (Fig. 9.1).

Case 9.2 Low-Grade SCC of Nose, Rhinectomy
Strategy: transcutaneous bone anchorage using epiplating bridges, episthesis fixation via magnets (Figs. 9.2 and 9.3).

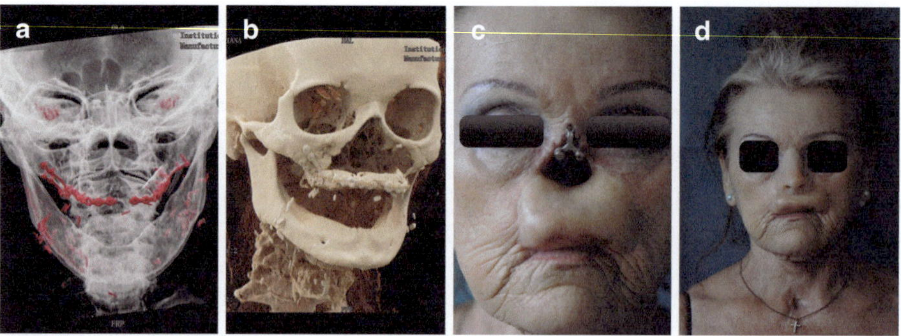

Fig. 9.1 (**a**) CT scan with Ti-plates coloration, (**b**) CT 3D reconstruction, (**c**) defect area with transcutaneous epiplating bridge anchored to nasal bone, (**d**) silicone prosthesis fixed via magnets onto the bridge

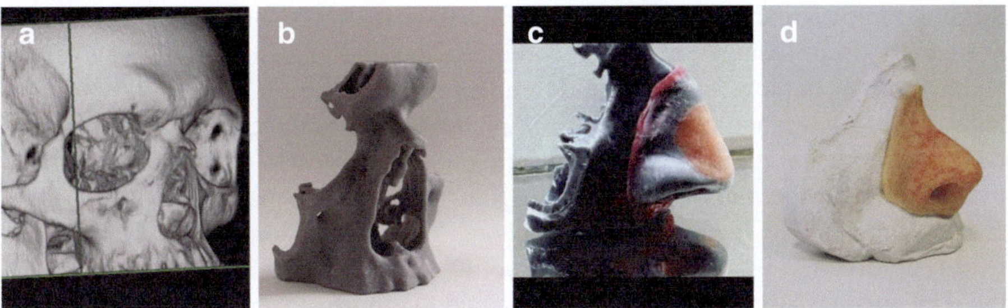

Fig.9.2 (**a**) CT scan 3c reconstruction, (**b**) 3d print, (**c**) print model, (**d**) silicone prototype

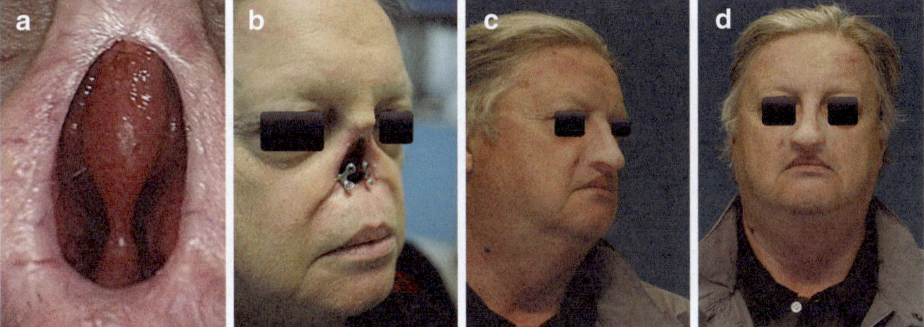

Fig. 9.3 (**a**) defective area, (**b**) transcutaneous bone anchored epiplating bridges, (**c**, **d**) silicone prosthesis fixed with magnets onto the bridge

9.4 Retention

To obtain a successful outcome of the prosthetic rehabilitation, the most important features required are appropriate retention, stability, and support of the epitheses. There are four main solutions that allow proper attachment of a midfacial epitheses: *mechanically* by anchoring the epithesis to spectacle frames or rubber bands, *anatomically* by clamping the epithesis into existing structures, *chemically* by using adhesive materials, or by *bone anchorage* exploiting the process of bone integration of titanium implants. There are some disadvantages to using an adhesive. It can damage both the skin, causing contact dermatitis especially if used for a long time, and the epitheses surface during insertion and removal. Therefore, adhesives should be carefully selected as they may adversely affect the physical and optical properties of the maxillofacial elastomers, may cause a change in the color of the epitheses, and can disrupt the structure and abrade the edges. All adhesive systems are inadequate to ensure the rigid fixation of facial prostheses, as they do not provide sufficient adhesion against gravity, sweating, and tissue movement. If thicker prosthetic margins are used in order to facilitate the application of adhesives, both an increase in microorganism colonization and aesthetic damage may happen. Medical adhesives include double-sided tape, glue, sprayers, pastes, and liquid systems. Due to difficult removal and unpleasant odor, both latex-based pats and surgical cement are not widely used. Double-sided tape is more widely adopted as it is easier to apply and to remove, but low flexibility and frequent loss of adhesion are known disadvantages [44]. Skin-penetrating titanium implants were developed as an extension of the titanium dental implant, since this technology emerged as a reliable reconstruction method for the maxillofacial/oral region, to overcome the limitations of adhesives. While at the beginning, some concern regarding long-term stability and recurrent infection was vocalized by some, work in the late 1970s and early 1980s by Tjellstrom, Albrektsson, Branemark, and Lindstrom proved that titanium implants were a reliable and safe technique for prosthetic reconstruction of extraoral defects. Implants can be isolated bone-anchored screws or grouped screws with plates (Epiplating) or grids (Epitec) to better distribute the weight. Short-length craniofacial implant fixtures tolerate placement in areas with insufficient bone [45]. In the midface area, the only locations for screw implant placement are the glabella and the upper (basal) alveolar crest of the maxilla; therefore, axial bone supply is rather limited, and anchorage of screw-type implants might be difficult. If vertical or even horizontal bone dimensions are limited in the alveolar crest because of atrophy or after resection, axial implants often cannot be used. The use of orthopedic (disk) implants via basal osseointegration in compact bone that is resistant to resorption represents in the latter cases another option that has the advantage of having a cortical anchorage, allows the insertion of more bone screws for better stabilization, has modest demand for vertical (axial) bone, and is highly infection-resistant. Today, the technique that is gaining popularity consists of the fabrication of a customized mesostructure by computer-designing a metal structure obtained with laser synthesis or milling machines. This is fixed with screws and to which the new nose obtained from the presurgical anatomy is attached. Facial prostheses can be retained with the aid of a bar-and-clip mechanism or magnetic attachments, thus making it possible to use large devices resting on movable tissues [46]. Independently from the retain system, nasal epitheses seem to be well tolerated, but there seems to be a general preference of patients for implant-retained epitheses over adhesive-retained epitheses probably over stability concerns [16, 38, 47–49].

9.5 Complications

Even if some authors reported low or extremely low complication rates and exceptional implant survival rates [50, 51], according to a recent systematic review by Chrcanovic et al. [52], the probability of failure of a craniofacial implant is 5.5% overall and 12.2% specifically for the nasal region. Interestingly follow-up time did not seem to impact the proportion of failures. Most of the reported complications are soft tissue adverse reactions, but skin infections (4 on the scoring system developed by Holgers et al. [53]) only accounted for 0.4% of observations or 0.3% of implants evaluated depending on the reporting method used by the authors. Soft-tissue breakdown at the abutment interface has been reported too [54]. Tissue adverse reactions seem to be related to implant care and hygiene with worse problems in adult patients [55], Korfage et al. reported that 65.2% of their patients needed repeated hygiene instructions [49]. The review by Chrcanovic et al., citing other works [56, 57], suggested an impact of both difficult access for placement and difficult maintenance of the implant as the factor responsible for the worse failure rate of nasal implants and poor implant stability due to the loose trabecular bone structure of the nasal floor [58]. However, both access and subsequent maintenance can be improved by modification of the nasal defect [59]. Other factors seemingly involved in implant success are smoking, extent of rhinectomy, length (shorter implants failing more frequently) and location of the implant (with implants placed in the orbital rims and maxilla failing more frequently than implants placed in the zygoma, floor of the nose, and glabella), and type of retention (bars for retention are associated with an increased frequency of failure compared with magnets) [49, 57, 59–61]. Korfage et al. reported clips' damage in 30.4% of patients and surgical aftercare with subcutaneous tissue reduction in 7.1% of patients [49]. Papaspyrou reported one case of dura mater perforation requiring duraplasty [62]. Other complications have been reported for extra-oral implants, including osteoradionecrosis [63], hemorrhage, and nerve lesions and infections [64–66], but these did not specifically involve nasal epitheses.

Radiotherapy, and in particular external beam radiotherapy, is another factor at play when considering implant failure rates of the nasal region, and the perfect timing of implant placement (before or after radiotherapy) is still debated, but an early implant positioning during the ablative surgery seems to be preferable [57, 61, 67]. Some of the published data show that implants are impacted by the adverse effects of radiotherapy, even if the reported impact is subject to variability, with some reporting no impact at all [38, 49, 50, 56, 59, 61, 62, 66, 68–74]. A systematic review performed by Chrcanovic et al. confirmed a significant impact of radiotherapy on craniofacial implants (OR 5.80, 95%CI 3.77–8.92, $P < 0.00001$) [52]. As suggested by the same group of authors in another paper [75] citing previous work [76], such negative impact might be related to the long-term negative effects of radiotherapy on local tissue vascularization. Impact of hyperbaric oxygen on adverse effects related to radiotherapy is still debated [59, 68, 75, 77–79].

9.6 Reported Functional, Cosmetic Results, and QOL

Not many studies cover functional, cosmetic results and quality-of-life measures with reliable and established tools [80, 81], and the different tools used in the published studies make it difficult to compare results; however, interest in this kind of measures is growing to facilitate patient-centered care and to highlight physical and psychological problems and progression other time [82–85]. Interesting information about quality of life in treated patients can be picked up from a paper published by Atay and colleagues in 2013 [23]. They surveyed 72 patients (equally distributed in three groups according to the type of epitheses: auricular, ocular, nasal) and 27 controls with the World Health Organization Quality-of-Life Instrument that measures physical, social, and psychosocial well-being as perceived by the subject. They found that patients with nasal epitheses scored lower than patients with auricular epitheses in the psychological, social, and overall QOL domains. Only patients with nasal epitheses scored lower than the control group in the social relationship domain (along with all the other domains). Both sociodemographic and clinical characteristics were associated with the patient's reported QOL. These results underline the greater impact of nasal epitheses when compared with controls and other types of facial epitheses. The authors explain such results with the prominent position of the nose and more problems with the epitheses especially with hot-cold weather, sports, more difficult camouflaging, and allergies. It should be noted that given the nature of QOL scores, the results are influenced by the social and cultural context and thus not necessarily identical everywhere [16, 86]. Becker and colleagues reported QOL data coming from University of Washington quality-of-life questionnaire [87] compiled by 43 of their patients [47]. Activity and mood domains were the most affected in patients with nasal epitheses. Interestingly, the impact on QOL was lower than expected, and the mean score for the domain "appearance" reported (67.44) ranged between the answers: "my appearance bothers me but I remain active" (50) and "the change in my appearance is minor" (75). Appearance was also only the third most important domain after "activity" and "mood," and in particular, activity was interpreted as a possible hint of the fear of instability of the epitheses. Interestingly, the authors reported on the QOL of the same group of patients along with functional results obtained with another specifically built questionnaire [88], a modified version of "The Nasal Appearance and Function Evaluation Questionnaire" [89]. Results highlighted a high score for overall function and a high average usage of the epitheses (17.4 h). The domains with the best results were function, appearance, and fit, while the most impacted were breathing, smelling, crusts, nose bleed, speech, and stability, nasal crusts being the item with the lowest score. The authors interpreted the scores for breathing and smelling and their high variability as a sign of possible occurrence of the "empty nose syndrome" in patients who underwent particularly demolitive surgery. The item "nose bleed" was impacted by time since demolitive surgery (higher early after surgery). The item "self-confidence" was impacted by sex (most impacted female subjects) and both "self-confidence" and "stability during sport activities" were impacted by age, the same items along with income impacted respectively on "environmental health" and "social relationships" in the study by Atay and colleagues [23]. Interestingly, the comparison with the UWQOL compiled by the same patients revealed that the item "satisfaction with function" had the most influence on the UWQOL domains. Nearly all of the surveyed patients stated that they would recommend prosthetic rehabilitation after rhinectomy, and the results for "appearance" were comparable to those obtained after surgical reconstruction [90]. Interestingly, 42.9% of the not retired patients had a significant impact on their career and opted for early retirement, confirming the socioeconomic impact of the disease [91], an issue brought up also by Markt and colleagues [92]. In 2001, an article reporting the opinions of 76 respondents to a survey sent out to patients who underwent extraoral maxillofacial prosthetic rehabilitation at the M. D. Anderson Cancer Center was published [92]. Patients were administered a 52-question survey specifically designed, 36% of the respondents had prosthetic noses. Among various aspects, the questionnaire explored the perceptions of self-image, self-consciousness, socialization frequency before and after prosthetic rehabilitation. In total, 79% of respondents reported a routine use of their epitheses and an average daily use of 14.34 h. Most of the patients rated positively (4–5 on a 5-point scale) the fit (80%), comfort (85%), shape (85%), and look (71%) of the epitheses. Only 20% of patients reported a change in their social life, including both patients that sow a decrement and an increment of it. Interestingly, most of the patients felt confident enough to show themselves to someone without the epitheses (55%) and to go anywhere without it (65%). D'heygere et al. recently published a study covering all their reconstructive procedures after total rhinectomy over a period of 3 years, for a total of 16 patients, all of whom compiled a FACE-Q questionnaire [50, 93]. Their patients were generally satisfied with the appearance of the epitheses, but had lower scores related to the general facial appearance (58/100). Social and psychological scores, albeit not critical, were still seriously impacted (but above 60/100). Slightly better results regarding self-perception and social life were reported in a small group of patients treated with bone-anchored epitheses by Wagenblast and colleagues [51]. Korfage et al., with a more simple 10-point scale, found that their patients' satisfaction score had a median result of 8. An interesting insight on the different impact that maxillofacial epitheses have on psychosocial well-being and perceived appearance between cancer patients and patients with congenital/post-traumatic defects comes from two papers from Sela and Lowental. The first one focused on psychosocial well-being [94] and showed how cancer patients had the least relevant psychosocial impact (if at all) from the maxillofacial prosthesis restoration. The authors interpreted these data as a sign of the inner feeling of being "doomed" of cancer patients. The second one compared patients' and external evaluation of cosmetic results [95]. While subjective improvement did not vary among different diagnostic categories (average 38.6%), the external evaluation of a prosthodontist, a physician, and a sculptor scored lower in the improvements in cancer patients compared to injury and congenital defect patients. Chang and colleagues published a comparison between various QOL aspects in patients with implant-retained, adhesive-retained, or with experience with both types of epitheses [48]. They administered a specifically developed 28 items questionnaire investigating comfort, appearance, fit, irritation, daily usage, and treatment value, with answers chosen from a 5-point scale. Both types of epitheses were generally well tolerated and appreciated by their patients (including 37% with a nasal epitheses), but implant-retained epitheses scored higher values even if significance was reached only for some items including ease in placement, ease in removal, frequency of wear at home, retention during regular home activities and during perspiration and sneezing/coughing. Around 90% of patients with implant-retained and adhesive-retained epitheses considered the treatment worthwhile and recommendable, but patients carrying both types of prostheses considered more worthwhile the implant-retained one (100% versus 42%), a piece of data supported also by the work of Schoen and colleagues (albeit not including nasal epitheses) [38].

9.7 Future Perspectives

Alongside 3D scanning, 3D printing techniques involving synthetic materials, and computer modeling, other advancements are growing into clinically applicable techniques. Bioprinting and biofabrication allow the combination of cells, growth factors, and biomaterials to fabricate 3D cellularized constructs with a layer-by-layer approach based on CAD models. Such an approach might involve direct creation of finalized 3D structures or creation of biocompatible and absorbable scaffolds injected with bioinks containing hydrogels and cells that will grow and integrate with existing tissues [96]. Many technical issues currently hinder routine clinical application of biofabrication techniques in the maxillofacial field, including finding a reliable cell source, production of ear-shaped cartilage with a pre-designed 3D shape, and satisfying mechanical properties and unfavorable host response to the engineered graft [97–101]. However, thanks in particular to bioprinting, some of these limitations have been overcome, and attempts have been made to translate these advances in the clinical practice [98, 102–104]. Future applications alone or in hybrid solutions with synthetic components should be expected. Such techniques could be further enhanced in the future by 3D printing of organic semiconductors and piezoelectric materials. The implementation of this technique will allow for direct manufacturing of bionic and sensate epitheses and for overall lower costs for such technologies [42]. A proof of concept of such technique has been recently proposed by Jodat and colleagues, who described an odor-perceptive nose-like hybrid, composed of a cartilage-like construct and a biocompatible biosensing platform [105].

References

1. Turkyilmaz I. Implant dentistry: a rapidly evolving practice. BoD—Books on Demand; 2011.
2. Singh V. Sushruta: The father of surgery. Natl J Maxillofac Surg. 2017;8:1–3.
3. Paré A. De chirurgie, ende opera van alle de wercken. 1649.
4. Wilson G. Great men of science: their lives and discoveries. 1932.
5. van Doorne JM. Extra-oral prosthetics: past and present. J Invest Surg. 1994;7:267–74.
6. Delabarre CF. Traite de la partie mecanique de l'art du chirurgien-dentiste. 1820.
7. Kazanjian VH, Rowe AT, Young HA. Prosthesis of the mouth and face. J Dent Res. 1932;12:651–93. https://doi.org/10.1177/00220345320120050101.
8. Tjellström A, Lindström J, Hallén O, Albrektsson T, Brånemark PI. Osseointegrated titanium implants in the temporal bone. A clinical study on bone-anchored hearing aids. Am J Otol. 1981;2:304–10.
9. Dey JK, Ishii LE, Joseph AW, Goines J, Byrne PJ, Boahene KDO, et al. The cost of facial deformity: a health utility and valuation study. JAMA Facial Plast Surg. 2016;18:241–9.
10. Valente SM. Visual disfigurement and depression. Plast Surg Nurs. 2009;29:10–6; quiz 17–8.
11. Ishii L, Carey J, Byrne P, Zee DS, Ishii M. Measuring attentional bias to peripheral facial deformities. Laryngoscope. 2009;119:459–65.
12. Oh W-S, Roumanas E, Beumer J 3rd. Maxillofacial restoration after head and neck tumor therapy. Compend Contin Educ Dent. 2007;28:70–6; quiz 77, 101.
13. Lansdown R. Visibly different: coping with disfigurement. Boca Raton, FL: CRC; 1997.

14. Thompson A, Kent G. Adjusting to disfigurement: processes involved in dealing with being visibly different. Clin Psychol Rev. 2001;21:663–82.
15. Reich M, Leemans CR, Vermorken JB, Bernier J, Licitra L, Parmar S, et al. Best practices in the management of the psycho-oncologic aspects of head and neck cancer patients: recommendations from the European Head and Neck Cancer Society Make Sense Campaign. Ann Oncol. 2014;25:2115–24.
16. Klein M, Menneking H, Spring A, Rose M. Analysis of quality of life in patients with a facial prosthesis. Mund Kiefer Gesichtschir. 2005;9:205–13.
17. Levine E, Degutis L, Pruzinsky T, Shin J, Persing JA. Quality of life and facial trauma. Ann Plast Surg. 2005;54:502–10. https://doi.org/10.1097/01.sap.0000155282.48465.94.
18. Lim S-Y, Lee D, Oh KS, Nam B, Bang S-I, Mun G-H, et al. Concealment, depression and poor quality of life in patients with congenital facial anomalies. J Plast Reconstr Aesthet Surg. 2010;63:1982–9.
19. Sousa AD, De Sousa A. Psychological issues in acquired facial trauma. Indian J Plast Surg. 2010;43:200–5. https://doi.org/10.1055/s-0039-1699436.
20. Callahan C. Facial disfigurement and sense of self in head and neck cancer. Soc Work Health Care. 2004;40:73–87.
21. Newton JT, Fiske J, Foote O, Frances C, Loh IM, Radford DR. Preliminary study of the impact of loss of part of the face and its prosthetic restoration. J Prosthet Dent. 1999;82:585–90.
22. De Sousa A. Psychological issues in oral and maxillofacial reconstructive surgery. Br J Oral Maxillofac Surg. 2008;46:661–4.
23. Atay A, Peker K, Günay Y, Ebrinç S, Karayazgan B, Uysal Ö. Assessment of health-related quality of life in Turkish patients with facial prostheses. Health Qual Life Outcomes. 2013;11:11.
24. Walker-Smith GJ, Gale AG, Findlay JM. Eye movement strategies involved in face perception. Perception. 2013;42:1120–33.
25. Godoy A, Ishii M, Byrne PJ, Boahene KDO, Encarnacion CO, Ishii LE. How facial lesions impact attractiveness and perception: differential effects of size and location. Laryngoscope. 2011;121:2542–7.
26. Stanley RJ, Olsen KD. Rhinectomy for malignant disease. A 20-year experience. Arch Otolaryngol Head Neck Surg. 1988;114:1307–11.
27. Jeannon J-P, Riddle PJ, Irish J, O'sullivan B, Brown DH, Gullane P. Prognostic indicators in carcinoma of the nasal vestibule. Clin Otolaryngol. 2007;32:19–23.
28. Gion GG. Surgical versus prosthetic reconstruction of microtia: the case for prosthetic reconstruction. J Oral Maxillofac Surg. 2006;64:1639–54. https://doi.org/10.1016/j.joms.2006.03.050.
29. Bou C, Pomar P, Miquel JL, Poisson P. Maxillo-facial prostheses: an issue in public health. Odontostomatol Trop. 2006;29:34–40.
30. Weiss MG, Ramakrishna J, Somma D. Health-related stigma: rethinking concepts and interventions. Psychol Health Med. 2006;11:277–87.
31. Patel RG. Nasal anatomy and function. Facial Plast Surg. 2017;33:3–8.
32. Serletti J, Taub P, Wu L. Current reconstructive surgery. New York, NY: McGraw Hill Professional; 2012.
33. Atay A. Overview of maxillofacial prosthetics. Mississauga, ON: Nova Biomedical; 2013.
34. Teichgraeber JF, Goepfert H. Rhinectomy: timing and reconstruction. Otolaryngol Head Neck Surg. 1990;102:362–9.
35. Miles BA, Sinn DP, Gion GG. Experience with cranial implant-based prosthetic reconstruction. J Craniofac Surg. 2006;17:889–97.
36. Becker C, Kayser G, Pfeiffer J. Squamous cell cancer of the nasal cavity: new insights and implications for diagnosis and treatment. Head Neck. 2016;38(Suppl 1):E2112–7.
37. Thornton JF, Griffin JR, Constantine FC. Nasal reconstruction: an overview and nuances. Semin Plast Surg. 2008;22:257–68.

38. Schoen PJ, Raghoebar GM, van Oort RP, Reintsema H, van der Laan BF, Burlage FR, et al. Treatment outcome of bone-anchored craniofacial prostheses after tumor surgery. Cancer. 2001;92:3045–50.
39. Peled IJ, Wexler MR, Ticher S, Sela M. Silicone ectoprostheses for correction of facial defects. Isr J Med Sci. 1983;19:165–8.
40. Brenner P, Berger A. Epitheses of the face. Handchir Mikrochir Plast Chir. 1992;24:88–92.
41. Faris C, Heiser A, Quatela O, Jackson M, Tessler O, Jowett N, et al. Health utility of rhinectomy, surgical nasal reconstruction, and prosthetic rehabilitation. Laryngoscope. 2020;130:1674–9.
42. Powell SK, Cruz RLJ, Ross MT, Woodruff MA. Past, present, and future of soft-tissue prosthetics: advanced polymers and advanced manufacturing. Adv Mater. 2020;32:e2001122.
43. Rosen EB, Golden M, Huryn JM. Fabrication of a provisional nasal prosthesis. J Prosthet Dent. 2014;112:1308–10.
44. Diken Türksayar AA, Saglam SA, Bulut AC. Retention systems used in maxillofacial prostheses: a review. Niger J Clin Pract. 2019;22:1629–34.
45. Konstantinović VS, Lazić VM, Stefan I. Nasal epithesis retained by basal (disk) implants. J Craniofac Surg. 2010;21:33–6.
46. Sinn DP, Bedrossian E, Vest AK. Craniofacial implant surgery. Dent Clin N Am. 2011;55:847–69.
47. Becker C, Becker AM, Pfeiffer J. Health-related quality of life in patients with nasal prosthesis. J Craniomaxillofac Surg. 2016;44:75–9.
48. Chang T-L, Garrett N, Roumanas E, Beumer J 3rd. Treatment satisfaction with facial prostheses. J Prosthet Dent. 2005;94:275–80.
49. Korfage A, Raghoebar GM, Noorda WD, Plaat BE, Vissink A, Visser A. Recommendations for implant-retained nasal prostheses after ablative tumor surgery: minimal surgical aftercare, high implant survival, and satisfied patients. Head Neck. 2016;38(Suppl 1):E619–24.
50. D'heygere V, Mattheis S, Stähr K, Bastian T, Höing B, Lang S, et al. Epithetic nasal reconstruction after total rhinectomy: oncologic outcomes, immediate and long-term adverse effects, and quality of life. J Plast Reconstr Aesthet Surg. 2021;74:625. https://doi.org/10.1016/j.bjps.2020.10.013.
51. Wagenblast J, Baghi M, Helbig M, Arnoldner C, Bisdas S, Gstöttner W, et al. Craniofacial reconstructions with bone-anchored epithesis in head and neck cancer patients—a valid way back to self-perception and social reintegration. Anticancer Res. 2008;28:2349–52.
52. Chrcanovic BR, Nilsson J, Thor A. Survival and complications of implants to support craniofacial prosthesis: a systematic review. J Craniomaxillofac Surg. 2016;44:1536–52.
53. Holgers KM, Tjellstrom A, Bjursten LM, Erlandsson BE. Soft tissue reactions around percutaneous implants: a clinical study on skin-penetrating titanium implants used for bone-anchored auricular prostheses. Int J Oral Maxillofac Implants. 1987;2:35–9.
54. Alvi R, McPhail J, Hancock K. Closed-field titanium magnets for the retention of complex craniofacial prostheses. Br J Plast Surg. 2002;55:668–70.
55. Granström G, Bergström K, Tjellström A. The bone-anchored hearing aid and bone-anchored epithesis for congenital ear malformations. Otolaryngol Head Neck Surg. 1993;109:46–53.
56. Lundgren S, Moy PK, Beumer J 3rd, Lewis S. Surgical considerations for endosseous implants in the craniofacial region: a 3-year report. Int J Oral Maxillofac Surg. 1993;22:272–7.
57. Roumanas E, Nishimura RD, Beumer J, Moy PK, Weinlander M, Lorant J. Craniofacial defects and osseointegrated implants: six-year follow-up report on the success rates of craniofacial implants at UCLA. Int J Oral Maxillofac Implants. 1994;9:579–85.
58. Jensen OT, Brownd C, Blacker J. Nasofacial prostheses supported by osseointegrated implants. Int J Oral Maxillofac Implants. 1992;7:203–11.
59. Ethunandan M, Downie I, Flood T. Implant-retained nasal prosthesis for reconstruction of large rhinectomy defects: the Salisbury experience. Int J Oral Maxillofac Surg. 2010;39:343–9.
60. Scott N, Kittur MA, Evans PL, Dovgalski L, Hodder SC. The use of zygomatic implants for the retention of nasal prosthesis following rhinectomy: the Morriston experience. Int J Oral Maxillofac Surg. 2016;45:1044–8.

61. Roumanas ED, Freymiller EG, Chang T-L, Aghaloo T, Beumer J 3rd. Implant-retained prostheses for facial defects: an up to 14-year follow-up report on the survival rates of implants at UCLA. Int J Prosthodont. 2002;15:325–32.
62. Papaspyrou G, Schick B, Schneider M, Al Kadah B. Epithetic nasal reconstruction for nasal carcinoma: retrospective analysis on 22 patients. Eur Arch Otorhinolaryngol. 2017;274:867–72.
63. Curi MM, Oliveira MF, Molina G, Cardoso CL, Oliveira LDG, Branemark P-I, et al. Extraoral implants in the rehabilitation of craniofacial defects: implant and prosthesis survival rates and peri-implant soft tissue evaluation. J Oral Maxillofac Surg. 2012;70:1551–7.
64. Federspil PA. Implant-retained craniofacial prostheses for facial defects. GMS Curr Top Otorhinolaryngol Head Neck Surg. 2009;8:Doc03.
65. Scolozzi P, Jaques B. Treatment of midfacial defects using prostheses supported by ITI dental implants. Plast Reconstr Surg. 2004;114:1395–404.
66. Leonardi A, Buonaccorsi S, Pellacchia V, Moricca LM, Indrizzi E, Fini G. Maxillofacial prosthetic rehabilitation using extraoral implants. J Craniofac Surg. 2008;19:398–405.
67. Dings JPJ, Maal TJ, Muradin MS, Ingels KJ, Klevering BJ, Koole R, et al. Extra-oral implants: insertion per- or post-ablation? Oral Oncol. 2011;47:1074–8.
68. Abu-Serriah MM, McGowan DA, Moos KF, Bagg J. Extra-oral craniofacial endosseous implants and radiotherapy. Int J Oral Maxillofac Surg. 2003;32:585–92.
69. Wolfaardt JF, Wilkes GH, Parel SM, Tjellström A. Craniofacial osseointegration: the Canadian experience. Int J Oral Maxillofac Implants. 1993;8:197–204.
70. Parel SM, Tjellström A. The United States and Swedish experience with osseointegration and facial prostheses. Int J Oral Maxillofac Implants. 1991;6:75–9.
71. Tolman DE, Desjardins RP, Jackson IT, Brånemark PI. Complex craniofacial reconstruction using an implant-supported prosthesis: case report with long-term follow-up. Int J Oral Maxillofac Implants. 1997;12:243–51.
72. Flood TR, Russell K. Reconstruction of nasal defects with implant-retained nasal prostheses. Br J Oral Maxillofac Surg. 1998;36:341–5.
73. Klein M. Prosthetic management of tumor-induced nasal defects. HNO. 1999;47:623–8.
74. Visser A, Raghoebar GM, van Oort RP, Vissink A. Fate of implant-retained craniofacial prostheses: life span and aftercare. Int J Oral Maxillofac Implants. 2008;23:89–98.
75. Chrcanovic BR, Albrektsson T, Wennerberg A. Dental implants in irradiated versus nonirradiated patients: a meta-analysis. Head Neck. 2016;38:448–81.
76. Yerit KC, Posch M, Seemann M, Hainich S, Dörtbudak O, Turhani D, et al. Implant survival in mandibles of irradiated oral cancer patients. Clin Oral Implants Res. 2006;17:337–44.
77. Donoff RB. Treatment of the irradiated patient with dental implants: the case against hyperbaric oxygen treatment. J Oral Maxillofac Surg. 2006;64:819–22.
78. Granström G. Radiotherapy, osseointegration and hyperbaric oxygen therapy. Periodontol 2000. 2003;33:145–62.
79. Granström G. Placement of dental implants in irradiated bone: the case for using hyperbaric oxygen. J Oral Maxillofac Surg. 2006;64:812–8.
80. Goiato MC, de Carvalho Dekon SF, de Faria Almeida DA, Sánchez DMIK, dos Santos DM, Pellizzer EP. Patients' satisfaction after surgical facial reconstruction or after rehabilitation with maxillofacial prosthesis. J Craniofac Surg. 2011;22:766–9.
81. Goiato MC, Pesqueira AA, Ramos da Silva C, Gennari Filho H, Micheline Dos Santos D. Patient satisfaction with maxillofacial prosthesis. Literature review. J Plast Reconstr Aesthet Surg. 2009;62:175–80.
82. Lohr KN, Zebrack BJ. Using patient-reported outcomes in clinical practice: challenges and opportunities. Qual Life Res. 2009;18:99–107. https://doi.org/10.1007/s11136-008-9413-7.
83. Snyder CF, Aaronson NK, Choucair AK, Elliott TE, Greenhalgh J, Halyard MY, et al. Implementing patient-reported outcomes assessment in clinical practice: a review of the options and considerations. Qual Life Res. 2012;21:1305–14. https://doi.org/10.1007/s11136-011-0054-x.

84. Rogers SN, Lowe D. Screening for dysfunction to promote multidisciplinary intervention by using the University of Washington Quality of Life Questionnaire. Arch Otolaryngol Head Neck Surg. 2009;135:369. https://doi.org/10.1001/archoto.2009.7.

85. Penner JL. Psychosocial care of patients with head and neck cancer. Semin Oncol Nurs. 2009;25:231–41. https://doi.org/10.1016/j.soncn.2009.05.008.

86. Group W, Whoqol Group. Development of the WHOQOL: rationale and current status. Int J Mental Health. 1994;23:24–56. https://doi.org/10.1080/00207411.1994.11449286.

87. Hassan SJ, Weymuller EA. Assessment of quality of life in head and neck cancer patients. Head Neck. 1993;15:485–96. https://doi.org/10.1002/hed.2880150603.

88. Becker C, Becker AM, Dahlem KKK, Offergeld C, Pfeiffer J. Aesthetic and functional outcomes in patients with a nasal prosthesis. Int J Oral Maxillofac Surg. 2017;46:1446–50.

89. Moolenburgh SE, Mureau MAM, Duivenvoorden HJ, Hofer SOP. Validation of a questionnaire assessing patient's aesthetic and functional outcome after nasal reconstruction: the patient NAFEQ-score. J Plast Reconstr Aesthet Surg. 2009;62:656–62. https://doi.org/10.1016/j.bjps.2007.07.024.

90. Moolenburgh SE, Mureau MAM, Hofer SOP. Aesthetic outcome after nasal reconstruction: patient versus panel perception. J Plast Reconstr Aesthet Surg. 2008;61:1459–64.

91. Whitney RL, Bell JF, Reed SC, Lash R, Bold RJ, Kim KK, et al. Predictors of financial difficulties and work modifications among cancer survivors in the United States. J Cancer Surviv. 2016;10:241–50.

92. Markt JC, Lemon JC. Extraoral maxillofacial prosthetic rehabilitation at the M. D. Anderson Cancer Center: a survey of patient attitudes and opinions. J Prosthet Dent. 2001;85:608–13.

93. Klassen AF, Cano SJ, Scott A, Snell L, Pusic AL. Measuring patient-reported outcomes in facial aesthetic patients: development of the FACE-Q. Facial Plast Surg. 2010;26:303–9.

94. Sela M, Lowental U. Therapeutic effects of maxillofacial prostheses. Oral Surg Oral Med Oral Pathol. 1980;50:13–6.

95. Lowental U, Sela M. Evaluating cosmetic results in maxillofacial prosthetics. J Prosthet Dent. 1982;48:567–70.

96. Moroni L, Burdick JA, Highley C, Lee SJ, Morimoto Y, Takeuchi S, et al. Biofabrication strategies for 3D in vitro models and regenerative medicine. Nat Rev Mater. 2018;3:21–37.

97. Haisch A. Ear reconstruction through tissue engineering. Adv Otorhinolaryngol. 2010;68:108–19.

98. Jessop ZM, Javed M, Otto IA, Combellack EJ, Morgan S, Breugem CC, et al. Combining regenerative medicine strategies to provide durable reconstructive options: auricular cartilage tissue engineering. Stem Cell Res Ther. 2016;7:19.

99. Nayyer L, Patel KH, Esmaeili A, Rippel RA, Birchall M, O'Toole G, et al. Tissue engineering: revolution and challenge in auricular cartilage reconstruction. Plast Reconstr Surg. 2012;129:1123–37.

100. Yanaga H, Imai K, Tanaka Y, Yanaga K. Two-stage transplantation of cell-engineered autologous auricular chondrocytes to regenerate chondrofat composite tissue: clinical application in regenerative surgery. Plast Reconstr Surg. 2013;132:1467–77.

101. Yanaga H, Imai K, Fujimoto T, Yanaga K. Generating ears from cultured autologous auricular chondrocytes by using two-stage implantation in treatment of microtia. Plast Reconstr Surg. 2009;124:817–25.

102. Zhou G, Jiang H, Yin Z, Liu Y, Zhang Q, Zhang C, et al. In vitro regeneration of patient-specific ear-shaped cartilage and its first clinical application for auricular reconstruction. EBioMedicine. 2018;28:287–302.

103. Fulco I, Miot S, Haug MD, Barbero A, Wixmerten A, Feliciano S, et al. Engineered autologous cartilage tissue for nasal reconstruction after tumour resection: an observational first-in-human trial. Lancet. 2014;384:337–46.

104. Hong CJ, Giannopoulos AA, Hong BY, Witterick IJ, Irish JC, Lee J, et al. Clinical applications of three-dimensional printing in otolaryngology-head and neck surgery: a systematic review. Laryngoscope. 2019;129:2045–52.

105. Jodat YA, Kiaee K, Vela Jarquin D, De la Garza Hernández RL, Wang T, Joshi S, et al. A 3D-printed hybrid nasal cartilage with functional electronic olfaction. Adv Sci. 2020;7:1901878.

External Beam Radiotherapy for Nose Vestibule Malignancies

10

Ida D'Onofrio, Roberto Gallus, Fabrizio Sanna, Dalila Di Mario, Emilia Degni, Salvatrice Campoccia, Luca Tagliaferri, and Yun Gan Tao

10.1 Introduction

Squamous cell carcinoma of the nasal vestibule (NV), which is the most common NV cancer, is relatively rare (<1% of H&N cancer), even if probably its incidence is underestimated, and presents, as described in the previous chapters, several anatomical clinical and histological peculiarities when compared with malignancies of the nasal cavity proper and skin (see Chap. 3) [1, 2]. In general, the prognosis is

I. D'Onofrio
Radiation Oncology, Ospedale del Mare, ASL Napoli 1 Centro, Naples, Italy
e-mail: ida.donofrio@aslnapoli1centro.it

R. Gallus (✉)
Otolaryngology, Mater Olbia Hospital, Olbia, Italy
e-mail: roberto.gallus@materolbia.com

F. Sanna · D. Di Mario
Institute of Radiological Sciences, Azienda Ospedaliero Universitaria, Sassari, Italy
e-mail: fabrizio.sanna@aouss.it; dalila.dimario@aouss.it

E. Degni
Otolaryngology Division, Azienda Ospedaliero Universitaria, Sassari, Italy
e-mail: emilia.degni@aouss.it

S. Campoccia
Radioterapia Oncologica, Ospedale "San Francesco", Nuoro, Italy
e-mail: salvatrice.campoccia@aslnuoro.it

L. Tagliaferri
UOC Radioterapia Oncologica, Dipartimento di Diagnostica per Immagini, Radioterapia Oncologica ed Ematologia, Fondazione Policlinico Universitario A. Gemelli, IRCCS, Rome, Italy
e-mail: luca.tagliaferri@policlinicogemelli.it

Y. G. Tao
Department of Oncology-Radiotherapy, Gustave Roussy, Villejuif, France
e-mail: Yungan.tao@gustaveroussy.fr

© Springer Nature Switzerland AG 2023
F. Bussu (ed.), *Malignancies of the Nasal Vestibule*,
https://doi.org/10.1007/978-3-031-32850-3_10

considered favorable, with 3-year locoregional control and overall survival rates ranging from 67% to 92% and from 50% to 90%, respectively [3–5].

The most frequent presenting symptoms and signs are not specific, including nasal airway obstruction, associated with epistaxis and rhinorrhea, and this causes a delay of the diagnosis. Also, as the most frequent presenting site is the perinasal skin, these cases are often primarily referred to plastic surgeons and dermatologists, which misclassify them as primary skin cancer with improper primary definition of the extension and of the origin of the tumor [6].

Due to the rarity of the condition and to the lack of randomized/prospective studies, a class I evidence is missing. The therapeutic decision is based on a retrospective series with a limited number of patients, enrolled over a long period of time.

10.1.1 Potential Predictive Factors, Data to Guide Treatment Recommendation

The series describing NV SCC are few and generally small. Different authors describe different putative predictive factors with the potential to guide treatment decisions. No definitive conclusion can currently be drawn on the subject.

The *tumor extension* can have an impact on the treatment choice: septum invasion has been reportedly associated with a significantly higher risk of recurrence [7, 8]. In particular, the involvement of deep tissues of the septum and the columella, especially around the anterior nasal spine, had been described to have a worse prognosis when treated with radiotherapy alone [9].

Tumors of the floor of the vestibule, extending into the upper lip, and of the alar wall, invading the underlying cartilage, have been often considered unsuitable for surgery, due to poor cosmetic results, difficult to correct even with complex reconstructions [10]. The *tumor size* seems to have an impact on local control (LC) as well [4, 11]. Wong et al. [12] found that tumor size of 2 cm or more and the involvement of the lip, the columella, and the skin of the *ala nasi* were associated with a worse LC rate. Wray et al. found that patients who received radiotherapy alone had an excellent disease control except for tumors with a maximum diameter of more than 4 cm [4]. Compared with similarly sized T1-T2, T4 cancers according to AJCC, with a diameter of less than 4 cm, had no higher risk of local recurrence [13]. No difference was found in the probability of LC after radiotherapy of newly diagnosed primary lesions compared to that of *recurrences* after previous surgery [4]. Tumor diameter >1.5 cm and T2 stage are associated with a decreased regional control [14]. Poor *histologic differentiation* is a risk factor for poor LC [15]. Not surprisingly, patients with clinically metastatic neck lymph nodes (cN+) have a poor prognosis and might have benefits from more aggressive/combined treatment [11]. In our opinion, neck dissection remains the mainstay of treatment for patients with metastatic lymph nodes in the neck.

In any case, clear evidence supporting one treatment modality versus another is lacking, and the choice of the treatment is described more extensively in other chapters of this monograph. The foregoing chapter will focus on technical aspects and clinical outcomes of external beam radiotherapy (EBRT) for nasal vestibule cancers.

10.1.2 EBRT

Radiotherapy has a role as primary treatment for early-stage nasal vestibule cancer and in the postoperative setting for advanced lesions. Radiotherapy modalities vary among different treatment centers from external irradiation alone, interstitial brachytherapy alone, or combinations of external irradiation and brachytherapy (BRT).

EBRT alone is indicated for small primaries with cN0 necks, cT3 (according to Wang classification) and/or cN+ cases are often treated with concomitant chemotherapy (usually cisplatin).

In any case, it is hard to compare the different series for several reasons: (1) no universally recognized classification (see Chaps. 4 and 5), (2) different radiation treatment modalities and schedules used across the years, (3) radiotherapy treatment often highly individualized without clear definition of the criteria and available guidelines.

10.1.2.1 Early Stage (T1–T2 According to Wang)

In early stages, radiotherapy or surgery could result in equally good oncological outcomes [16] producing LC rates of 90% or more. Choice of treatment is based on size, extension, and anticipated cosmetic outcomes. Surgery is a good option for small, well-delineated, and superficial lesions [17], usually not invading the skin [10]. Several reports proposed radiotherapy as primary treatment in early stages for its better cosmetic results compared to surgery [3, 12, 13, 16, 18, 19].

In a retrospective study by Langendijk et al. [3], primary EBRT (with or without endocavitary brachytherapy boost) is the standard treatment for T1 and T2 patients, according to the WANG system. The choice of radiation technique depended on tumor extension and radiation oncologist's experience. Specifically, EBRT alone was reserved for tumors involving the upper lip. Primary radiotherapy was considered effective for early stage tumors, resulting in 2-year LC of 80%, with a 2-year ultimate LC rate of 95%, after salvage surgery.

In fact, in another retrospective study, Levandang et al. [11] reported only 3% of recurrence in patients treated by brachytherapy alone versus 13% and 38% in EBRT only and combined EBRT-brachytherapy groups, respectively, which may be due to selection bias (the majority of T2 stage was treated with combined modality).

In a report by Vanneste et al. [20], patients with T1 or selected T2 (no bulky, no invasion of upper lip or nasal septum) were treated with interstitial brachytherapy. Other T2 and T3 patients were treated with EBRT. LC rate for T1 was extremely high (97% at 5 years). For T2, recurrences were observed only in the EBRT group, probably attributable to the selection bias. This report confirmed that higher T class was associated with poorer LC (only 53% for cT3 tumors according to Wang's classification).

In fact, in a multivariate analysis, Wray et al. [4] found no significant differences between radiation treatment modalities (BRT alone, EBRT alone, or combined BRT-EBRT) in terms of LC, local-regional control (LRC), distant metastases (DM), overall survival (OS), and cause-specific survival (CSS). On a stage-by-stage basis, the overall LC in early-stage tumors was 100% with BRT alone, 88% and 86% with combined EBRT-BRT and EBRT alone, respectively.

No specific parameters contraindicating radiotherapy as primary modality were found in retrospective studies. Mccollough [13] noted that cartilage invasion was not associated with worse LC rates in patients treated with radiotherapy alone.

However, a recent multicentric analysis [14] describes that BRT provided higher 3-year LC and nose preservation rate, compared with EBRT (95% vs. 71%), also in multivariable risk-stratified analysis, in cT1-T2 (according to Wang) NV carcinomas. This would confirm studies reporting lower survival and worse LC rates of EBRT compared to brachytherapy or surgery [11, 19].

10.1.2.2 Advanced Stage (T3 According to WANG or More Than 4 cm)

In a definitive radiotherapy setting, EBRT treatment combined with chemotherapy has been recommended in large size and/or deep infiltrating tumors, solely or in combination with brachytherapy as a boost. Anyway, it is difficult to obtain LC of advanced tumors, and there is a high tendency to relapse after irradiation. Therefore, tumors larger than 4 cm and/or with bone invasion are unsuitable for either radiation therapy or surgery alone but should rather be treated with a combination of these two modalities [19, 21]. A retrospective study of the DAHANCA group reported very poor results in Wang cT3 tumors, mainly treated by EBRT: 39% 5-year disease-specific survival (DSS) and 0% 5-year OS, which suggested the necessity of the combination with a surgical approach [17]. In fact, in advanced stages, the surgical resection associated with postoperative EBRT offered higher LC rates [4].

In general, in the postoperative setting, adjuvant EBRT is indicated in case of advanced tumors (classified as T3 WANG or T4 AJCC), involved or unclear margin, nodal involvement, or perineural invasion [4, 17].

In some reports, the use of preoperative (in case of neoadjuvant irradiation, but mostly in case of recurrence after definitive EBRT) radiotherapy appeared to be associated with a greater risk of *sequelae* such as bone exposure or wound complication when patients are submitted to ablative surgery [4, 22].

10.2 Role of Chemotherapy

There are few data on the role of chemotherapy in NV cancer treatment, as NV cancer is generally considered as more similar to the skin than to mucosal malignancies, even if this is not demonstrated by evidence. Therefore, the choice of chemotherapy is left to the discretion of the clinician, based on the stage and risk factors. cT3 according to Wang and clinical nodal involvement can be considered parameters to indicate concomitant chemotherapy in cases treated primarily by EBRT.

On the other hand, in the postoperative setting, extensive neck involvement, namely pN2-3 (according to eighth AJCC classification), and incomplete resection (R1) usually indicate adjuvant concomitant chemoradiotherapy in other head and neck subsites and can be considered valid criteria also for operated NV carcinomas.

Table 10.1 analytically describes the results of the main studies reporting the outcomes of radiotherapy for treatment of nose vestibule carcinomas.

10.3   EBRT Techniques

EBRT is the most common modality of radiotherapy, which delivers radiation beams from a source external to the patient.

Megavoltage (MV) photons and electron beams are generated from linear accelerators. MV electron beams represent an important radiation treatment modality often providing a unique option in the treatment of superficial targets. This is possible because the electron beam exhibits a higher surface dose than MV photon beams. The electron beam has a sharp fall-off of the dose sparing deeper tissues. The depth of penetration may be adjusted by varying the energy of the electron beam. On the contrary, megavoltage photons are more penetrating, and their slow fall-off is an issue in case of superficial lesions as most often nose vestibule cancers are.

Using a lead cut-out, the electron field can be easily adapted to the area to treat, although the wide penumbra of the electron beam requires a larger margin (1.5 cm) than that is required for photons treatments [23].

Historical series describe widely 2D conventional/3D conformal techniques for EBRT treatment of NV carcinoma. Over the last decades, intensity-modulated radiation therapy (IMRT) has become the standard treatment in head and neck cancers, improving conformability and homogeneity of dose distribution to the planning target volume (PTV) and sparing the adjacent structures at risk. Nowadays, modern techniques that include IMRT and volumetric-modulated radiation therapy (VMAT) are routinely used in most centers.

10.3.1   Positioning and Immobilization

10.3.1.1   3D Conformal Radiotherapy

Historically, EBRT treatment for nasal vestibule cancers consists of a combination of anterior fields using 20-MeV electrons and 6-MV photons weighted 4–1. Patient is immobilized in supine position using a thermoplastic mask, with the head +/− shoulder slightly flexed. Placing a customized lead shield directly on the patient's skin, the electron field can be shaped to fit the treatment area, reducing the penumbra of the electron beam and sparing critical tissues as the nasolacrimal duct and the eye (Fig. 10.1).

To increase the dose delivery to the skin near the gross tumor volume (GTV) region, bolus material (0.5–1 cm thickness) is often used for the electron portion of

Table 10.1 Results of the main studies reporting the outcomes of radiotherapy for treatment of nose vestibule carcinomas

Author, Year Institution	No pts	Classification	Primary RT	RT Technique	Local control (%)	Overall survival (%)	Regional control (%)	Note	Late side effects
Langendijk et al. (2004) [3] VU University Medical Center Amsterdam	56 (1980–2000)	WANG (only T1-T2)	100%	47 EBRT + Endocavitary BRT	2 years LC 79%	5 years OS 66%	2 years RC 87%	No statistically significant differences between RT modalities	Rhinorrea (45%)
				9 EBRT alone (if upper lip involvement)	LC (after surgery) 95%	5 years DSS 87%	2 years RC 97%		Nasal dryness (39%)
									Epistaxis (15%)
									Adhesions (4%)
									Skin necrosis (5%)
									1 Post-Rt sarcoma
Vanneste et al. (2016) [20] The Nederlands Cancer institute Amsterdam	81 (1977–2012)	WANG	100%	T1-T2 = IRT	5 years LC	5 years OS 59%	5 years LCR 68%	All recurrences among EBRT pts	Epistaxis (11%)
				T2 Bulky: EBRT	T1 = 97%	5 years PFS 57%	10% Node Recurrence		Persistent crust formation (28%)
				T3: EBRT	T2 Bulky = 55%				Perforated septum (3%)
					T3 = 53%				Severe Stenosis (2%)

Author, Year Institution	No pts	Classification	Primary RT	RT Technique	Local control (%)	Overall survival (%)	Regional control (%)	Note	Late side effects
Wray et al. (2016) [4]	99 (1970–2013)	Sixth AJCC skin cancer	86%	15 BRT	5 years LC: 100%	5 years OS: 77%	5 years RC in N0 pts: 87%	No statistically significant differences between RT modalities in term of LC, LCR OS, CSS, M+	One second cancer (Small cell carcinoma) in treatment field
University of Florida				39 EBRT	5 years LC: 84%	5 years CSS: 94%	10 years RC in N0 pts: 87%		Severe complication only in surgical patients
				45 EBRT + BRT	5 years LC: 86%	10 years OS: 51%			
						10 years CSS: 94%			
Levendag et al. (1990) [11]	59 (1978–1988)	WANG (only T1-T2-N0)	100%	36 BRT	90%	65%	4/56 node recurrence (7%)	Influence of size on local tumor control	No data
Hospital Dijkzigt Rotterdam				15 EBRT					
				6 EBRT + BRT					

(continued)

Table 10.1 (continued)

Author, Year Institution	No pts	Classification	Primary RT	RT Technique	Local control (%)	Overall survival (%)	Regional control (%)	Note	Late side effects
Wong et al. (1986) [12] (1958–1983) Princess Margaret Hospital	56	Tumor size	100%	EBRT	<2 cm = 97% >2 cm = 54%	66%	3/54 node recurrence	size >2 cm or more and involvement of lip, columella and skin of ala nasi is associated with worse local control rate	Maxillary ostheonecrosis (3%) Epistaxis (2%) Nasal stenosis (2%)
Horsman et al. (1999) [8] Odense University Hospital, Denmark	41 (1878–1992)	WANG	66%	EBRT (Electrons)	68%	48%		No significant differences in survival or recurrence comparing primary surgery to primary EBRT. Septal location is a risk factor for local recurrence	
Dowley et al. (2008) [9] University Hospital Nottingham	26 (1988–2008)	WANG	54%	Not recorded	50%	57%	90%	T2-T3 lesion are best managed by surgery	One patient had reconstructive surgery for radionecrosis

Author, Year / Institution	No pts	Classification	Primary RT	RT Technique	Local control (%)	Overall survival (%)	Regional control (%)	Note	Late side effects
Agger et al. (2009) [17] DAHANCA database	174 (1993–2002)	WANG	70%	120 EBRT				In T1-EBRT treated group, OS was better in 54 Gy/18 fractions rather than 66 Gy/33 fractions	
				28 Surgery + EBRT					
				22 Surgery alone					
				T1 stage:					
				63 EBRT	61	49			
				22 Surgery + EBRT	87	53			
				17 Surgery alone	94	57			
Czerwinski et al. (2021) [14]	225 (2010–2016)	WANG (only T1-T2)	100%	153 BRT	3-year 95%	3-year 82%	3-year 89%	BRT provided higher 3-year survival with preserved nose compared with EBRT (82% vs. 61%, $p < 0.01$).	5-year incidence of grade ≥2 toxicity was higher after BRT (20% vs. 3%, $p = 0.03$). Mostly radiation ulcers.
6 Dutch Institutions				65 EBRT	3-year 71%	3-year 82%	3-year 89%		Radiation ulcers (24%)
									Septal defects (10%)
									Chondronecrosis (4%)

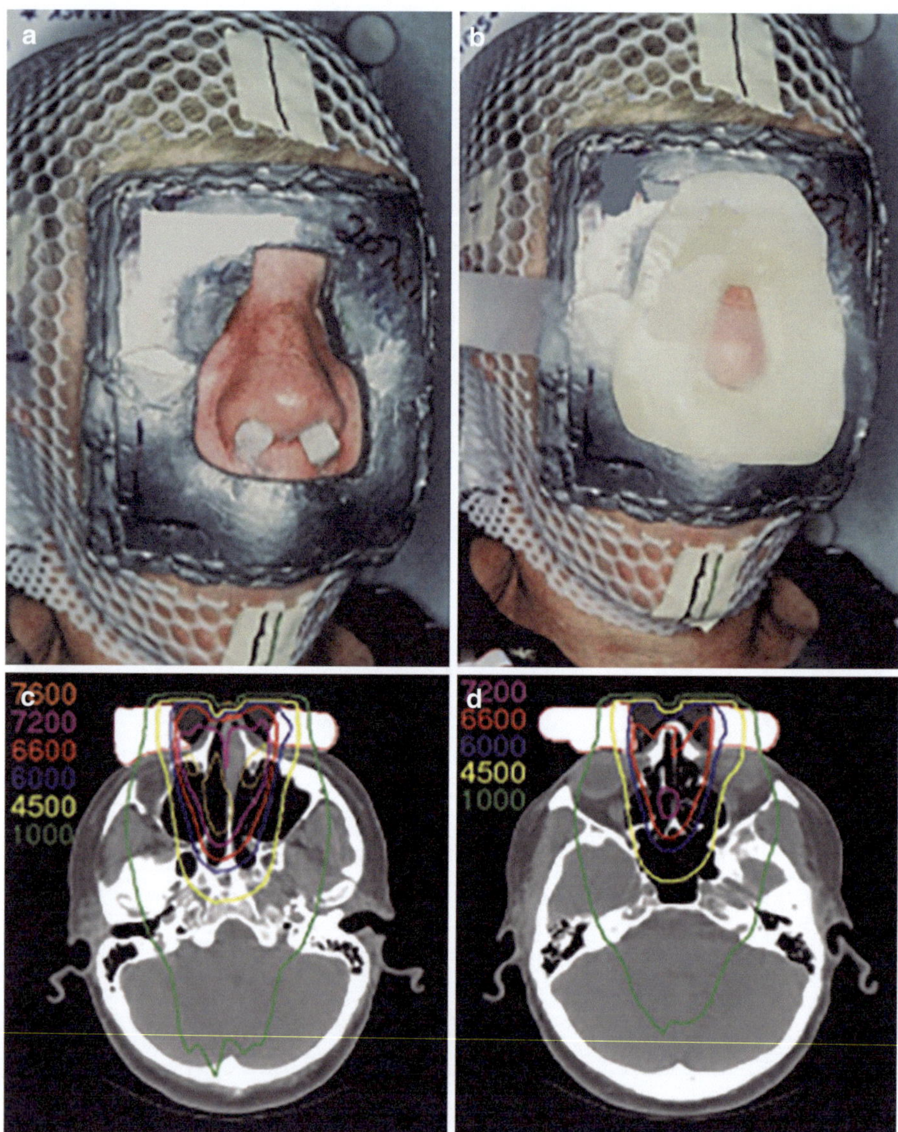

Fig. 10.1 (**a–d**) Placing a customized lead shield directly on the patient's skin, the electron field can be shaped to fit the treatment area, reducing the penumbra of the electron beam and sparing critical tissues as the nasolacrimal duct and the eye

the treatment. It can help to "smooth" irregular surface contours, optimizing the electron beam dose distribution. For a simple skin dose built up on a reasonably flat surface, a layer of superflab of appropriate thickness is sufficient. For surface contour modification, a custom-made beeswax bolus may be preferred [24]. Bolus material can be used also in the postoperative setting, on postoperative defects or skin scars.

A stent can be placed over the upper alveolar processes to open the mouth and separate the lips, excluding the lower lip from the radiation field and displacing the tongue posteriorly to prevent irradiation of the gingiva, the part of the stent that is between the upper lip and the alveolar ridge can be filled with Cerrobend [25] (Fig. 10.2).

Nasal packing may be used, to reduce/avoid build up effect and to improve dose homogeneity.

10.3.1.2 IMRT/VMAT

IMRT with Simultaneous Integrated Boost technique (SIB-IMRT) allows the delivery of different daily doses to different target volumes within a single fraction of treatment: large fields and boost can be integrated in the same plan and treated simultaneously. Recently, only few studies have investigated the IMRT role in nasal cavity and NV cancer treatment [26].

Given the close proximity of the target volume to critical structures such as naso-lacrimal duct, eyes, and oral cavity, the IMRT may represent an opportunity to spare structures at risk and reduce acute and late toxicities.

In the first published SIB-IMRT series treating patients with nasal vestibule cancer (5 pts, 33%), Janssen et al. [27] reported outcomes comparable with the historic series in terms of LC and OS and good clinical and aesthetic results, with few late sequelae of grade II or higher.

For the IMRT/VMAT technique, the patient is immobilized in a supine position, with a thermoplastic head and shoulder mask fixed on a carbon fiber base plate with a foam head support. Superficial lesions/scars are often marked with a radio-opaque thread. A bolus could be placed around the nasal structure to superficialize the dose

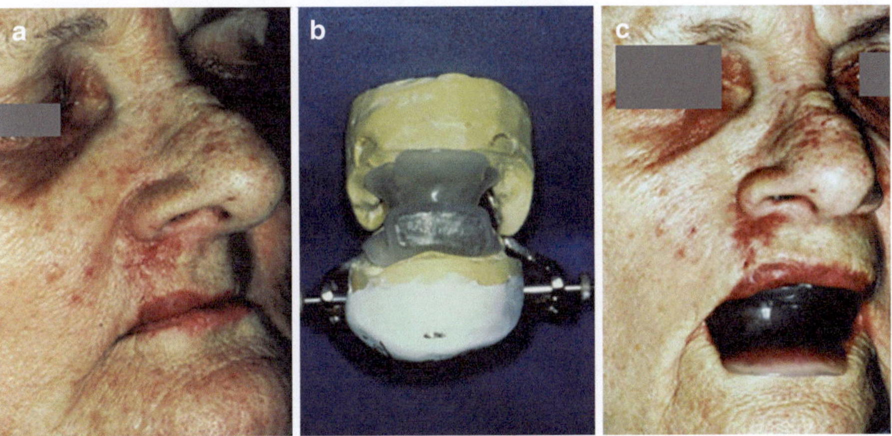

Fig. 10.2 (**a–c**) Nasal packing may be used, to reduce/avoid build up effect and to improve dose homogeneity

and achieve a better coverage of superficial targets. The personalized bolus is typically made of wax-like material, which can be shaped to fit into the surface. To date, several studies have examined the use of 3D-printed boluses, which adhere to the skin surface more accurately, minimizing air gaps and improving daily reproducibility.

A bolus material is used to fill the nares. An intraoral device is commonly used to push the tongue posteriorly, out to the treatment field. A thermoplastic mask is placed on the top of the inserted bolus to immobilize the patient [28, 29] (Figs. 10.3 and 10.4).

The Radiation Oncologist should evaluate the positioning and immobilization devices, patient weight, and bolus positioning through two orthogonal exposures with a planar view EPID (6 MV) or cone beam CT (CBCT), as deemed appropriate.

10.3.2 Definition of Target Volume

We can identify different target volumes. The gross tumor volume (GTV) is defined as the gross palpable or visible extent of the tumor. It may consist of a primary tumor or lymphadenopathy. The delineation of GTV is possible if the tumor is demonstrable through CT and/or magnetic resonance (MR) imaging and positron

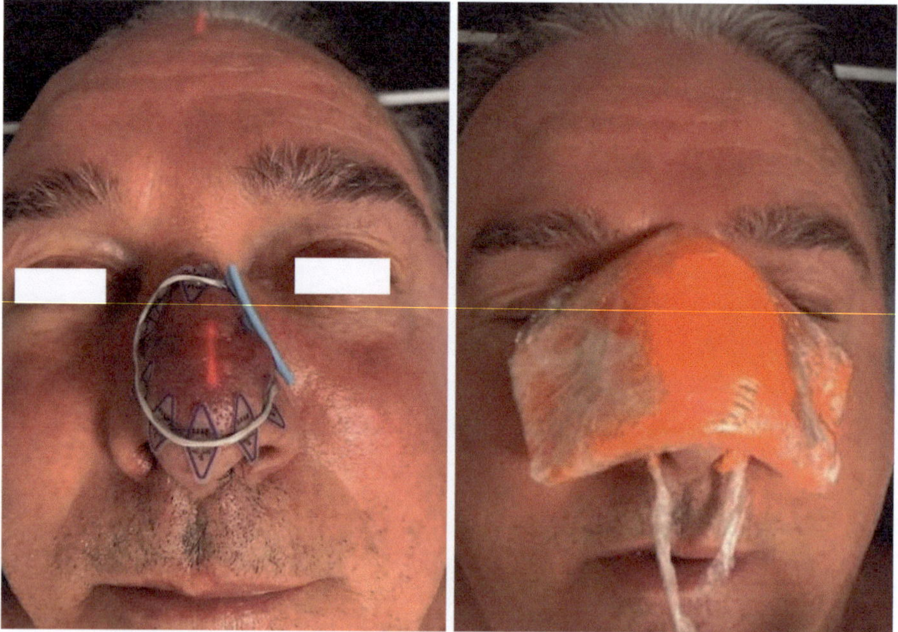

Fig. 10.3 A bolus material is used to fill the nares. An intraoral device is commonly used to push the tongue posteriorly, out to the treatment field

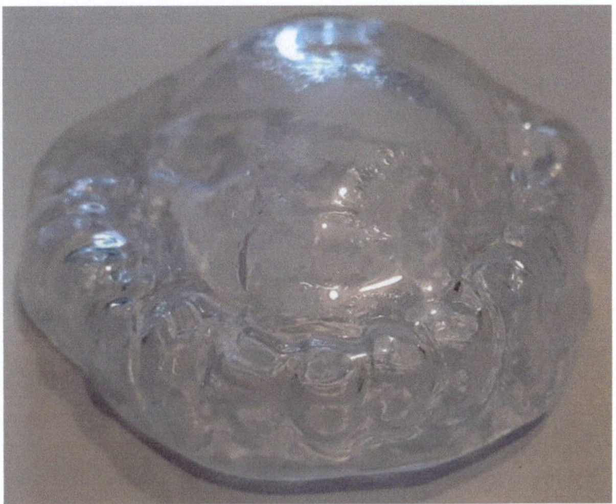

Fig. 10.4 A thermoplastic mask is placed on the top of the inserted bolus to immobilize the patient

emission tomography (PET). GTV cannot be delineated if the tumor has been surgically removed.

The clinical target volume (CTV) is defined as the volume that contains the GTV and subclinical microscopic disease. Three different levels of dose corresponding to the risk of microscopic disease can be distinguished as follows: CTV high-risk (CTV HR), CTV intermediate-risk (CTV IR), and CTV low-risk (CTV LR). The use of SIB-IMRT technique enables dose escalation to GTV, while maintaining relatively low doses to CTV IR and CTV LR, without affecting the overall treatment time (OTT).

Target volumes include the initial (LOW RISK) CTV and the boost (HIGH RISK) CTV. The initial (LOW RISK) CTV (CTV1) includes high-risk areas with further margin taking account of potential microscopic diseases. For *well-differentiated* early-stage tumors (with diameters of 2 cm or less without extension into adjacent structures), the volume is GTV + 1 cm margin, based on the proximity to critical structures such as the eyes and the optic nerves. For *poorly differentiated* tumors of any size or *well-differentiated* tumors >2 cm in diameter without palpable nodes (N0), the volume is GTV + 2 cm margin and all areas considered at risk for potential microscopic diseases. The Boost (HIGH RISK) CTV (CTV2) includes the GTV with 5–10 mm margins in case of curative EBRT or high-risk postoperative areas in case of adjuvant treatment [24]. Adaptive replanning may be considered during treatment if there is change in aeration in response to radiotherapy given the proximity to critical structures. The postoperative CTV includes the entire surgical bed based on preoperative imaging studies fused with postoperative computed tomography. Optional boost could be delineated on high-risk areas.

Basing on the considerations concerning the typical spread patterns from the three walls of the vestibule (see Chap. 3), we propose enlarging the margins of the CTV2 along the main axis of the spread (the septum for lesions involving the colu-mella, the superior lip for lesions involving the inferior wall, the nasal skin for lesions involving the lateral wall). In the presence of risk factors for lymph node metastasis (as bone invasion, T3/WANG scale or T4/AJCC scale) inclusion of bilateral facial lymphatics ("Manchu Moustache Area"), level IB (submandibular) and level IIA (subdigastric), and level III nodes could be considered. Patients with involved node(s) also receive irradiation to the level III and IV nodes. In case of macroscopic/multiple microscopic perineural invasion, the inclusion of nerve paths (in particular the nasociliary nerve (V1) and the infraorbital nerve (V2)) for at least 30 mm in low-risk volume should be considered [30].

Postoperative radiation therapy is indicated for close/positive margins, perineural invasion, T3-T4 patients, and positive lymph nodes. The CTV1 includes a surgical bed with 1–1.5 cm margin. Neck irradiation depends on whether the neck dissection was carried out, on the presence of lymph node diseases or other risk factors.

The PTV margin is based on institutional setup and verification protocols. PTV margins of 3–5 mm are commonly applied in head and neck radiotherapy.

With the increasing use of image-guided radiotherapy (IGRT), setup uncertainties can be assessed and corrected during the treatment, enabling a reduction of the PTV margin.

10.3.3 Dose

Small lesions (1.5 cm or less): 50 Gy in 25 fractions followed by 16–20 Gy in 8–10 fractions boost, by external irradiation. Larger lesions (more than 1.5 cm): 50 Gy in 25 fractions followed by 20 Gy in 10 fractions boost. In case of IMRT: definite RT or chemo-RT: CTV HR to 66–70 Gy (depending on tumor size, smaller than 1.5 cm or larger lesion); CTV IR to 60–63 Gy, CTV LR 54–57 Gy to elective neck, in 33 or 35 fractions.

When EBRT and brachytherapy are combined, approximately 50 Gy is usually administered with EBRT and the remainder with a brachytherapy boost. The interval between EBRT and brachytherapy is usually 1–2 weeks.

Elective treatment of the facial (moustache area) and the upper neck nodes (level IB and level IIA nodes): 50 Gy in 25 fractions. Palpable nodes receive a total dose of 66–70 Gy, depending on their size.

A total dose of 60 Gy is usually prescribed in adjuvant settings. For cases with involved margins or residual disease, the dose might be increased to 66–70 Gy (IMRT: CTV IR to 60 Gy with optional CTV HR to 66 Gy to high risk areas as involved margins, ECE, PNI. CTV LR to 50–54 Gy to elective neck).

The prescribed dose for SIB-IMRT/VMAT is 54–60 Gy in 33 Fractions for CTV1 and 66–70 Gy in 33 Fractions for CTV2.

10.3.4 Side Effects and Cosmetic Results

The acute morbidity with EBRT is usually mild and well tolerated. Patients often show radio-dermatitis and moist skin desquamation, radio-mucositis and crust in nasal vestibule and nasal cavity [3, 11, 13, 19, 21, 31]. Nasal epistaxis is rarely reported. Nasal douche with saline and nasal dilatation with lubricated cotton-swab applicators following irradiation are recommended to avoid synechiae, crusting, and subsequent nasal stenosis [13, 21, 31]. Late complications such as telangiectasia and fibrosis are less frequently described. Side effects exceeding grade III are very rare and reported only by the earliest series [32]. Skin ulceration and septal perforation have been rarely described, probably depending on the tumor origin [3, 20]. More serious late complications have been reported after combined surgery and radiotherapy, as naso-buccal fistula [33] and bone exposure [4]. Published data reported two cases of a second tumor, several years after completing the radiation treatment [3, 4]. Previous studies indicated a 3% incidence of maxilla osteonecrosis [12, 34]. In the last decades, the improvement of radiotherapy techniques and the introduction of oral hygiene measures had decreased the risk of this major complication.

Janssen reported very satisfying cosmetic outcomes and no grade II or more late sequelae in patients with cancer in the nasal cavity/vestibule treated with IMRT [27]. In particular, no severe side effects concerning vision or lacrimal glands had been reported. The cosmetic outcomes in patients treated with definitive EBRT are usually very good [22, 35]. Substantial changes of the nasal shape have not been described, except for large tumors, which have caused tissue destruction. Late complications such as mild skin fibrosis and telangiectasia have been reported, especially if a bolus material was used to skin dose build-up [12].

The main toxicities after EBRT for nose lesions affect nose mucosa function with an impact on smell and most of all mucociliary clearance [36]. The impact on quality of life can be very relevant with a significant impairment of nose function.

10.4 Conclusions

In summary, external beam radiotherapy has an acknowledged role in the treatment strategy of nasal vestibule cancer. Indications for adjuvant radiation are positive or close resection margins, perineural invasion, or regional lymph node metastases. Advocates of EBRT as primary treatment for NV cancers (excluding T3 according to Wang) outline the good cosmetic results without compromising the oncological outcomes [10]. The main cons are lower local and regional control rates in some series and the long-term impact on nose function [1].

References

1. Bussu F, Tagliaferri L, Piras A, Rizzo D, Tsatsaris N, De Corso E, Parrilla C, Paludetti G. Multidisciplinary approach to nose vestibule malignancies: setting new standards Approccio multidisciplinare ai tumori maligni del vestibolo del naso: verso la definizione di nuovi standard Acta Otorhinolaryngologica Italica 2021;41(Suppl. 1):S158–S165. https://doi.org/10.14639/0392-100X-suppl.1-41-2021-16.

2. Bussu F, Tagliaferri L, Crescio C, Rizzo D, Gallus R, Parrilla C, Fionda B, Lancellotta V, Mattiucci GC, Galli J. New standards for the management of nose vestibule malignancies Acta Oto-Laryngologica 2023;143(3):215–22. https://doi.org/10.1080/00016489.2023.2179662.

3. Langendijk JA, Poorter R, Leemans CR, de Bree R, Doornaert P, Slotman BJ. Radiotherapy of squamous cell carcinoma of the nasal vestibule. Int J Radiat Oncol Biol Phys. 2004;59(5):1319–25. https://doi.org/10.1016/j.ijrobp.2004.01.007.

4. Wray J, Morris CG, Kirwan JM, Amdur RJ, Werning JW, Dziegielewski PT, et al. Radiation therapy for nasal vestibule squamous cell carcinoma: a 40-year experience. Eur Arch Otorhinolaryngol. 2016;273(3):661–9. https://doi.org/10.1007/s00405-015-3603-z.

5. Levendag PC, Nijdam WM, van Moolenburgh SE, Tan L, Noever I, van Rooy P, et al. Interstitial radiation therapy for early-stage nasal vestibule cancer: a continuing quest for optimal tumor control and cosmesis. Int J Radiat Oncol Biol Phys. 2006;66(1):160–9. https://doi.org/10.1016/j.ijrobp.2006.03.041.

6. Beatty CW, Pearson BW, Kern EB. Carcinoma of the nasal septum: experience with 85 cases. Otolaryngol Head Neck Surg. 1982;90(1):90–4. https://doi.org/10.1177/019459988209000116.

7. Mak AC, van Andel JG, van Woerkom-Eijkenboom WM. Radiation therapy of carcinoma of the nasal vestibule. Eur J Cancer. 1980;16(1):81–5. https://doi.org/10.1016/0014-2964(80)90111-5.

8. Horsmans JD, Godballe C, Jørgensen KE, Bastholt L, Løntoft E. Squamous cell carcinoma of the nasal vestibule. Rhinology. 1999;37(3):117–21. https://www.ncbi.nlm.nih.gov/pubmed/10567990.

9. Dowley A, Hoskison E, Allibone R, Jones NS. Squamous cell carcinoma of the nasal vestibule: a 20-year case series and literature review. J Laryngol Otol. 2008;122(10):1019–23. https://doi.org/10.1017/S0022215108002259.

10. Goepfert H. The vex and fuss about nasal vestibule cancer. Head Neck. 1999;21(5):383–4. https://doi.org/10.1002/(sici)1097-0347(199908)21:5<383::aid-hed1>3.0.co;2-#.

11. Levendag PC, Pomp J. Radiation therapy of squamous cell carcinoma of the nasal vestibule. Int J Radiat Oncol Biol Phys. 1990;19(6):1363–7. https://doi.org/10.1016/0360-3016(90)90345-k.

12. Wong CS, Cummings BJ, Elhakim T, Briant TD. External irradiation for squamous cell carcinoma of the nasal vestibule. Int J Radiat Oncol Biol Phys. 1986;12(11):1943–6. https://doi.org/10.1016/0360-3016(86)90129-x.

13. McCollough WM, Mendenhall NP, Parsons JT, Mendenhall WM, Stringer SP, Cassisi NJ, et al. Radiotherapy alone for squamous cell carcinoma of the nasal vestibule: management of the primary site and regional lymphatics. Int J Radiat Oncol Biol Phys. 1993;26(1):73–9. https://doi.org/10.1016/0360-3016(93)90175-u.

14. Czerwinski MD, Jansen PP, Zwijnenburg EM, Al-Mamgani A, Vergeer MR, Langendijk JA, et al. Radiotherapy as nose preservation treatment strategy for cancer of the nasal vestibule: the Dutch experience. Radiother Oncol. 2021;164:20–6. https://doi.org/10.1016/j.radonc.2021.08.018.

15. Pantelakos ST, McGuirt WF, Nussear DW. Squamous cell carcinoma of the nasal vestibule and anterior nasal passages. Am J Otolaryngol. 1994;15(1):33–6. https://doi.org/10.1016/0196-0709(94)90037-x.

16. Wong CS, Cummings BJ. The place of radiation therapy in the treatment of squamous cell carcinoma of the nasal vestibule. A review. Acta Oncol. 1988;27(3):203–8. https://doi.org/10.3109/02841868809093526.

17. Agger A, von Buchwald C, Madsen AR, Yde J, Lesnikova I, Christensen CB, et al. Squamous cell carcinoma of the nasal vestibule 1993-2002: a nationwide retrospective study from DAHANCA. Head Neck. 2009;31(12):1593–9. https://doi.org/10.1002/hed.21132.

18. Wang CC. Treatment of carcinoma of the nasal vestibule by irradiation. Cancer. 1976;38(1):100–6. https://doi.org/10.1002/1097-0142(197607)38:1<100::aid-cncr2820380118>3.0.co;2-9.

19. Wallace A, Morris CG, Kirwan J, Amdur RJ, Werning JW, Mendenhall WM. Radiotherapy for squamous cell carcinoma of the nasal vestibule. Am J Clin Oncol. 2007;30(6):612–6. https://doi.org/10.1097/COC.0b013e31815aff1f.

20. Vanneste BGL, Lopez-Yurda M, Tan IB, Balm AJM, Borst GR, Rasch CR. Irradiation of localized squamous cell carcinoma of the nasal vestibule. Head Neck. 2016;38(Suppl 1):E1870–5. https://doi.org/10.1002/hed.24337.

21. Mendenhall NP, Parsons JT, Cassisi NJ, Million RR. Carcinoma of the nasal vestibule treated with radiation therapy. Laryngoscope. 1987;97(5):626–32. https://doi.org/10.1288/00005537-198705000-00018.

22. Mendenhall WM, Stringer SP, Cassisi NJ, Mendenhall NP. Squamous cell carcinoma of the nasal vestibule. Head Neck. 1999;21(5):385–93. https://doi.org/10.1002/(sici)1097-0347(199908)21:5<385::aid-hed2>3.0.co;2-r.

23. Wu Q, Manning M, Schmidt-Ullrich R, Mohan R. The potential for sparing of parotids and escalation of biologically effective dose with intensity-modulated radiation treatments of head and neck cancers: a treatment design study. Int J Radiat Oncol Biol Phys. 2000;46(1):195–205. https://doi.org/10.1016/s0360-3016(99)00304-1.

24. Kian Ang K, Garden AS. Radiotherapy for head and neck cancers: indications and techniques. Philadelphia, PA: Wolters Kluwer Health/Lippincott Williams & Wilkins; 2012. 292 p. https://play.google.com/store/books/details?id=qEJGYgEACAAJ.

25. Kaanders JH, Fleming TJ, Ang KK, Maor MH, Peters LJ. Devices valuable in head and neck radiotherapy. Int J Radiat Oncol Biol Phys. 1992;23(3):639–45. https://doi.org/10.1016/0360-3016(92)90023-b.

26. Mukai Y, Janssen S, Glanzmann C, Holzmann D, Studer G. Local control and intermediate-term cosmetic outcome following IMRT for nasal tumors: an update. Strahlenther Onkol. 2017;193(4):295–304. https://doi.org/10.1007/s00066-016-1083-8.

27. Janssen S. IMRT for nasal tumors – local control and cosmetic outcome. J Nucl Med Rad Ther. 2014;5:1. https://doi.org/10.4172/2155-9619.1000170.

28. Canters RA, Lips IM, Wendling M, Kusters M, van Zeeland M, Gerritsen RM, et al. Clinical implementation of 3D printing in the construction of patient specific bolus for electron beam radiotherapy for non-melanoma skin cancer. Radiother Oncol. 2016;121(1):148–53. https://doi.org/10.1016/j.radonc.2016.07.011.

29. Dipasquale G, Poirier A, Sprunger Y, Uiterwijk JWE, Miralbell R. Improving 3D-printing of megavoltage X-rays radiotherapy bolus with surface-scanner. Radiat Oncol. 2018;13(1):203. https://doi.org/10.1186/s13014-018-1148-1.

30. Biau J, Dunet V, Lapeyre M, Simon C, Ozsahin M, Grégoire V, et al. Practical clinical guidelines for contouring the trigeminal nerve (V) and its branches in head and neck cancers. Radiother Oncol. 2019;131:192–201. https://doi.org/10.1016/j.radonc.2018.08.020.

31. Mendenhall NP, Parsons JT, Cassisi NJ, Million RR. Carcinoma of the nasal vestibule. Int J Radiat Oncol Biol Phys. 1984;10(5):627–37. https://doi.org/10.1016/0360-3016(84)90293-1.

32. Haynes WD, Tapley N. Proceedings: radiation treatment of carcinoma of the nasal vestibule. Am J Roentgenol Radium Therapy, Nucl Med. 1974;120(3):595–602. https://doi.org/10.2214/ajr.120.3.595.

33. Poulsen M, Turner S. Radiation therapy for squamous cell carcinoma of the nasal vestibule. Int J Radiat Oncol Biol Phys. 1993;27(2):267–72. https://doi.org/10.1016/0360-3016(93)90237-p.

34. Chobe R, McNeese M, Weber R, Fletcher GH. Radiation therapy for carcinoma of the nasal vestibule. Otolaryngol Head Neck Surg. 1988;98(1):67–71. https://doi.org/10.1177/019459988809800112.

35. Turner SL, Lochrin CA, Dische S, Saunders MI, Maher EJ. Continuous hyperfractionated accelerated radiotherapy in the treatment of carcinoma of the columella and vestibule of the nose. Eur J Cancer B Oral Oncol. 1995;31B(6):368–72. https://doi.org/10.1016/0964-1955(95)00029-1.
36. Bussu F, Tagliaferri L, De Corso E, Passali GC, Lancellotta V, Mattiucci GC, Gambacorta MA, Rizzo D, Di Cintio G, Salvati A, Paludetti G, Valentini V, Galli J. Functional results of exclusive interventional radiotherapy (brachytherapy) in the treatment of nasal vestibule carcinomas Brachytherapy 2021;20(1):178–84. https://doi.org/10.1016/j.brachy.2020.08.008.

Interventional Radiotherapy (Brachytherapy) for the Treatment of Primary Lesions in Nasal Vestibule Malignancies

Tagliaferri Luca, Lancellotta Valentina, Bruno Fionda, De Luca Laura Maria, Parrilla Claudio, Jose Luis Guinot, Rafael Martinez-Monge, Rembielak Agata, Di Stefani Alessandro, Vincenzo Valentini, György Kovács, and Francesco Bussu

T. Luca · L. Valentina · B. Fionda · V. Valentini
UOC Radioterapia Oncologica, Dipartimento di Diagnostica per Immagini, Radioterapia Oncologica ed Ematologia, Fondazione Policlinico Universitario A. Gemelli, IRCCS, Rome, Italy
e-mail: luca.tagliaferri@policlinicogemelli.it; valentina.lancellotta@policlinicogemelli.it; vincenzo.valentini@unicatt.it

D. L. L. Maria (✉)
Otolaryngology Division, Azienda Ospedaliero Universitaria di Sassari, Sassari, Italy

P. Claudio
Institute of Otorhinolaryngology, "A. Gemelli" Polyclinic, Catholic University "Sacro Cuore", Rome, Italy
e-mail: claudio.parrilla@unicatt.it

J. L. Guinot
Department of Radiation Oncology, Fundacion Instituto Valenciano de Oncologia (I.V.O.), Valencia, Spain
e-mail: jguinot@fivo.org

R. Martinez-Monge
Department of Oncology, Clínica Universidad de Navarra, Pamplona, Spain
e-mail: rmartinezm@unav.es

R. Agata
Department of Clinical Oncology, The Christie NHS Foundation Trust, Manchester, UK

Division of Cancer Sciences, Faculty of Biology, Medicine and Health, University of Manchester, Manchester, UK
e-mail: agata.rembielak@christie.nhs.uk

© Springer Nature Switzerland AG 2023
F. Bussu (ed.), *Malignancies of the Nasal Vestibule*,
https://doi.org/10.1007/978-3-031-32850-3_11

D. S. Alessandro
Institute of Dermatology, Università Cattolica, Rome, Italy
e-mail: alessandro.distefani@policlinicogemelli.it

G. Kovács
Interdisciplinary Brachytherapy Unit, University of Lübeck/UKSH-CL, Lübeck, Germany
e-mail: gyorgy.kovacs@unicatt.it

F. Bussu
Department of Medicine, Surgery and Pharmacy, University of Sassari, Sassari, Italy

Otolaryngology Division, Azienda Ospedaliero Universitaria di Sassari, Sassari, Italy

11.1 Background

The aim of radiotherapy as a noninvasive treatment is to achieve the best oncologic outcome with low morbidity rates, excellent cosmesis, and maintained function. Due to the relatively low number of patients affected by primary nasal vestibule malignancies, there are no randomized controlled trials or prospective studies to define the best treatment for these patients. Treatment options vary across centers according to local expertise. Consequently, the management of patients with nasal vestibule malignancies should be guided by a multidisciplinary team in order to achieve best possible outcomes, both in terms of survival and cosmesis and to preserve organ (nose) function [1–3].

Radiotherapy, either in a definitive or postoperative setting, is an effective treatment for such patients [4]. It can be delivered as external beam radiation therapy (EBRT), high-dose-rate interventional radiotherapy (HDR-IRT), or as a combination of both.

Growing evidence supports HDR-IRT as the potential treatment of choice in patients with vestibular nose cancer [4–6]. It is usually delivered in a hypofractionated or hypofractionated-accelerated schedule—delivery of fewer, larger (>2 Gy) doses of radiotherapy—and associated with a high radiation dose conformity to the target volume, to a rapid dose fall-off in adjacent organs at risk, to a short treatment time, and to an excellent cosmetic and functional outcome.

11.2 History of Interventional Radiotherapy

In nasal vestibule tumors, interventional radiotherapy (IRT) can be performed with low dose rate (LDR—the patient is treated with a low dose of radiation for hours at a time) or high dose rate (HDR—a high dose of radiation is delivered to the tumor in a short burst in a few minutes. This treatment can be repeated several times in a day or last over one or more weeks) modality.

In the years that followed radium discovery, IRT was one of the most widely used noninvasive cancer therapies. The most common LDR-IRT radium applications were intracavitary implants for gynecological cancer, while interstitial implants were used for breast, head and neck, and skin malignancies. In LDR-IRT, radium constituted the gold standard. As new artificial radioactive sources have become available, the use of radium has steadily declined over the years and now completely ceased. Radium application was often done manually increasing risk of staff exposure to radiation. Such a technique has been replaced by manual and later remote afterloading, reducing any unnecessary radiation exposure. These systems administer a radioisotope directly to the tissue, thereby minimizing the radiation dose to surrounding tissue and eliminating the radiation exposure to hospital staff.

With the advent of remote afterloading machines, HDR has become more commonly used in clinical practice due to easier and safer application methodology. The first equipment for remote afterloading, a Cathetron Co 60 (TEM Instrument Ltd.), was installed in 1977. The Cathetron was replaced by a Selectron HDR Co 60 (Nucletron B.V.) in 1987, and in 1990, the equipment was supplemented by a MicroSelectron HDR Ir 192 (Nucletron B.V.). Radium has not been used for head and neck cancer since 1977. Instead, HDR-IRT is the most commonly used IRT method around the globe.

When planning systems were first introduced in IRT, orthogonal IRT was used for reconstruction of two-dimensional radiography information and for radiation dose calculation. Such reconstruction was suboptimal for adequate source configuration in relation to soft tissue anatomy. Therefore, even with best possible placement of catheters, the accuracy of dose calculations was suboptimal. As a result of such inaccuracy, isolated hot (hot spots are volume of tissue that would receive doses greater than the prescribed one as per the applicable constraints) or cold spots (cold spots are those locations that receive a dose less than the prescribed one) could not be monitored. Therefore, higher doses could have been delivered to the organ at risk such as nasal cartilage resulting in chronic painful chondritis and consequently in overall high toxicity of such treatment [7].

To improve dose personalization, image guidance for IRT was introduced, becoming soon a standard. The current state of the art in nasal vestibule IRT is described below.

11.3 IRT Techniques

HDR-IRT using the iridium-192 source delivered by a remote afterloading machine has become the most frequently used technique. For small and/or superficial lesions affecting nasal vestibule, the use of an intracavitary/contact mold may be adequate, while for more common larger and thicker lesions, interstitial implant should be used.

We recommend that all patients be evaluated for target definition with morphological imaging (magnetic resonance (MRI) or computed tomography), and in selected cases, to better define the tumor spread and, most of all, the nodal involvement, computed tomography–positron emission tomography (CT-PET). The discussion and treatment decision should always follow discussion at the relevant multidisciplinary team meeting.

11.3.1 Mold Technique/Superficial Application

Using an alginate paste, an impression of nasal vestibule along with the tumor, the nasal tip, and the upper lip is obtained. The impression should be large enough to improve placement of the mold and facilitate its fixation. The alginate model is duplicated in methyl methacrylate, in which different virtually planned plastic afterloading catheters are to be placed at a distance of 5–10 mm from each other. In each catheter, an active length is chosen in order to deliver an adequate dose to the target volume, including a 0.5–1 cm margin around the lesion to be treated. The treatment planning is performed in order to encompass the whole tumor with the prescription isodose. Subsequently, the mold is inserted in the patient's nasal cavity and fixed with adhesive tape for the duration of the radiation. It is removed after each fraction. Alternatively, a bi-component silicon compound can be used for modeling the individual nasal vestibule, which can be inserted as per computer-planned dose distribution (Fig. 11.1).

11.3.1.1 Contact Mold Preparation

A personalized double-layer mold of thermoplastic mask material is applied to the anatomical site of the skin tumor. If a skin tumor is invading through the ala nasi into the cavity, it could be treated with a contact mold from the outside. A bolus material of at least 3 mm thickness is used to separate skin from the plastic tubes, which were fixed in appropriate geometry over the target area with an interspacing distance of about 1 cm [8]. The clinical target volume (CTV) is marked on the mold surface by radiopaque material for lesion visualization for computerized tomography (CT) planning (Fig. 11.2).

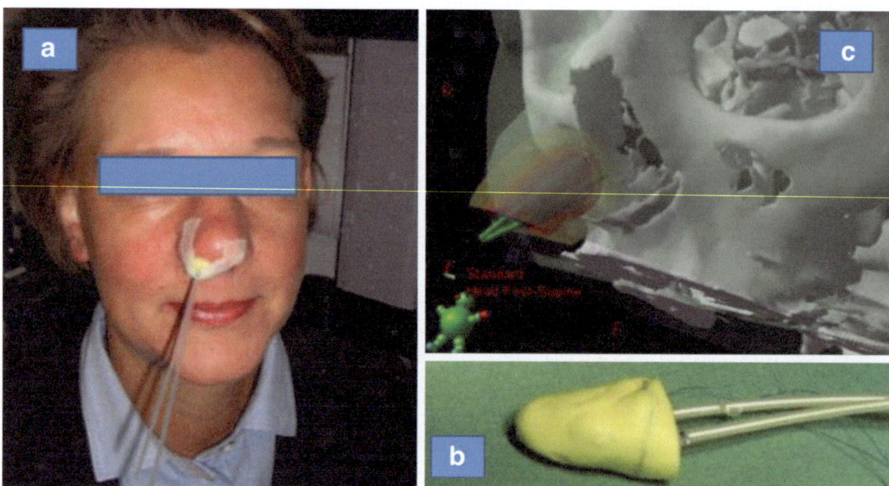

Fig. 11.1 A nose vestibule cT1 (according to Wang staging) squamous cell carcinoma (SCC) (**a, b**) bi-component silicon compound used for modelling the individual nasal vestibule, which can be implanted according to the virtual dose distribution plan treated by IRT (implants shown in **c**)

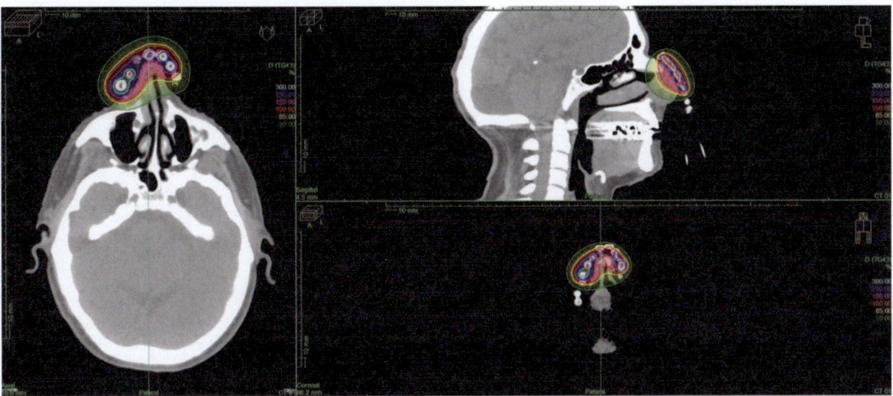

Fig. 11.2 Axial (**a**), sagittal (**b**), and coronal (**c**) view of computer-planned dose distribution with contact mold

11.3.2 Interstitial Implantation Technique

Interstitial HDR-IRT is a highly personalized treatment based on volume implants with multiple planes of needles to obtain a complete coverage of the target volume. To determine CTV, tumor projection is delineated on the skin, including a 0.5–1.0 cm margin in all directions with adequate correction for bone and air. Afterward, in accordance with the Paris system, flexible implant tubes are inserted, with an interspacing of 0.8–1.2 cm apart, following guide channels earlier guided by a metal needle. Final implant catheters are fixed by buttons sutured between them. The exact configuration and number of catheters are individually tailored to the extent, depth, and shape of the target lesion. The radiation dose is prescribed encompassing the full CTV and sparing as much as possible the surrounding healthy structures (Fig. 11.3).

For both HDR-IRT techniques (mold and interstitial), image-guided three-dimensional implant reconstructions are required. Dosimetry is done according to the TG-43 protocol [9]. Manual dwell-time adjustments are performed to personalize dose homogeneity and to avoid skin hotspots. From our experience, we have been applying the following dose constraints (restriction on the prospective doses to individuals, which may result from a defined source, for use at the planning stage in radiation protection whenever optimization is involved) in organs at risk: 54 Gy for both optic nerves and chiasma, 50 Gy for retina, and 12 Gy for lens. There are different recommended fractionations depending on the tumor size, delivered daily or twice a day for a total dose of 55–75 Gy (biologically equivalent total dose at 2 Gy/fraction (EQD2)) [10].

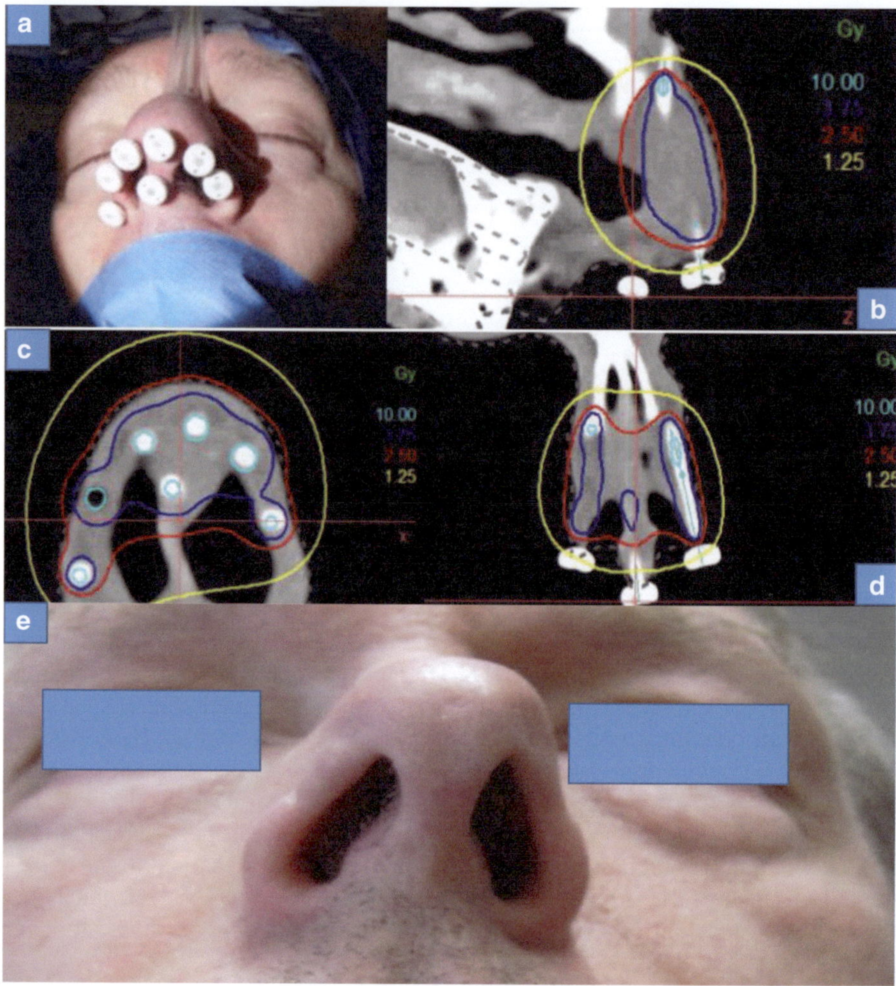

Fig. 11.3 Interstitial implant—at the time of neck surgery, plastic tubes were placed parallel along the main axis of the nose, with a complete cover of the tumor volume by the dose. Position of catheters at the time of surgical implantation (**a**), corresponding treatment plan views (sagittal (**b**), axial (**c**), coronal (**d**), and clinical result (**e**))

In our opinion and experience, interstitial implantation is more reliable and fit for a wide range of primary lesions arising in the vestibule, in particular when tumor depth is of concern. In mold technique, the limiting factor is often the maximum dose that can be deposited on the skin/nasal mucosa, similarly to maximum skin dose in IBT for skin cancer [8]. Extensive and high-volume primary lesions will undoubtedly require a high number of tubes, often in multiplanar configuration to cover the target volume. General anesthesia should be performed for interstitial implant application, which is usually done by an interventional radiation oncologist and ENT surgeon.

11.4   Outcomes of IRT

Despite lack of randomized studies, published evidence seems to confirm a better local control in primary vestibule lesions treated by HDR-IRT than in those treated by external beam radiotherapy (EBRT) [4] and similar local control (LC) and overall survival (OS) as in patients treated with surgery [1, 11–13].

LC in IRT ranges from 85% to 100% [10, 12, 14–17]. Many factors may contribute to such excellent outcomes. Firstly, image guidance, which has become a standard for modern IRT, allows for more precise delineation and better dose planning calculation (manual dwell-time adjustments), improving dose delivery to the tumor. Secondly, recent data demonstrate that excellent LC may be achieved with a radiation dose of 67.8 Gy EQD2. Wray et al. reported a 5-year LC of 100% with doses of 65–80 Gy [16]. Dose escalation over 67.8 Gy EQD2 seems unnecessary and may lead to increased treatment-related toxicity. On the other hand, studies employing doses of 60 Gy EQD2 achieved lower 5-year LC rates of 83%–92% [11, 12]. Yet, limited dose de-escalation could be considered in small, low-risk tumors and after surgical excision (adjuvant treatment). Probably nasal tumors treated with IRT alone respond better compared to postoperative IRT following incompletely excised tumors [18], and generally in oncology, a single modality treatment is preferable to multimodality treatment, as long as oncological outcomes are not different. Also, the high LC achieved by HDR-IRT can be due to higher localized doses and shorter overall treatment duration compared to EBRT [19, 20]. As for OS, the studies report a range between 65% and 85% [7, 10, 12–14, 18–23] for nose vestibule SCC cases whose primary lesions were treated by IRT. Acute side effects during HDR-IRT are moderate desquamation of the skin of the nose and nasal mucosa. Most frequent late effects are dryness and crusting of the nasal cavity, which are anyway significantly milder than in EBRT cases [22]. The risk of serious complications after HDR-IRT, such as cosmetic deformity or pain due to tissue necrosis, is less than 5% [11–13, 16]. Relatively low toxicity correlates with good/excellent patient satisfaction, nasal function, and aesthetic outcomes as reported in many investigations [11, 12, 16, 24] (see Chap. 13).

Despite the outstanding results of IRT reported in literature, only a few centers use IRT to routinely treat primaries located in the nose vestibule. Lack of experience, specific expertise required, and treatment complexity are among factors hampering the use of IRT in the clinical routine. The most decisive issue is the need for an efficient and expert multidisciplinary cooperation. An experienced IRT multidisciplinary team plays a fundamental role in management of patients with nasal vestibule requiring IRT. Such a team needs to include a radiation oncologist with experience in IRT, as well as medical physicists and radiographers/dosimetrists, radiology and pathology experts [25, 26] who should closely cooperate with ENT surgeons. Each staff member must be accredited according to individual country's regulations, and radiation oncologist/clinical oncologist must have adequate training in IRT [27–29].

In view of limited literature data, larger studies with meta-analysis and ideally randomized studies are required to confirm the best management strategy in nasal vestibule neoplasms. Since randomized trials are lacking [30] and their implementation is complicated by low number of cases, the creation of a large international database could be helpful in validating IRT as the standard for the treatment of nose vestibule primaries [31, 32]. In such a setting, the definition of reliable prognostic models and/or of nomograms may further improve management and treatment personalization [33]. Anyway, basing on the current data, nose vestibule malignancies appear the most relevant field of application for IRT in the head and neck, and most evidences support HDR IRT as the standard of care for primary lesions not involving the bone (T1 and T2 according to Wang's classification) [34–36].

References

1. Waldman A, Schmults C. Cutaneous squamous cell carcinoma. Hematol Oncol Clin North Am. 2019;33:1–12.
2. Siegel RL, Miller KD, Jemal A. Cancer statistics, 2018. CA Cancer J Clin. 2018;68:7–30.
3. Fleming ID, Cooper JS, Henson DE, Hutter RVP, Kennedy BJ, Murphy GP, et al. American Joint Committee: Cancer manual for staging of cancer. Chicago, IL: AJCC; 1997.
4. Czerwinski MD, Jansen PP, Zwijnenburg EM, Al-Mamgani A, Vergeer MR, Langendijk JA, Wesseling FWR, Kaanders JHAM, Verhoef CG. Radiotherapy as nose preservation treatment strategy for cancer of the nasal vestibule: the Dutch experience. Radiother Oncol. 2021;164:20–6.
5. Bussu F, Tagliaferri L, Piras A, Rizzo D, Tsatsaris N, De Corso E, Parrilla C, Paludetti G. Multidisciplinary approach to nose vestibule malignancies: setting new standards. Acta Otorhinolaryngol Ital. 2021;41:S158–65.
6. New standards for the management of nose vestibule malignancies. Acta Oto-Laryngologica. 2023;143(3):215–22. https://doi.org/10.1080/00016489.2023.2179662.
7. Lipman D, Verhoef LC, Takes RP, Kaanders JH, Janssens GO. Outcome and toxicity profile after brachytherapy for squamous cell carcinoma of the nasal vestibule. Head Neck. 2015;37:1297–303.
8. Ciérvide R, Ramos L, Aristu JJ, Montesdeoca N, Martínez-Monge R. Use of customized-mold brachytherapy in the management of malignancies arising in the maxillary antrum after maxillectomy: a dosimetric analysis. Brachytherapy. 2011;10:159–62.
9. Rivard MJ, Coursey BM, DeWerd LA, Hanson WF, Huq MS, Ibbott GS, Mitch MG, Nath R, Williamson JF. Update of AAPM Task Group No. 43 report: a revised AAPM protocol for brachytherapy dose calculations. Med Phys. 2004;31:633–74.
10. Mazeron J-J, Ardiet J-M, Haie-Méder C, Kovács G, Levendag P, Peiffert D, Polo A, Rovirosa A, Strnad V. GEC-ESTRO recommendations for brachytherapy for head and neck squamous cell carcinomas. Radiother Oncol. 2009;91:150–6.
11. Czerwinski MD, van Leeuwen RGH, Kaanders JHAM, Zwijnenburg EM, Lipman D, Takes RP, Verhoef CG. Image guided brachytherapy for cancer of the nasal vestibule: local control and cosmesis. Int J Radiat Oncol Biol Phys. 2019;103:913–21.
12. Bussu F, Tagliaferri L, Mattiucci G, et al. Comparison of interstitial brachytherapy and surgery as primary treatments for nasal vestibule carcinomas. Laryngoscope. 2016;126:367–71.
13. Levendag PC, Nijdam WM, van Moolenburgh SE, Tan L, Noever I, van Rooy P, Mureau MAM, Jansen PP, Munte K, Hofer SOP. Interstitial radiation therapy for early-stage nasal vestibule cancer: a continuing quest for optimal tumor control and cosmesis. Int J Radiat Oncol Biol Phys. 2006;66:160–9.

14. Vanneste BGL, Lopez-Yurda M, Tan IB, Balm AJM, Borst GR, Rasch CR. Irradiation of localized squamous cell carcinoma of the nasal vestibule. Head Neck. 2016;38(Suppl 1):E1870–5.
15. Bacorro W, Escande A, Temam S, et al. Clinical outcomes after interstitial brachytherapy for early-stage nasal squamous cell carcinoma. Brachytherapy. 2017;16:1021–7.
16. Wray J, Morris CG, Kirwan JM, Amdur RJ, Werning JW, Dziegielewski PT, Mendenhall WM. Radiation therapy for nasal vestibule squamous cell carcinoma: a 40-year experience. Eur Arch Otorhinolaryngol. 2016;273:661–9.
17. Bussu F, Tagliaferri L, De Corso E, et al. Functional results of exclusive interventional radiotherapy (brachytherapy) in the treatment of nasal vestibule carcinomas. Brachytherapy. 2021;20:178–84.
18. Rio E, Bardet E, Ferron C, Peuvrel P, Supiot S, Campion L, De Montreuil CB, Mahe MA, Dreno B. Interstitial brachytherapy of periorificial skin carcinomas of the face: a retrospective study of 97 cases. Int J Radiat Oncol Biol Phys. 2005;63:753–7.
19. The European society for Therapeutic Radiology and Oncology ESTRO. The GEC ESTRO handbook of brachytherapy. Washington, DC: ACCO; 2002.
20. Rutkowski T. The role of tumor volume in radiotherapy of patients with head and neck cancer. Radiat Oncol. 2014;9:23.
21. Talmi YP, Ferlito A, Takes RP, Strojan P, Langendijk JA, Shaha AR, Rinaldo A. Lymph node metastasis in nasal vestibule cancer: a review. Head Neck. 2011;33:1783–8.
22. Baris G, Visser AG, van Andel JG. The treatment of squamous cell carcinoma of the nasal vestibule with interstitial iridium implantation. Radiother Oncol. 1985;4:121–5.
23. Ang KK, Jiang GL, Frankenthaler RA, Kaanders JH, Garden AS, Delclos L, Peters LJ. Carcinomas of the nasal cavity. Radiother Oncol. 1992;24:163–8.
24. Mukai Y, Janssen S, Glanzmann C, Holzmann D, Studer G. Local control and intermediate-term cosmetic outcome following IMRT for nasal tumors: an update. Strahlenther Onkol. 2017;193:295–304.
25. Lettmaier S, Strnad V. Intraluminal brachytherapy in oesophageal cancer: defining its role and introducing the technique. J Contemp Brachyther. 2014;6:236–41.
26. Rodrigo JP, Shah JP, Silver CE, Medina JE, Takes RP, Robbins KT, Rinaldo A, Werner JA, Ferlito A. Management of the clinically negative neck in early-stage head and neck cancers after transoral resection. Head Neck. 2011;33:1210–9.
27. Nag S, Dally M, de la Torre M, Tatsuzaki H, Kizilbash N, Kurusun S, Pinillos L, Pokrajac B, Sur R, Levin V. Recommendations for implementation of high dose rate 192Ir brachytherapy in developing countries by the Advisory Group of International Atomic Energy Agency. Radiother Oncol. 2002;64:297–308.
28. Kovács G, Tagliaferri L, Valentini V. Is an Interventional Oncology Center an advantage in the service of cancer patients or in the education? The Gemelli Hospital and INTERACTS experience. J Contemp Brachyther. 2017;9:497–8.
29. Tagliaferri L, Kovács G, Aristei C, et al. Current state of interventional radiotherapy (brachytherapy) education in Italy: results of the INTERACTS survey. J Contemp Brachyther. 2019;11:48–53.
30. Tagliaferri L, Fionda B, Bussu F, et al. Interventional radiotherapy (brachytherapy) for squamous cell carcinoma of the nasal vestibule: a multidisciplinary systematic review. Eur J Dermatol. 2019;29:417–21.
31. Tagliaferri L, Budrukkar A, Lenkowicz J, et al. ENT COBRA ONTOLOGY: the covariates classification system proposed by the Head & Neck and Skin GEC-ESTRO Working Group for interdisciplinary standardized data collection in head and neck patient cohorts treated with interventional radiotherapy (brachytherapy). J Contemp Brachyther. 2018;10:260–6.
32. Tagliaferri L, Carra N, Lancellotta V, et al. Interventional radiotherapy as exclusive treatment for primary nasal vestibule cancer: single-institution experience. J Contemp Brachyther. 2020;12:413–9.

33. Lancellotta V, Guinot JL, Fionda B, et al. SKIN-COBRA (Consortium for Brachytherapy data Analysis) ontology: the first step towards interdisciplinary standardized data collection for personalized oncology in skin cancer. J Contemp Brachyther. 2020;12:105–10.
34. Bussu F, Tagliaferri L, Mattiucci G, et al. HDR interventional radiotherapy (brachytherapy) in the treatment of primary and recurrent head and neck malignancies. Head Neck. 2019;41(6):1667–75.
35. Bussu F, Tagliaferri L, Piras A, Rizzo D, Tsatsaris N, De Corso E, Parrilla C, Paludetti G. Multidisciplinary approach to nose vestibule malignancies: setting new standards Approccio multidisciplinare ai tumori maligni del vestibolo del naso: verso la definizione di nuovi standard Acta Otorhinolaryngologica Italica 2021;41(Suppl. 1):S158–S165. https://doi.org/10.14639/0392-100X-suppl.1-41-2021-16.
36. Bussu F, Tagliaferri L, Crescio C, Rizzo D, Gallus R, Parrilla C, Fionda B, Lancellotta V, Mattiucci GC, Galli J. New standards for the management of nose vestibule malignancies Acta Oto-Laryngologica 2023;143(3):215–22. https://doi.org/10.1080/00016489.2023.2179662.

Brachytherapy for Nose Vestibule Malignancies: Functional Results

12

Jacopo Galli, Francesco Bussu, Giulio Cesare Passali, Eugenio De Corso, Davide Rizzo, Caterina Kihlgren, Luca Tagliaferri, V. Valentini, and G. Paludetti

J. Galli
Department of Head-Neck and Sensory Organs, Università Cattolica del Sacro Cuore, Rome, Italy

Unit of Otorhinolaryngology, "A. Gemelli" University Hospital Foundation, IRCCS, Rome, Italy
e-mail: Jacopo.Galli@unicatt.it

F. Bussu · D. Rizzo (✉)
Otolaryngology Division, Sassari University Hospital, Sassari, Italy

Department of Medicine, Surgery and Pharmacy, University of Sassari, Sassari, Italy
e-mail: fbussu@uniss.it; davide.rizzo@aouss.it; drizzo@uniss.it

G. C. Passali
Division of Otorhinolaryngology, Multidisciplinary Gemelli Group for HHT, Fondazione Policlinico Universitario Agostino Gemelli, Università Cattolica del Sacro Cuore School of Medicine, IRCCS, Rome, Italy

E. De Corso
Unit of Otorhinolaryngology, "A. Gemelli" University Hospital Foundation, IRCCS, Rome, Italy

C. Kihlgren
Otolaryngology Division, Sassari University Hospital, Sassari, Italy

L. Tagliaferri
UOC di Radioterapia Oncologica, Dipartimento di Diagnostica per Immagini, Radioterapia Oncologica ed Ematologia, Fondazione Policlinico Universitario A. Gemelli, IRCCS, Rome, Italy
e-mail: luca.tagliaferri@policlinicogemelli.it

V. Valentini
UOC di Radioterapia Oncologica, Dipartimento di Diagnostica per Immagini, Radioterapia Oncologica ed Ematologia, Fondazione Policlinico Universitario A. Gemelli, IRCCS, Rome, Italy

Istituto di Radiologia, Università Cattolica del Sacro Cuore, Rome, Italy

G. Paludetti
Department of Aging, Neurologic, Orthopedic and Head-Neck Sciences, Otorhinolaryngology Unit, Fondazione Policlinico Universitario A. Gemelli, IRCCS, Rome, Italy

© Springer Nature Switzerland AG 2023
F. Bussu (ed.), *Malignancies of the Nasal Vestibule*,
https://doi.org/10.1007/978-3-031-32850-3_12

12.1 Physiology of the Nose and Paranasal Sinuses

The nose as part of the rhino-pharyngeal-tubal unit performs important and essential functions for the physiology of the entire respiratory system (Fig. 12.1):

12.1.1 Ventilatory Function

The nose represents the first part of the respiratory tract, and it is thanks to the play of the nasal muscles that the air is compacted at the level of the nasal valve and passes further, recalled by the negative pressure of the lower airways, at the speed of 2–3 m/s. At the beginning the flow is laminar, but the presence of the turbinates changes it in micro-turbulences (Fig. 12.2). In particular, after the nasal valve, the flow is divided into three components: the upper one directed toward the olfactory cleft, the middle one running through the middle meatus, and the lower one, proceeding along the floor of the nasal cavities. In this way, the air–mucous contact surface is greatly amplified, and the air heating and humidification mechanisms are more efficient.

The air that is channeled into the nasal passages at each respiratory act is of the most importance not only for the gaseous exchanges at pulmonary level but also for the ventilation of the paranasal sinuses [1]; in fact, during inspiration, the pressure gradient between the two structures forces the air into the nasal cavities; on the contrary, during the expiratory act, the pressure inside the nasal fossae drops below that of the sinuses with consequent escape of air from them (Fig. 12.3). The perfect functioning of this process also depends on the size of the ostium: if, for example, the ostium of the maxillary sinus has a diameter of less than 2.4 mm, the pO_2 inside

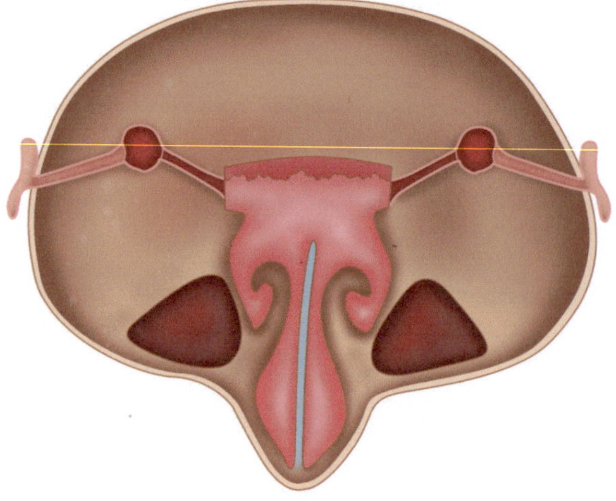

Fig. 12.1 Schematic representation of the rhino-pharyngo-tubal unit. (Courtesy of Prof. D. Passali)

Fig. 12.2 Schematic representation of the nasal air flows. (Courtesy of Prof. D. Passali)

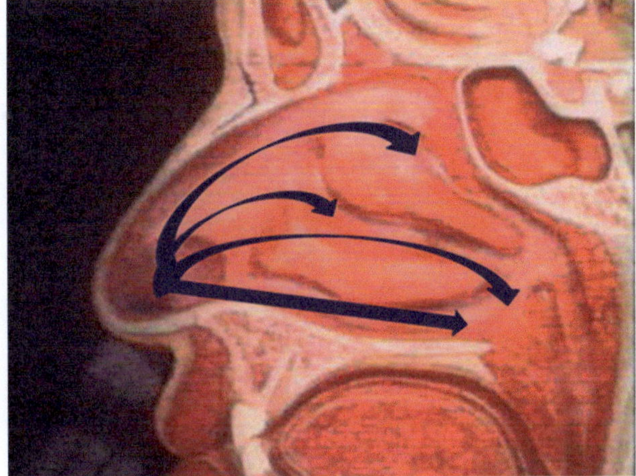

Fig. 12.3 Schematic representation of the sinus ventilation. (Courtesy of Prof. D. Passali)

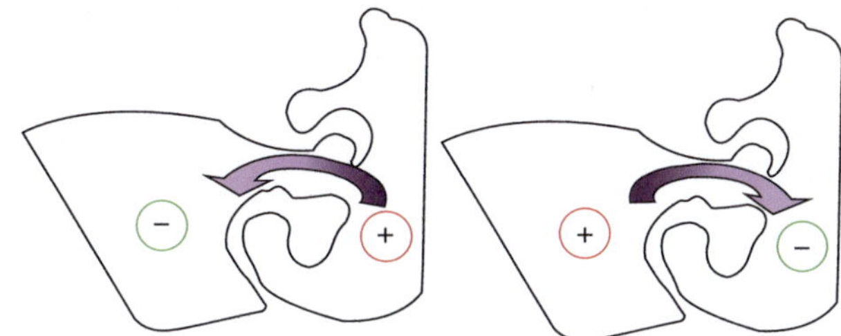

the same, falls below the critical value of 116 mmHg; the simultaneous increase in pCO_2 promotes bacterial proliferation and inflammation, which with its edematogenic component aggravates the ostial obstruction.

12.1.2 Air-Conditioning Function

Conditioning means humidification and heating, which must take place simultaneously and which are essential to avoid damages to the lower respiratory tract. These processes take place not only thanks to the airway micro-turbolences already mentioned but also by means of a complex system of neurovegetative reflexes on the rich vascularization of the nasal mucosa and the specific organization of the submucosal vessel network; these reflexes are activated by the temperature of the inspired air: if this is cold or hot, we will expect, respectively, an opening or a closing of the arterovenous shunts to allow more or less heat to flow (Fig. 12.4). Thanks to this process, the air reaches the glottis at constant temperature of 31–32 °C independently from the environmental temperature. Even the humidification of the air is regulated by a reflex, in fact, if the air is too dry, a parasympathetic reflex is activated, which stimulates the secretion of the serous glands that are located in the

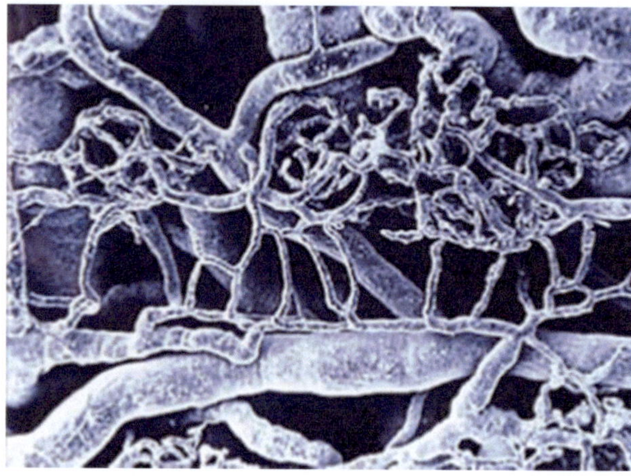

Fig. 12.4 Electronic microscopy view of the arteriovenous shunts. (Courtesy of Prof. D. Passali)

front of the nasal cavities. A saving of water, fundamental for humidification, also occurs thanks to the fact that the nasal fossae have a temperature of about 2 °C lower than that of the lower airways. This gradient allows the exhaled air to condense. Thanks to these two mechanisms, the air reaches the glottis always at a relative humidity of 95–98%.

12.1.3 Defense Function

Research studies, addressed to clarify the mechanisms at the origin of the airways inflammatory pathologies, have recently pointed the attention on the role of the respiratory epithelium as a barrier against any kind of injury.

The first, coarse, defense attempt is carried out by the vibrissae, which, however, simply retain the larger particles (>50 μm).

Subsequently, the epithelial cells attached to their neighbors by different kind of cell–cell junctions form an impermeable and effective mechanical barrier, which allows the maintenance of an ionic gradient for directional secretion of many substances [2].

The physicochemical barrier is represented by the mucociliary transport: approximately 90% of inhaled particles are entrapped and transported with mucus by the beats of cilia present on the surfaces of airway epithelial cells (Figs. 12.5, 12.6, and 12.7). The airway mucus is a viscoelastic gel with a complex composition in which almost 200 different proteins have been identified, such as antimicrobial substances (lysozyme and defensins), cytokines, and antioxidant proteins. It is secreted continuously by intraepithelial goblet cells and by mucous cells of submucosal glands toward the surface of the epithelium. The airway mucus is a viscoelastic gel with a complex composition in which almost 200 different proteins have been identified, such as antimicrobial substances (lysozyme and defensins), cytokines, and antioxidant proteins. It is secreted continuously by intraepithelial goblet cells and by

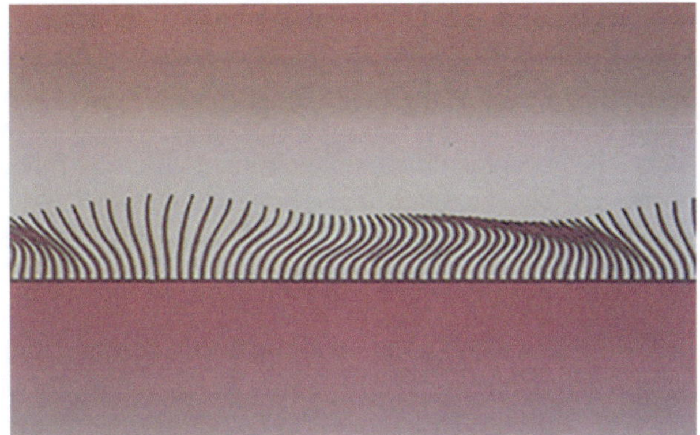

Fig. 12.5 Metacronal movement of ciliated epithelium. (Courtesy of Prof. D. Passali)

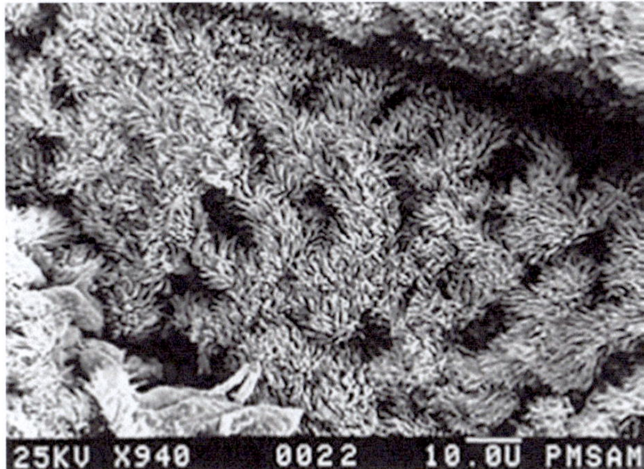

Fig. 12.6 Electronic microscopy view of the ciliated epithelium. (Courtesy of Prof. D. Passali)

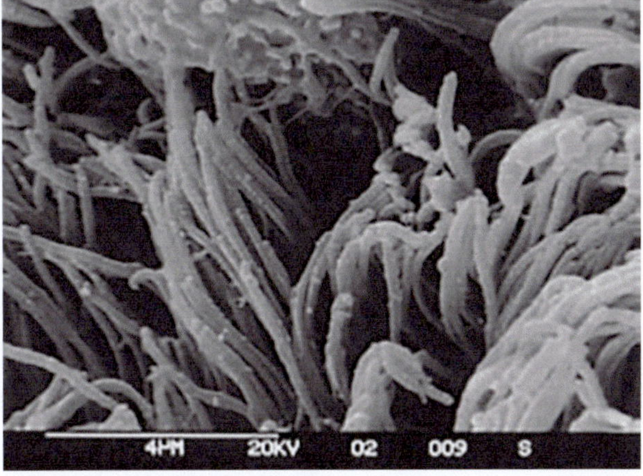

Fig. 12.7 Electronic microscopy view of the ciliated epithelium. (Courtesy of Prof. D. Passali)

mucous cells of submucosal glands toward the surface of the epithelium. Detailed study of the components of the mucociliary system has revealed a surfactant-like substance (SLS) distributed between the sol and gel layers of the mucous lining. By virtue of the bipolarity of its phospholipid molecules, the SLS promotes flow of the mucus layer on the ciliate epithelium, facilitating mucociliary transport. The composition of SLS includes lipids, proteins, and a small quantity of carbohydrates. The lipid component is by far the largest, with phospholipids constituting 65–85%. The protein components consist of at least three proteins (SP-A, SP-B, SP-C). Studies involving structural and functional characterization of these proteins have suggested that SP-A and SP-D are potent innate immune molecules that are involved in viral neutralization, clearance of bacteria, fungi, apoptotic and necrotic cells, downregulation of allergic reaction, and resolution of inflammation [3].

The acquired immune defense takes place thanks to the presence of the lymphoid tissue associated with the mucosa (NALT, Nose-Associated Lymphoid Tissue), which includes antigen-presenting cells (A.P.C.), T and B lymphocytes. All together, these cells are able to recognize and present the antigens to both lymphocytes and macrophages, for the purpose of stimulating immunoglobulin production. Actually, the specific antibody defense assumes peculiar characteristics at mucosal level. The SIgA (secretory IgA) (Fig. 12.8), the prevalent immunoglobulin in nasal secretion, is a dimer in which the two monomers are held together by labile S-S bonds and stabilized by the J (joining) polypeptide chain; in turn, the dimeric SIgA is coupled with a glycoprotein of epithelial origin, the secretory component (S.C.). At the end of this veritable "assembly chain," the SIgA is distributed in the gel stratum of the mucous secretion acting as a protective film or trap for microbes, certainly playing a very important role in different pathologies as demonstrated by their variable concentration in atopic subjects or in patients affected by chronic inflammatory processes of the nose and paranasal sinuses [4].

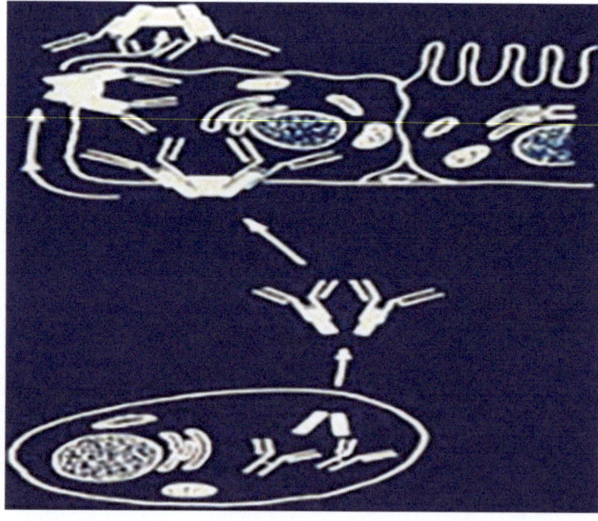

Fig. 12.8 Schematic representation of the IgAs secretion. (Courtesy of Prof. D. Passali)

Interestingly, a daily fluctuation of the SIgA concentrations in nasal secretion can be observed in normal subjects with the greatest values at 4.00 a.m. and the lowest at 10.00 a.m. Circadian changes of the MCT times are also shown. Moreover, the comparison of the data pertaining to these two parameters shows opposite patterns: when the mucociliary transport speed decreases, the secretory immunoglubulins reach the highest levels. The phase displacement of the two functions thus makes it possible to compensate cyclic impairments of one activity with contemporary improvement of the other [5, 6].

12.1.4 Olfactory Function

The olfactory mucosa occupies an area of about 5 cm^2 on the vault of the nasal fossae in correspondence with the lamina cribra descending for 2 cm on the septum and on the lateral walls; it consists of non-ciliated pseudostratified epithelium, devoid of a basal membrane and resting directly on the chorion, where the Bowman glands (tubule-acinose serous) are contained. The sensorineural cells (Schulze cells) end with the olfactory termination, which are the real cornerstone of the olfactory sensation.

The olfactory sensation is generated by the stimulation of the olfactory receptors by odorous molecules present in the inspired air. The odorous molecules must have peculiar characteristics such as: size, water, and fat solubility. More specifically, the dimensions must be between 14 and 300 Da and must be able to distribute themselves in the mucus but also to mediate the interaction with the lipoprotein phase of the neuroreceptor membranes. The mucus layer covering the olfactory mucosa consists of two phases: a thin, aqueous surface layer secreted by the Bowmann glands and a deep, mucoid, viscous layer produced by the support cells. The distal tract of the olfactory cilia is located at the interface of the two layers so that the odorous molecules must go beyond the aqueous layer to reach the receptors and generate a difference in potential across of the olfactory mucosa; for this purpose, they must be soluble in water. Therefore, it is believed that the physicochemical characteristics of the olfactory mucus, and in particular the pH, can play an important role in the olfactory function. In basal conditions, pH of the nasal secretions is more acidic than that of the blood. In bacterial infections, it is moved toward alkalinity, in allergic rhinitis, especially in the untreated perennial form, it is moved toward acid values. All this explains why this sensation does not depend only on the nasal patency, the airflow, and the concentration of odorous molecules reaching the olfactory receptors but also on the physicochemical characteristics of the nasal secretion.

The odorous molecules reach the olfactory mucosa both anteriorly during inspiration across the nasal fossae and posteriorly during exhalation and swallowing, through the choanas.

During normal inspiration, the olfactory mucosa is reached directly by a laminar air flow, which describes a semilunar trajectory into the nasal fossae.

The speed of the air flow has considerable importance on the olfactory stimulus, which depends on the number of molecules that reach the mucous membrane in the time unit.

In humans, in normal breathing, the inspired air flow is about 100 mL/s. The sniffing attitude increases the speed and diverts the direction of flow toward the vault of the nasal fossae, increasing the quantity of air at the level of the olfactory cleft and consequently the perception. Therefore, normal breathing allows to identify the smell, and the nose allows the distinction.

The sense of smell is also influenced by humidification and heating of the air. Excessive humidity obviously leads to a greater dilution of the odorous substances, while too low humidity does not allow their optimal diffusion. In addition, the heating of the inspired air increases the diffusion of odorous substances, promoting their perception and at the same time protecting the sensory epithelium from excessive thermal changes [7].

The odorous molecules, coming into contact with Schultze's sensorineural cells, determine the triggering of action potentials that are transmitted to the olfactory glomeruli, and from there, through the fibers of the olfactory nerve, they reach the olfactory cortical areas (pre-piriformes peri-amigdaloidea). The support cells of the olfactory epithelium are also in contact with myelinated fibers belonging to the trigeminal, and moreover, vagal and glossopharyngeal afferents from the olfactory cortex reach these cells. It is precisely for this reason that the trigeminal, vagus, and glossopharyngeal can be considered as accessory olfactory nerves, with the specific function of integrating the pure olfactory sensation with other afferents.

Olfactory substances are classified on the basis of excited nerve termination; so we can recognize:

1. Pure olfactory substances: rose water, lavender, anise, coffee, etc.
2. Trigeminal sense of smell: menthol, thymol, ether, ammonia, etc.
3. Olfactory-gustatory substances: vanilla
4. Olfactory-trigeminal-gustatory substances: chloroform.

12.1.5 Resonance Function

Physiologically, the nasal phonemes can be enriched with new frequencies thanks to the resonance offered by the nasal cavities [8].

12.1.6 Impact of Irradiation on Nasal Function

Basing upon this general overview about the multiple and articulated functions of nose and paranasal sinuses, it is easy to imagine as the treatment of squamous cell carcinoma (SCC) of the nasal vestibule (NV) is still a challenge not only for the oncological but also for the functional aspects.

Surgery, External Beam RadioTherapy (EBRT) and Interventional RadioTherapy (IRT, BrachyTherapy BT) are the current therapeutic options in clinical practice [9–11] (see Chap. 6). When choosing one of these treatment modalities for vestibule

SCCs, as for the other head and neck malignancies, functional issues are being currently taken into increasing consideration.

Among such functional issues, there is for sure the aesthetic appearance, which can be deeply impacted by any therapeutic procedure involving the nose and the nose vestibule in particular.

Also, disruption of any of the above-cited physiologic functions can be secondary to gross anatomic variations, as after oncological surgery, or to other pathological processes involving and impairing one or more of the above-cited mechanisms, mainly at the level of nose mucosa, as in case of irradiation.

Interstitial IRT has been demonstrated to be an oncologically effective local treatment of primary SCCs of the NV, with control rates comparable with surgery [9, 12–15]. A clearly better satisfaction in terms of esthetical appearance in patients treated for NV SCC by interstitial IRT than those treated by surgery has been demonstrated [13], which leads us to prefer the first modality to treat the primary lesion in cT1 and cT2 cases according to Wang (see Chaps. 11 and 16). Furthermore, we do believe that an "anatomic" implantation technique, which avoids piercing perichondrium and cartilage, can better preserve the nose function as well [14].

For the same reasons also external beam radiotherapy, with similar survival figures than IRT [12, 14, 15], is considered a valid alternative option also under an esthetical point of view [10, 16–19] and is probably the most frequently recommended primary treatment in Western countries at present [10, 18].

However, external beam radiotherapy harbors well-known acute and, most of all, late, toxicities. The nasal functions are notoriously affected by irradiation [20–22], and many complaints, such as crusting [21], dry nose and obstruction [23], dysosmia [22, 24], dysgeusia [22], in patients with a previous irradiation of nasal region are clearly linked to the disruption of physiological mechanisms by mucosal toxicity of radiotherapy [23, 25, 26].

On the contrary, one can postulate that the rapid dose fall off of brachytherapy, with a drastic reduction of the irradiated mucosal surface inside the nasal/paranasal cavities, may help functional preservation.

12.2 Personal Experience

To better understand the functional impact of radiation therapy delivered by either external beam or IRT on the nose of patients affected by squamous cell carcinomas of the nose vestibule, we compared for the first time nose functional parameters of primarily treated by exclusive interstitial IRT with matched healthy controls and with patients treated with External Beam Intensity-Modulated RadioTherapy (IMRT) [27].

We evaluated nose function in ten patients without evidence of disease 24 months after the completion of IRT. Median follow-up in IRT group has been 34 months (range 24–70). We compared the functional results of group 1 with eight patients irradiated by intensity-modulated external photon beams between 2007 and 2012, with a dose of at least 40 Gy in the area of nose vestibulum for nasal/ethmoid/vestibular malignancies (Group 2—EB cases) and with ten sex and age matched healthy subjects, with no history of rhinosinusitis or nasal symptoms (healthy controls).

All the patients and controls underwent nasal function tests including clinical evaluation, Mucociliary Transportation Time (MTC) [28], nasal citology, rhinomanometry, and olfactometry.

1. Clinical evaluation including NOSE SCALE questionnaire and nasal endoscopy. Patients were asked to complete a NOSE Scale questionnaire [29]. We obtained for every patient a total NOSE scale score from 0 to 20; rigid nasal endoscopy was performed in all subjects under local anesthesia with topical application of 2% xylocaine and using 0° and 30°, 4 mm diameter rigid nasal endoscope (Karl Storz, Germany). Nasal endoscopy was done by using the standard three-pass technique as described by Kennedy.

2. Mucociliary Transportation Time (MTC). We used the method devised by Passali [28], we put a mixture of an insoluble substance (vegetable carbon powder) and a soluble one (saccharin, which is however subjectively detected by the sweet taste) on the nasal mucosa at the level of the head of the inferior turbinate; we considered as tTMC the time from the moment of deposition of the tracer to that of its appearance in the pharynx.

3. Nasal citology was performed on scraped nasal tissue, obtained from the inferior turbinate bilaterally. Scraping was performed using Rhinoprobe® (Farmark s.n.c, Milan, Italy). The sample was gently spread on glass slides and immediately fixed in 95% ethyl alcohol and stained with May-Grunwald-Giemsa. The slides were examined under oil immersion by light microscopy at a magnification of ×1000. Cells were counted and categorized as neutrophils, eosinophils, mast cells, basophils, lymphocytes, epithelial cells, and goblet cells. Cells counts were expressed as percentage of the total cells, at high power field, as the mean of at least ten fields observed. The mean percentage of the cell type per 100 cells is reported. Neutrophilic flogosis was defined if neutrophils were >50% of total cells. Eosinophilic flogosis was defined if eosinophils were >20% of total cells. Nasal mucosa metaplasia was defined when we observed a rearrangement of the epithelium in favor of mucous-secreting cells (mucous-secreting metaplasia). In this case, an increase of mucous-secreting cells and a decrease of ciliated cells were observed [30, 31].

4. Active Anterior Rinomanometry (AAR) and nasal decongestion test (NDT). We performed AAR following the modalities codified by the Standardization Committee on Objective Assessment of the Nasal Airway (SCOANA) [32]. Active anterior rhinomanometry with a mask is our method of choice. The nasal mask was well adherent to the face without modifying the nasal structures. Baseline test and nasal decongestion test were performed. The baseline test allows the objective exploration of the nasal respiratory function, through the measurement of airflow and resistance to the passage of air through the nasal cavities. For the execution of the examination, the patients were asked to suspend at least 1 week before any nasal topical therapy. The nasal decongestion test was performed by nebulizing two puffs per nostril of a nasal decongestant with a short latency of action. We waited 5 min and repeated the administration of the drug. The test closes with a new rhinomanometric evaluation after another 5 min of waiting.

5. Olfactometry: All patients were studied through the Sniffin' Sticks® olfactory test (Burghart instruments, Wedel, Germany), performing the threshold, detection, and identification tests, as previously published [33]. All these tests were preceded by anterior active rhinomanometry (AAR), to measure the airflow and resistance of sinonasal cavities, and sensitized with nasal decongestion (realized by spraying two puffs per nostril of a nasal decongestant with short latency of action, naphazoline), in order to allow a correct odorants' diffusion to olfactory epithelium. Odorants were presented in felt tip pens. For odor presentation, the cap was removed for 3 s, and the pen's tip was placed at a distance of approximately 2 cm from both nostrils. Odor thresholds for n-butanol were assessed using a single staircase, three alternative forced choice (3-AFC) procedure. Sixteen dilutions were prepared in series starting from a 4% n-butanol solution (dilution ratio 1:2 in deionized water as solvent). Three pens were presented in randomized order, two containing the solvent and the third the odorant. Patients had to identify the odor containing pen. Triplets were presented at intervals of approximately 20 s. Reversal of the staircase was triggered when the odor was correctly identified in two successive trials. Threshold was defined as the mean of the last four of eight staircase reversals. The subjects' scores ranged between 0 and 16. In the odor discrimination task, again using a 3 AFC, triplets of pens were presented in randomized order, with two containing the same, and one a different odorant. Subjects had to determine which of three pens smelled different. Triplets were subsequently presented with a 20–30 s interval between them; the interval between the presentation of individual pens was approximately 3 s. Because 16 triplets were tested, the subjects' scores ranged from 0 to 16. When measuring odor thresholds and odor discrimination, subjects were blindfolded to prevent visual identification. Odor identification was assessed for 16 common odors. Using a multiple choice task, identification of individual odors was performed through lists of four descriptors each. The interval between odor presentations was 20/30 s. Again, the subjects' scores ranged from 0 to 16. Finally, we calculated the TDI score (threshold discrimination identification), with a range from 0 to 48. TDI values <15 identify an anosmic subject while values <5 must not be considered as reliable.

Five-year disease-specific survival of the patients with nose vestibule SCC primarily treated by interstitial IRT was 92.3%, the only disease-related death occurring in the cT3 case who refused to undergo demolitive surgery and died 8 months after treatment. No long-term skin or cartilaginous toxicity is recorded in EB and IRT groups. In particular, no chondritis, chondronecrosis, nor septal/alar perforations can be evidenced in the IRT group, probably thanks to the anatomic implantation technique (see Chap. 13).

Descriptive statistics of the functional parameters in the three groups is given in Table 12.1.

Symptoms evaluation by NOSE scale score revealed that the mean NOSE scale score was significantly higher in patient of group II than in group I and healthy controls ($p < 0.05$).

Table 12.1 Clinical and functional parameters in the three groups under analysis

	Group I	Group II		
	IRT cases ($n = 10$)	EB cases ($n = 8$)	Healthy controls ($n = 10$)	Whole series ($n = 28$)
Age (years)				
Median	56	66	58	60
Range	53–79	58–79	50–76	50–79
Sex-no. (%)				
Male	6 (60%)	6 (75%)	7 (70%)	19 (68%)
Female	4 (40%)	2 (25%)	3 (30%)	9 (32%)
Karnofsky p.s.-no. (%)				
100	6 (60%)	4 (50%)	7 (70%)	17 (60%)
90	3 (30%)	3 (37.5%)	3 (30%)	9 (32%)
80	0	1 (12.5%)	0	1 (4%)
70	1 (10%)	0	0	1 (4%)
Time from treatment (in months)				
Median	34	64	–	45
Range	24–70	40–83	–	24–83
T stage-no. (%)	Acc. to Wang			
T1	3 (30%)	2 (25%)	–	5 (28%)
T2	7 (70%)	3 (37.5%)	–	10 (55%)
T3	0	2 (25%)	–	2 (11%)
T4a	0	1 (12.5%)	–	1 (6%)
N stage-no. (%)				
N0	9 (90%)	3 (37.5%)	–	11 (65%)
N1	0	1 (12.5%)	–	1 (6%)
N2a	0	1 (12.5%)		1 (6%)
N2b	1 (10%)	2 (25%)	–	3 (17%)
N2c	0	1 (12.5%)	–	1 (6%)
NOSE scale score				
Mean value ± SD	9.5 ± 1.2	16 ± 1.9	8.1 ± 1.1	33.6 ± 1.7
Rhinomanometry parameters				
Total Inspiratory Flows (mL/s) (mean ± SD)	739 ± 259	959 ± 222	642 ± 312	726 ± 293
Total Inspiratory Resistances (Pa/mL/s) (mean ± SD)	0.26 ± 0.12	0.16 ± 0.03	0.29 ± 0.14	0.25 ± 0.12
Total Expiratory Resistances (Pa/mL/s) (mean ± SD)	0.25 ± 0.12	0.14 ± 0.02	0.29 ± 0.12	0.25 ± 0.12
Other functional parameters				
Olfactometry (TDI) (mean ± SD)	22 ± 6	16 ± 8.6	26 ± 5	23 ± 6.6
Mucociliary clearance (min) (mean ± SD)	13 ± 5.8	32 ± 2	17 ± 3	18.5 ± 8
Nasal Cytology report-no. (%)				
Normal	7 (70%)	2 (25%)	6 (60%)	15 (54%)

Table 12.1 (continued)

	Group I	Group II		
	IRT cases ($n = 10$)	EB cases ($n = 8$)	Healthy controls ($n = 10$)	Whole series ($n = 28$)
Neutrophilic flogosis with muciparous metaplasia	0	4 (50%)	0	4 (14%)
Neutrophilic flogosis	2 (20%)	2 (25%)	3 (30%)	7 (25%)
Eosinophilic flogosis	1 (10%)	0	1 (10%)	2 (7%)

The results of rhinomanometry showed that patients in group 2 (treated with external beams) presented higher nasal flow and lower resistance than patients of group 1 and healthy controls ($p < 0.05$). In group I, nasal flow and resistance were quite similar to healthy control ($p > 0.05$).

The mucociliary clearance was significantly reduced in group 2 compared to group 1 and healthy control. The mean time for the transportation of the stained marker was more than double in the patients treated by EB than in those treated with IRT ($p < 0.001$ at ANOVA and Student's T test).

The olphactometry TDI is lower in Group 2 than in Group 1 and healthy control, and at Student's T test, a significant difference ($p < 0.05$) was detected.

The distribution of cytologic patterns resulted significantly different at contingency analysis ($p = 0.035$ at Likelihood Ratio test), with the mucous cell metaplasia being typical of the noses previously irradiated by EB, which display most often (75%) an abnormal cytology (Table 12.1).

12.3 Conclusion: Brachytherapy (IRT) Preserves Nose Function

We confirmed with specific tests that the nose after EB irradiation has lower resistances, slower mucociliary clearance, impaired olfaction, and typical cytological alterations as mucous cell metaplasia, when compared with controls. These data are suggestive of an atrophic condition of nasal mucosa that could explain also the paradoxical subjective sensation of nasal obstruction as demonstrated by the NOSE scale score data.

On the contrary, in patients treated with IRT, nasal function and cytological findings are substantially preserved when compared to healthy non-irradiated subjects. The rapid dose fall off of the IRT, with a drastic reduction of the irradiated mucosal surface inside the nasal/paranasal cavities, may be the game changers for the functional preservation.

Such evidence, together with the confirmation of oncological effectiveness, which remains of course the most relevant argument, and of the excellent cosmetic results (Fig. 12.9) supports the establishment of interstitial IRT as the new standard for the treatment of the primary lesion in (cT1 and cT2 according to the Wang, cT1, 2, 3 according to Bussu) NV SCCs [34–36].

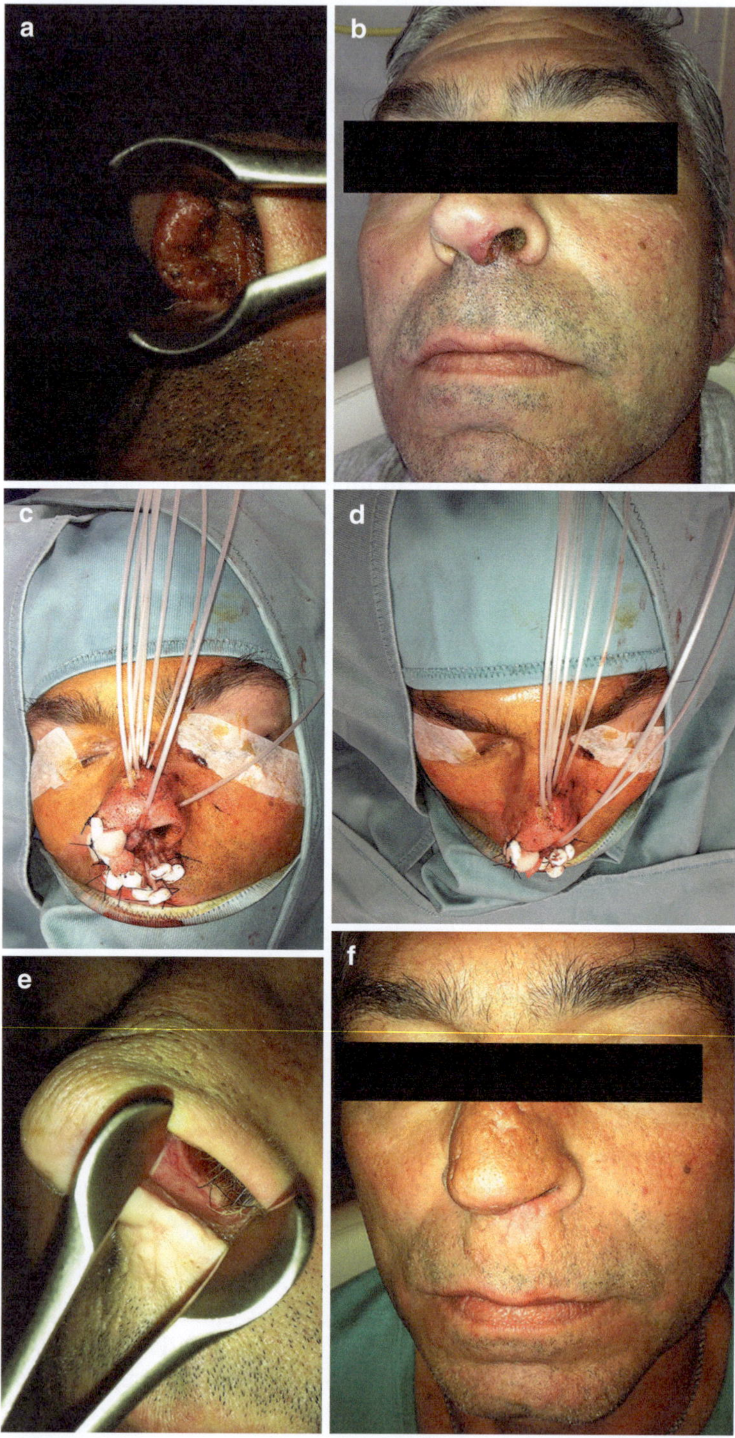

Fig. 12.9 A nose vestibule cT1 (according to Wang staging) SCC of the columella (**a**, **b**) treated by IRT (implants shown in **c**, **d**), with complete response and good cosmetic results 2 years after treatment (**e**, **f**)

References

1. Passàli D, Biagini C, Pedace E. [Presumed physiopathology of the nasal wall surgery and contemporary techniques of the inferior turbinates surgery]. Acta otorhinolaryngologica Italica: organo ufficiale della Societa italiana di otorinolaringologia e chirurgia cervico-facciale 1996;16(3):202–10.
2. Passali D, Bellussi L, Lauriello M. Diurnal activity of the nasal mucosa. Relationship between mucociliary transport and local production of secretory immunoglobulins. Acta Otolaryngol. 1990;110(5–6):437–42.
3. Passàli D, Bellussi L, Lauriello M. The rheological characteristics of nasal mucus in patients with rhinitis. Eur Arch Otorhinolaryngol. 1995;252(6):348–52.
4. Passàli D, Bellussi L. Circadian changes in the secretory activity of nasal mucosa. Acta Otolaryngol. 1988;106(3–4):281–5.
5. Passali D, Astore S, Boccuzzi S, Loglisci M, Cannatelli A, Passali GC, et al. Values of SP-a protein in the nasal mucosa. HNO. 2016;64(9):671–5.
6. Bellussi L, Cambi J, Passali D. Functional maturation of nasal mucosa: role of secretory immunoglobulin A (SIgA). Multidiscipl Respir Med. 2013;8(1):46.
7. L. Bellussi. Olfatto e Olfattometria. In: Lezioni di clinica otorinolaringoiatria 2 ed. I.G.C.; 1994.
8. Passali D. Around the nose. Firenze: Edizioni Conti tipocolor; 1988.
9. Levendag PC, Nijdam WM, van Moolenburgh SE, Tan L, Noever I, van Rooy P, et al. Interstitial radiation therapy for early-stage nasal vestibule cancer: a continuing quest for optimal tumor control and cosmesis. Int J Radiat Oncol Biol Phys. 2006;66(1):160–9.
10. Horsmans JD, Godballe C, Jørgensen KE, Bastholt L, Løntoft E. Squamous cell carcinoma of the nasal vestibule. Rhinology. 1999;37(3):117–21.
11. Guinot JL, Rembielak A, Perez-Calatayud J, Rodríguez-Villalba S, Skowronek J, Tagliaferri L, et al. GEC-ESTRO ACROP recommendations in skin brachytherapy. Radiother Oncol. 2018;126(3):377–85.
12. Vital D, Morand G, Huber GF, Studer G, Holzmann D. Outcome in squamous cell carcinoma of the nasal vestibule: a single center experience. Head Neck. 2015;37(1):46–51.
13. Bussu F, Tagliaferri L, Mattiucci G, Parrilla C, Dinapoli N, Miccichè F, et al. Comparison of interstitial brachytherapy and surgery as primary treatments for nasal vestibule carcinomas. Laryngoscope. 2016;126(2):367–71.
14. Lipman D, Verhoef LC, Takes RP, Kaanders JH, Janssens GO. Outcome and toxicity profile after brachytherapy for squamous cell carcinoma of the nasal vestibule. Head Neck. 2015;37(9):1297–303.
15. Koopmann M, Weiss D, Savvas E, Rudack C, Stenner M. Clinicopathological and immunohistochemical characteristics of surgically treated primary carcinoma of the nasal vestibule - an evaluation of 30 cases. Clin Otolaryngol. 2015;40(3):240–7.
16. Agger A, von Buchwald C, Madsen AR, Yde J, Lesnikova I, Christensen CB, et al. Squamous cell carcinoma of the nasal vestibule 1993-2002: a nationwide retrospective study from DAHANCA. Head Neck. 2009;31(12):1593–9.
17. Goepfert H. The vex and fuss about nasal vestibule cancer. Head Neck. 1999;21(5):383–4.
18. Mendenhall WM, Stringer SP, Cassisi NJ, Mendenhall NP. Squamous cell carcinoma of the nasal vestibule. Head Neck. 1999;21(5):385–93.
19. Langendijk JA, Poorter R, Leemans CR, de Bree R, Doornaert P, Slotman BJ. Radiotherapy of squamous cell carcinoma of the nasal vestibule. Int J Radiat Oncol Biol Phys. 2004;59(5):1319–25.
20. Kılıç C, Tunçel Ü, Cömert E, Kaya BV. The effect of radiotherapy on mucociliary clearance in patients with laryngeal and nasopharyngeal cancer. Eur Arch Otorhinolaryngol. 2015;272(6):1517–20.
21. Kamel R, Al-Badawy S, Khairy A, Kandil T, Sabry A. Nasal and paranasal sinus changes after radiotherapy for nasopharyngeal carcinoma. Acta Otolaryngol. 2004;124(4):532–5.

22. Álvarez-Camacho M, Gonella S, Campbell S, Scrimger RA, Wismer WV. A systematic review of smell alterations after radiotherapy for head and neck cancer. Cancer Treat Rev. 2017;54:110–21.
23. Surico G, Muggeo P, Mappa L, Muggeo V, Conti V, Lucarelli A, et al. Impairment of nasal mucociliary clearance after radiotherapy for childhood head cancer. Head Neck. 2001;23(6):461–6.
24. Hölscher T, Seibt A, Appold S, Dörr W, Herrmann T, Hüttenbrink KB, et al. Effects of radiotherapy on olfactory function. Radiother Oncol. 2005;77(2):157–63.
25. Stringer SP, Stiles W, Slattery WH III, Krumerman J, Parsons JT, Mendenhall WM, et al. Nasal mucociliary clearance after radiation therapy. Laryngoscope. 1995;105(4 Pt 1):380–2.
26. Riva G, Boita M, Ravera M, Moretto F, Badellino S, Rampino M, et al. Nasal cytological changes as late effects of radiotherapy for nasopharyngeal cancer. Am J Rhinol Allergy. 2015;29(2):e41–5.
27. Bussu F, Tagliaferri L, Mattiucci G, Parrilla C, Rizzo D, Gambacorta MA, et al. HDR interventional radiotherapy (brachytherapy) in the treatment of primary and recurrent head and neck malignancies. Head Neck. 2019;41(6):1667–75.
28. Passàli D, Bellussi L, Bianchini Ciampoli M, De Seta E. Experiences in the determination of nasal mucociliary transport time. Acta Otolaryngol. 1984;97(3–4):319–23.
29. Kahveci OK, Miman MC, Yucel A, Yucedag F, Okur E, Altuntas A. The efficiency of Nose Obstruction Symptom Evaluation (NOSE) scale on patients with nasal septal deviation. Auris Nasus Larynx. 2012;39(3):275–9.
30. de Corso E, Battista M, Pandolfini M, Liberati L, Baroni S, Romanello M, et al. Role of inflammation in non-allergic rhinitis. Rhinology. 2014;52(2):142–9.
31. De Corso E, Lucidi D, Battista M, Romanello M, De Vita C, Baroni S, et al. Prognostic value of nasal cytology and clinical factors in nasal polyps development in patients at risk: can the beginning predict the end? Int Forum Allergy Rhinol. 2017;7(9):861–7.
32. Ogura JH, Stokstead P. Rhinomanometry in some rhinologic diseases. Laryngoscope. 1958;68(12):2001–14.
33. Hummel T, Sekinger B, Wolf SR, Pauli E, Kobal G. 'Sniffin' sticks': olfactory performance assessed by the combined testing of odor identification, odor discrimination and olfactory threshold. Chem Senses. 1997;22(1):39–52.
34. Bussu F, Tagliaferri L, Piras A, Rizzo D, Tsatsaris N, De Corso E, Parrilla C, Paludetti G. Multidisciplinary approach to nose vestibule malignancies: setting new standards Approccio multidisciplinare ai tumori maligni del vestibolo del naso: verso la definizione di nuovi standard Acta Otorhinolaryngologica Italica. 2021;41(Suppl. 1):S158–65. https://doi.org/10.14639/0392-100X-suppl.1-41-2021-16.
35. Bussu F, Tagliaferri L, Crescio C, Rizzo D, Gallus R, Parrilla C, Fionda B, Lancellotta V, Mattiucci GC, Galli J.New standards for the management of nose vestibule malignancies Acta Oto-Laryngologica. 2023;143(3):215–22. https://doi.org/10.1080/00016489.2023.2179662.
36. Scheurleer WFJ, Tagliaferri L, Rijken JA, Crescio C, Rizzo D, Mattiucci GC, Pameijer FA, de Bree R, Fionda B, de Ridder M, Bussu F. Evaluation of Staging Systems for Cancer of the Nasal Vestibule Cancers. 2023;15(11):3028. https://doi.org/10.3390/cancers15113028.

A Novel Approach to Interventional Radiotherapy (Brachytherapy) in Nose Vestibule. From Paris System Rules to Anatomic Implantation

13

Francesco Bussu, Luca Tagliaferri, Laura Maria De Luca, Bruno Fionda, Nicola Tsatsaris, Claudia Crescio, Davide Rizzo, Alberto Artuso, Gyorgy Kovacs, and Jacopo Galli

F. Bussu · D. Rizzo
Otolaryngology Division, Azienda Ospedaliera Universitaria di Sassari, Sassari, Italy

Department of Medical, Surgical and Experimental Science, University of Sassari, Sassari, Italy
e-mail: davide.rizzo@aouss.it; drizzo@uniss.it

L. Tagliaferri · B. Fionda
UOC Radioterapia Oncologica, Dipartimento di Diagnostica per Immagini, Radioterapia Oncologica ed Ematologia, Fondazione Policlinico Universitario A. Gemelli, IRCCS, Rome, Italy

Institute of Otorhinolaryngology, "A. Gemelli" Polyclinic, Catholic University "Sacro Cuore", Rome, Italy
e-mail: luca.tagliaferri@policlinicogemelli.it; bruno.fionda@policlinicogemelli.it

L. M. De Luca (✉) · C. Crescio
Otolaryngology Division, Azienda Ospedaliera Universitaria di Sassari, Sassari, Italy
e-mail: claudia.crescio@aousassari.it; ccrescio1@uniss.it

N. Tsatsaris
Section of Neurosurgery, Department of Neurological and Movement Sciences, University of Verona, Verona, Italy

A. Artuso
Otolaryngology Division, Mater Olbia Hospital, Olbia, Italy

G. Kovacs
Gemelli-INTERACTS, Università Cattolica del Sacro Cuore, Rome, Italy
e-mail: gyorgy.kovacs@unicatt.it

J. Galli
Department of Head-Neck and sensory organs, Università cattolica del Sacro Cuore, Rome, Italy

Unit of Otorhinolaryngology, "A Gemelli", Unit University Hospital foundation, IRCCS, Rome, Italy
e-mail: jacopo.galli@unicatt.it

© Springer Nature Switzerland AG 2023
F. Bussu (ed.), *Malignancies of the Nasal Vestibule*,
https://doi.org/10.1007/978-3-031-32850-3_13

13.1 General Considerations

When performing an implantation for Interventional Radiotherapy (IRT) on the nose vestibule, the exact configuration and number of catheters are tailored to the extent, depth, and shape of the lesion and to the anatomy of the site. However, the implant geometry has always to support a personalized volume and an optimized dose planning and dose delivery [1]. For the IRT cases described in this chapter, interstitial 6F bottom-end Flexible Implant Tubes were mostly used.

13.2 Oncological Considerations

In Chap. 3, the most typical patterns of spread of nose vestibule epithelial malignancies have been described. They must be kept clearly in mind when a radical treatment is being planned, through whichever modality (surgery, external beam irradiation, IRT, combined treatments). More in detail, it means that in primaries arising along the lateral wall of the nose vestibule, the skin of the ala must be most often included in the resection and always included in the CTV (clinical target volume) in case of irradiation (both in case of external beams and brachytherapy) (Fig. 13.1a, b). Similarly, the cartilaginous septum and the superior lip should be included in the CTV in case of primaries of the columella/septal wall and of the inferior wall/floor of the nose, respectively [1] (Fig. 13.1c, d).

In case of primary IRT, the best way to incorporate a certain volume into the CTV is obviously the placement of plastic tubes within and around it, relying on intensity modulation possibilities offered by the stepping source technology in case of PDR/HDR (Pulsed-Dose-Rate/High-Dose-Rate) for further optimization of the dose distribution. The necessary CTV considered in the implantation pahse in case of IRT will therefore include the clinically evident disease (gross tumor volume, GTV) plus at least 1 cm margins, which should become 2 cm along the axis of the most typical tumor spread (skin of the ala for lateral wall, superior lip for inferior wall, cartilaginous septum for columella/septum). As primaries of the columella usually also have an extension toward the inferior wall of the vestibule, in these cases 2 cm of additional "coverage" should be warranted both along the cartilaginous septum and in the superior lip (Fig. 13.1c, d).

As a general rule, after a careful clinical and radiological assessment of the tumor spread, the implantation (including path, geometry, number of tubes, as well as the type of delivery which can be interstitial, endocavitary, or combined), as well as the strategy for fixation, must be carefully planned by radiation oncologists and surgeons in a multidisciplinary setting before bringing the patient to the surgical theater.

The criteria to be followed for such planning are, on the one hand, oncological, as described above, on the other hand, functional and cosmetic.

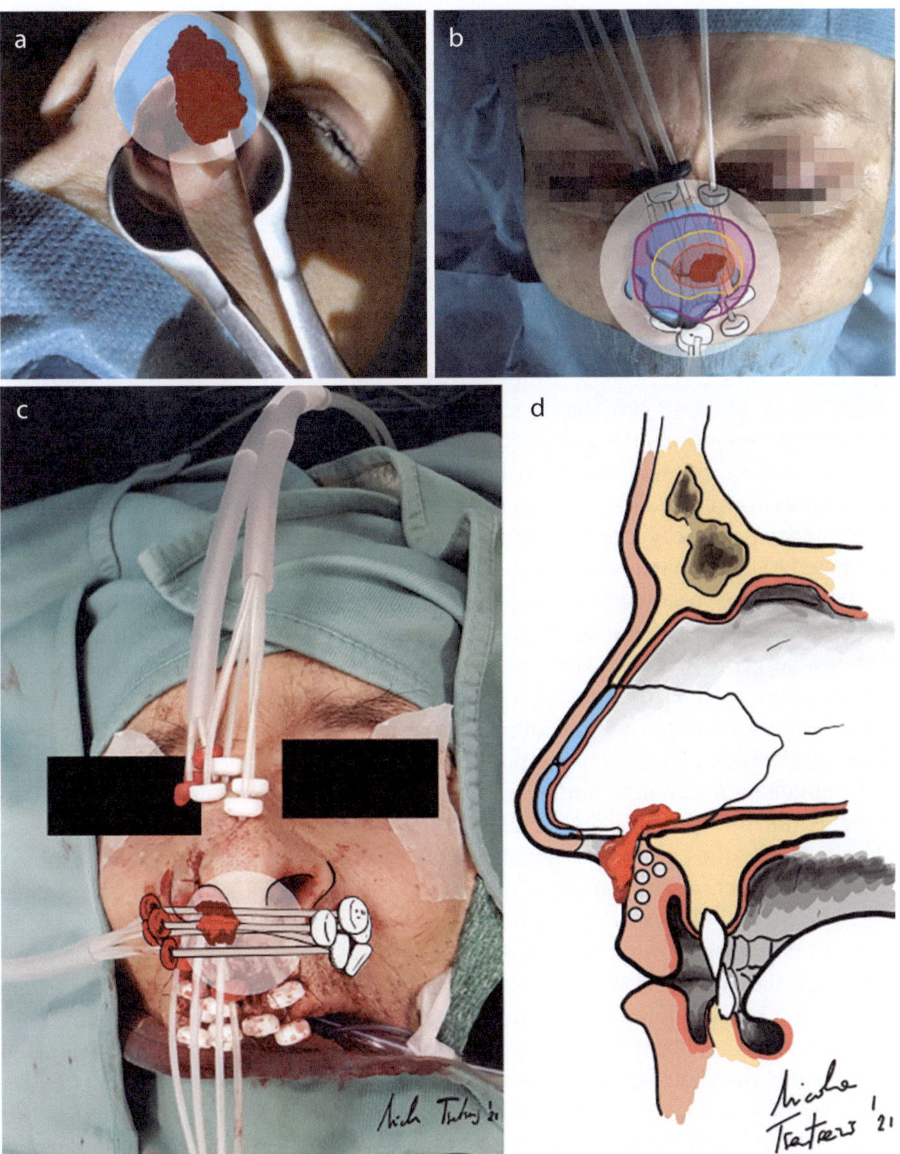

Fig. 13.1   The location of the tumor and the CTV for an adequate IRT treatment are shown in case of primaries of the lateral wall (**a**, **b**) and of the inferior/medial wall(s) (**c**, **d**) of the nose vestibule

13.3 Functional/Cosmetic Considerations

The aim of functional and, even more, cosmetic preservation of nose vestibule is best obtained through the preservation of the nose tip cartilaginous framework not already eroded by tumor growth. It is well known, also from laryngeal oncology [2], that the cartilage itself is particularly resistant to tumor invasion also because it is devoid of blood vessels and fed through the interstitium by direct diffusion from the vascularized perichondrium [3, 4]. When blood vessels are brought in by ossification, the probability of direct invasion by tumor cells drastically increases. However, nose cartilages, differently from laryngeal ones and thyroid cartilage in particular, do not usually get ossified even in the elderly, and in fact, as observed above, direct invasion is very late in nose vestibule SCCs. This aspect and the low toxicity of radiotherapy on nose cartilages [3, 5–9] are clear advantages for the purpose of cosmetic preservation after irradiation of nose vestibule malignancies.

Nevertheless, the main reported long-term toxicity of IRT in this site is notoriously chondronecrosis and consequent septal and even alar perforations [8]. These sequelae are reportedly more frequent when an interstitial dose delivery is chosen, if compared to endocavitary/mold technique [8]. This suggests that chondronecrosis is likely due to the mechanical damage and interruption of the perichondrium, which feeds the cartilage, by the implants rather than to the dose to the cartilage itself. Notably, surgeons with an experience in septoplasty and rhinoseptoplasty are completely aware that perforations of cartilages, and of the septum in particular, derive from the interruption of perichondral feeding because of tearing of mucoperichondrium itself. Based on these assumptions and awareness, we modified our interstitial IRT implantation technique for nose vestibule carcinomas following the principle to avoid as much as possible the piercing of the perichondrium and of the cartilages. Therefore, also the exposure of the plastic tubes inside the nasal cavity, which means tearing the perichondrium, must be avoided. To these aims, the implantation of nose vestibule SCCs belongs to skilled nose surgeons together with IRT experts who, in case of interstitial delivery, place the plastic tubes along the subperichondral planes, which are the main dissection routes of the functional and aesthetic surgery of the nose (Fig. 13.2). Therefore, the planes of the interstitial implants are ideally the subpericondral planes themselves, and the final geometry of the implants is dictated primarily by the anatomy of the nose tip (and not by the Paris system rules) [9, 10]. Such anatomic implantation technique resulted in no septal/alar perforation in our series, with markedly better anatomic and therefore cosmetic and functional results than in previous series [11–13]. The "anatomic" implantation technique, paired with the personalized, volume-optimized dose delivery, may contravene the "classical"

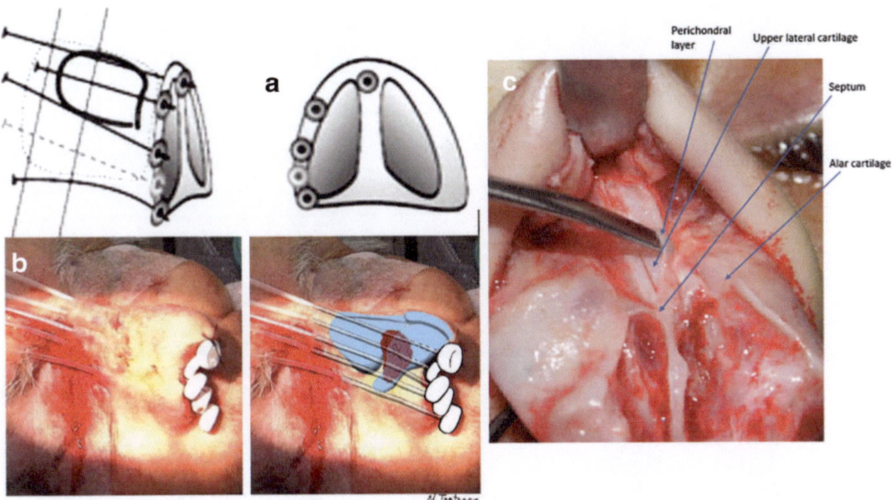

Fig. 13.2 The scheme of an implant for a SCC of the lateral wall of the nose vestibule is shown. Plastic tubes are placed parallel as much as possible (**a**), passing deep to the alar and superficial to the lateral cartilage (**b**), ideally in the planes between the perichondrium and the cartilages (**c**)

Paris system [14, 15], whose rules and principles remain valid to obtain an optimal dose distribution, especially with LDR linear sources. However, the stepping source-based potential of dose intensity modulation, combined with the image guidance, can improve the dose distribution in PDR/HDR IRT after "anatomic" implantation, in order to obtain optimal local control—which, in fact, is not inferior to other brachytherapy series [1, 8, 11, 12, 14–16] (Fig. 13.3).

Patient 1

Patient 2

Patient 3

Patient 4

Patient 5

Patient 6

Patient 7

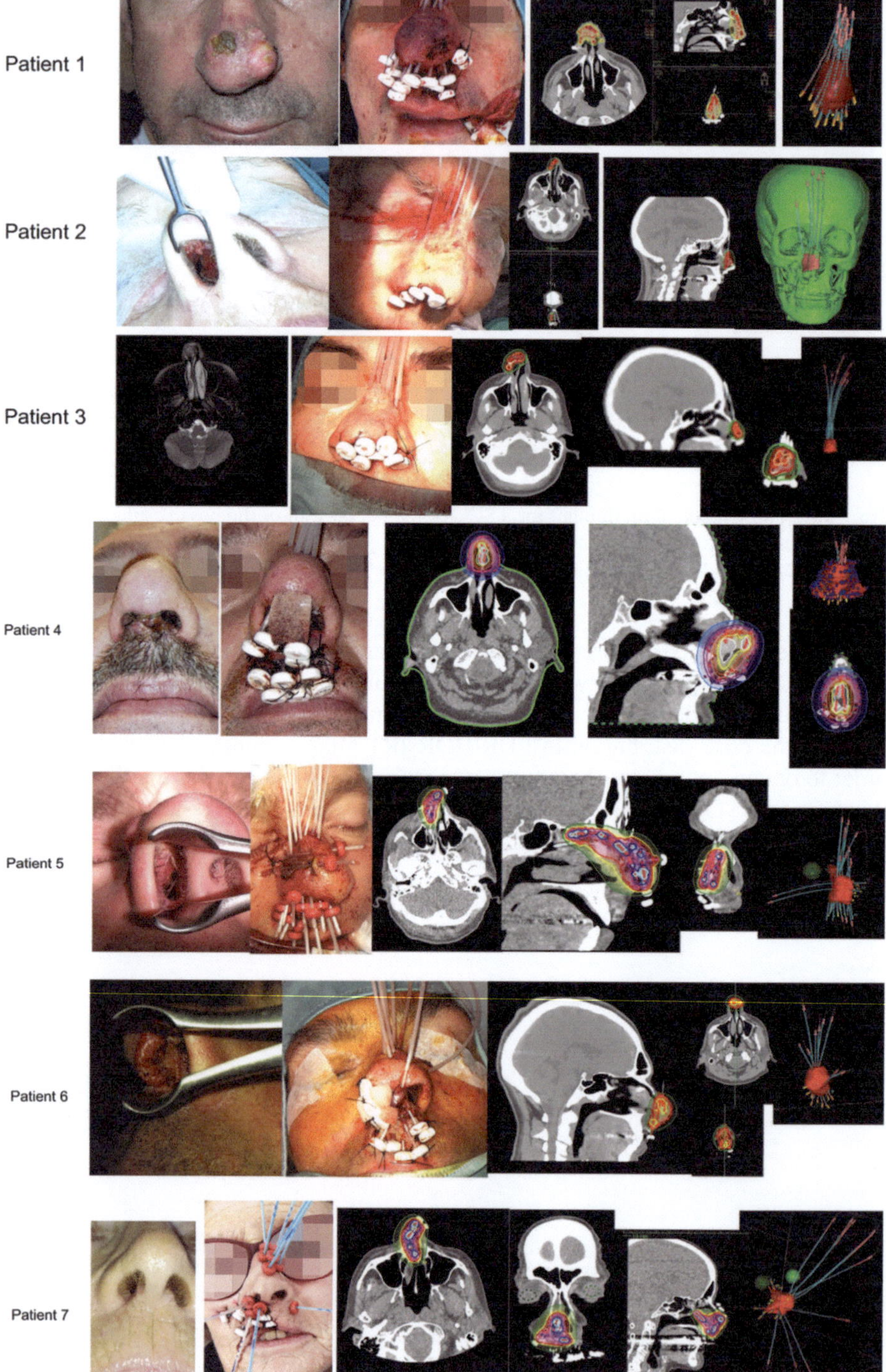

Fig. 13.3 A series of tumors, implants, and resulting clinical target volumes are shown. *Patient 1:* extensive invasion of the skin of the nose tip, multiple tubes are placed. Yellow line: 100% Isodose. *Patients 2 and 3:* Nose vestibule SCC spreading between alar and lateral cartilages. Plastic tubes follow the same path as the tumors themselves. Red line: 100% isodose. *Patient 4:* SCC of the medial wall (septum and columella). Violet line: 100% isodose. *Patient 5:* SCC of the lateral wall spreading between the lateral cartilage and the bone. Red line: 100% isodose. *Patient 6:* SCC of the medial wall (septum and columella). Red line: 100% isodose. *Patient 7:* SCC of the inferior wall. Red line: 100% isodose

13.4 Specific Considerations About Interstitial, Intracavitary, or Surface Dose Delivery

The above principles apply perfectly to the interstitial implantation: the CTV is covered by applicators placed inside and around the tumor, along the above-described planes, and the active part of the tubes is intramural ("buried"), a fundamental point for stabilization of the implant. The implants' geometry must be stable for the duration of the treatment—usually lasting at least 7 days in case of exclusive IRT for nose vestibule primaries (Chap. 12). The stability of the implant is of utmost importance for the reliability of the treatment plan, and it can be increased by keeping the plastic tubes' entrance and exit ("burial") points as far as possible from the CTV itself. This trick avoids changes of the entrance/exit points of the tubes and therefore their displacement, a probable event when they are very close or within the tumor, which can shrink or get ulcerated during the treatment, extruding the catheter(s). This is also one of the reasons why, in case of extensive involvement of the superior lip, we sometimes place tubes completely outside the subperichondral planes, yet fully interstitial, inside the superior lip itself, perpendicular to the main axis of the subperichondal route (Fig. 13.4). Another reason to follow this route is sometimes to warrant an adequate coverage and dose to the inferior nasal sill and to the area below and posterior to the anterior nasal spine, which could be more difficult to obtain with tubes following the subperichondal route.

In general, stability of the tubes and therefore reliability of the treatment plan as well as the low local toxicity rates are the main advantages of interstitial delivery, which, when feasible, in our opinion should be preferred for nose vestibule.

Nonetheless, in some situations, the CTV cannot be fully covered by an interstitial implant.

Among these situations, there is the event of a bulky, exophytic skin component. Superficial molds, which, in our opinion, have a limited role in nose vestibule IRT, may have a role in such an event. For the same goal, we also resort to contact delivery, mainly using tubes, in selected cases of exophytic skin involvements (Fig. 13.5).

Anyway, the most common situation when it can be impossible to cover the target volume with fully interstitial implants is a lesion extending beyond the plane tangential to the piriform opening (which we propose as a landmark both for the definition of the nose vestibule subsite, Chap. 1, and for the novel T classification,

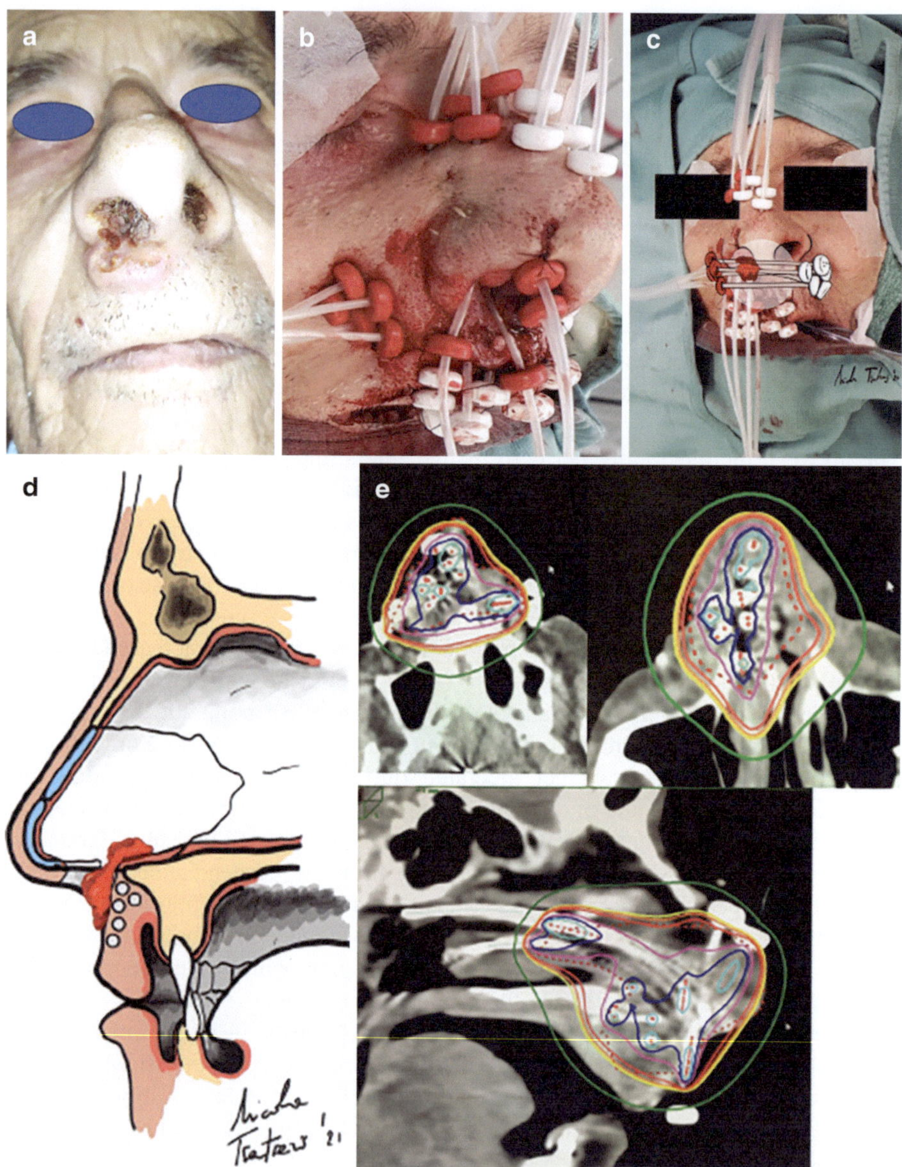

Fig. 13.4 A bulky lesion of the inferior wall of the vestibule extensively invaded the superior lip (**a**). Catheters were placed both along the "classical" subperichondral paths and perpendicular to them along the coronal main axis of the superior lip (**b**, **c**). This allowed to completely cover the target volume with a fully interstitial implant (**d**, **e**)

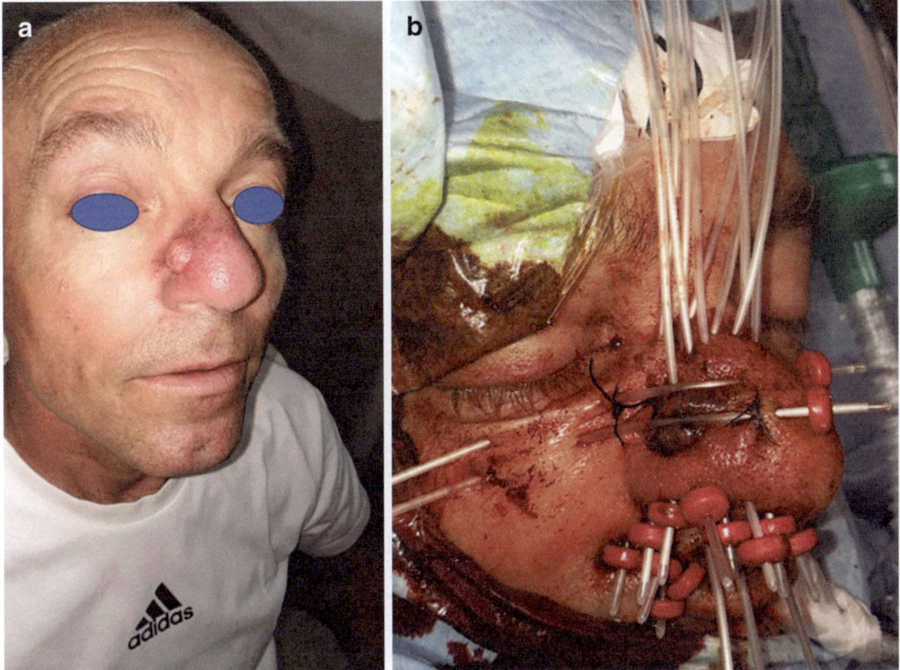

Fig. 13.5 The bulky skin component (**a**) could not be covered by "buried" subperichondral tubes. Two additional tubes (**b**) were placed externally and stabilized through a passage in the skin of the cheel and of the nasal dorsum

Chap. 5). In these cases, it must be kept in mind that the needles currently used for interstitial plastic tube placement badly tolerate bending and are to be considered practically straight (Fig. 13.6a). Therefore, the interstitially placed tubes, even if slightly bent, can barely overcome the plan of the pyriform opening (Fig. 13.6b). For tumors approaching such a plane, we use "combined" implants in which some tubes follow an interstitial route and others are endocavitary. A new standard for endocavitary nose and paranasal IRT implantation is the "endoscopy guided brachy-therapy" (IGBRT) [17] which allows more precise, targeted, and reliable tube place-ment and should be used, in case of posterior lesions of the nose vestibule, in combination with the interstitial implantation.

Nevertheless, the main issue of the endocavitary delivery in nose vestibule brachytherapy is stabilization of the catheters, which is always less reliable than in the interstitial one. Several tricks can be used to improve the stability and so the reliability of endocavitary implants. The most frequently used is the fixation to sponge packing of blind end tubes (Fig. 13.7), this is a simple and non-traumatic procedure, and the presence of the packing in the nasal cavity has the additional advantage to improve dose delivery by eliminating the interface with air.

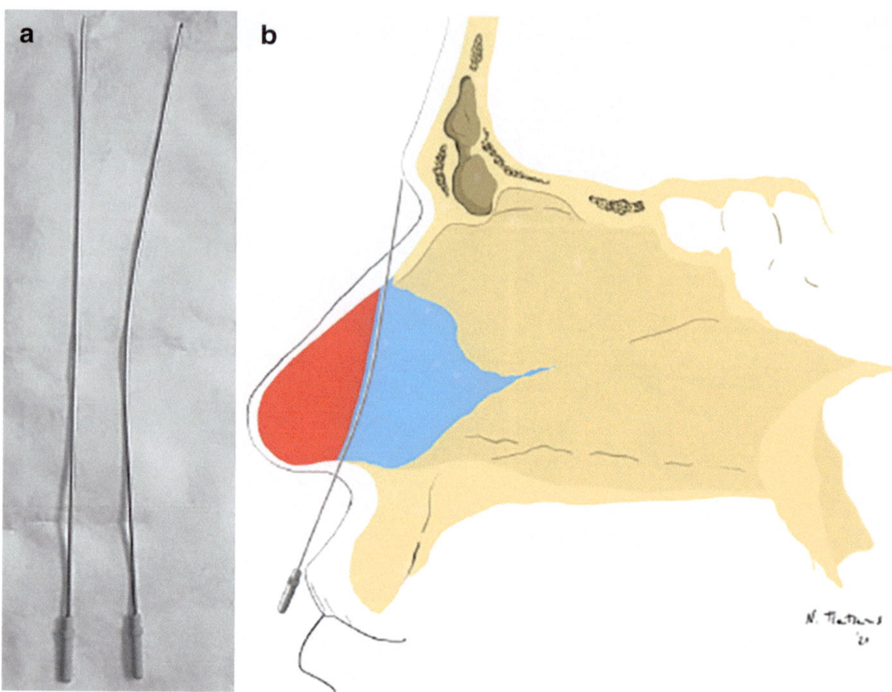

Fig. 13.6 Metal guides are provided straight and can be only slightly bended for the application of the plastic tubes (**a**). This implies that interstitial implants can only cover lesions confined to the nasal vestibule (considering the plane tangential to the pyriform opening as the posterior boundary of the nasal vestibule itself) (**b**)

Fig. 13.7 Plastic tubes are preliminarily fixed on nasal packing

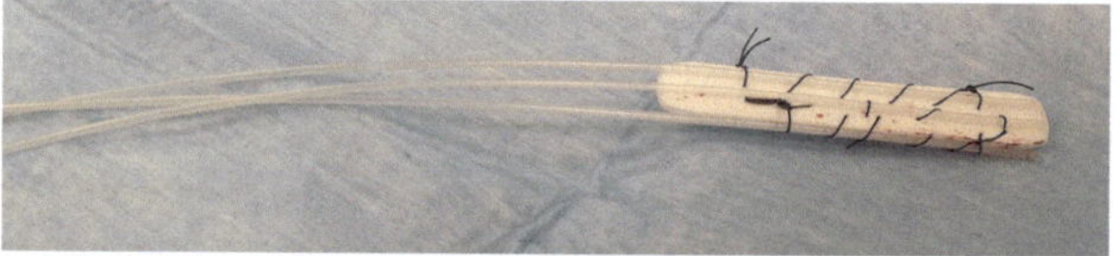

The administration of the dose through catheters fixed to nasal swabs is however affected by the following problems:

1. Fixation by stitches is not completely stable because tying is limited by the softness and friableness of sponge itself.
2. An overly tight stitch can "choke" the tube itself and compromise the passage of the source.
3. The placement under direct vision requires endoscopic aid [17], but the packing can move after retraction of the endoscope with unexpected paths (Fig. 13.8).

Another trick is to fix the tubes on the skin of the lip and nose using buttons to reduce the residual mobility (Fig. 13.9).

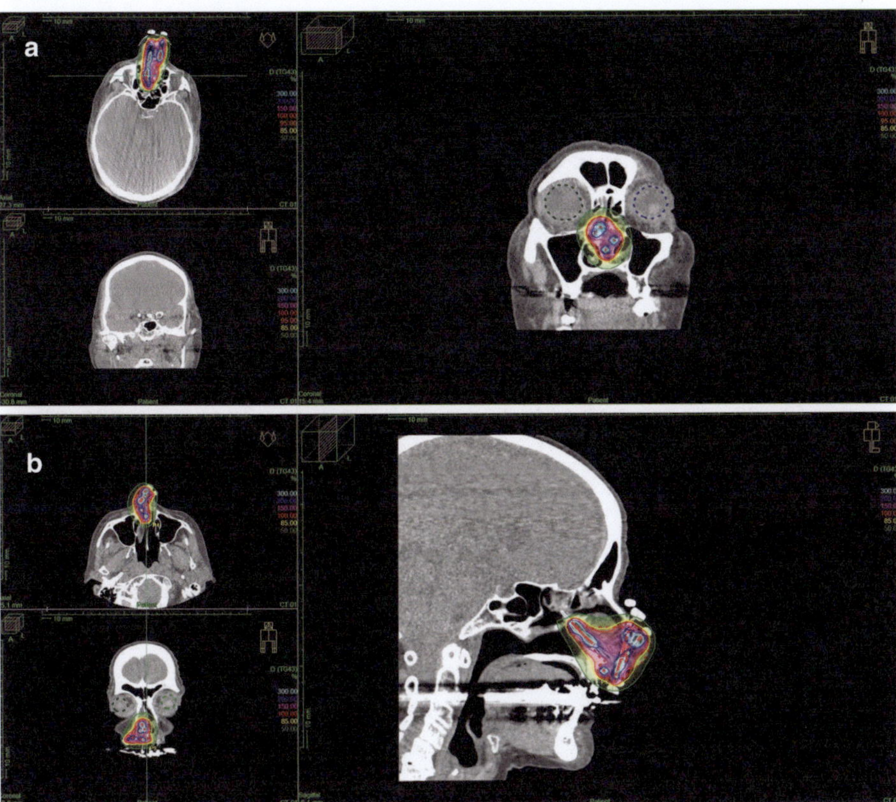

Fig. 13.8 (**a**) Endocavitary implant for a left septal primary involving the septum up to the level of ethmoid lamina. Septal deviation pushed the left packing towards the inferior choana, so that the CTV had to be covered exploiting the right nostril implant. This allowed local control with currently NED but required an increased dose on the right nasal fossa with turbinoseptal sinechas in the nasal fossa not originally affected by the tumor (see Fig. 13.12). (**b**) Inferior wall primary needed a mixed (interstitial and endocavitary) implant for an adequate coverage of the CTV, but the packing led the endocavitary tubes cranially, with dosimetric issues luckily solved through intensity modulation and adequate exploiting of all the implants, also in this case the local control has been obtained, and the patient is currently free of disease

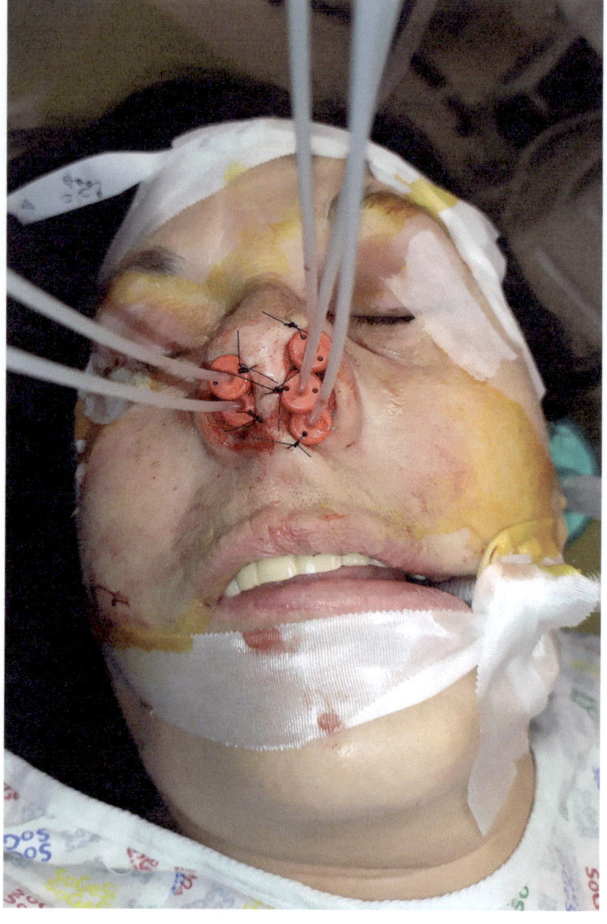

Fig. 13.9 Stabilization of implants through suture to the packing and buttons sutured to the skin, in an endocavitary implant for a septal primary extending beyond the piriform opening

Suturing the tubes to a silicon plate, which can be easily fixed on the nose/superior lip, is an alternative/additional method for implant stabilization. Such strategy (contrary to the packing) does not determine a complete nasal obstruction (Fig. 13.10).

All the above tricks can be variously combined according to the specific case to allow the optimal coverage of the target and the maximum stability of the tubes, privileging the interstitial modality as much as possible (Fig. 13.11).

The use of endocavitary molds has been suggested by Haynes [18] back in 1974, but poorly exploited, probably also for the lack of fast reliable polymers best suited for the scope and tolerable in the nasal cavity, which could allow tailoring of personalized molds.

We are currently evaluating such a hypothesis and in particular the feasibility of removable endocavitary molds made by polymers to be placed in the cavity

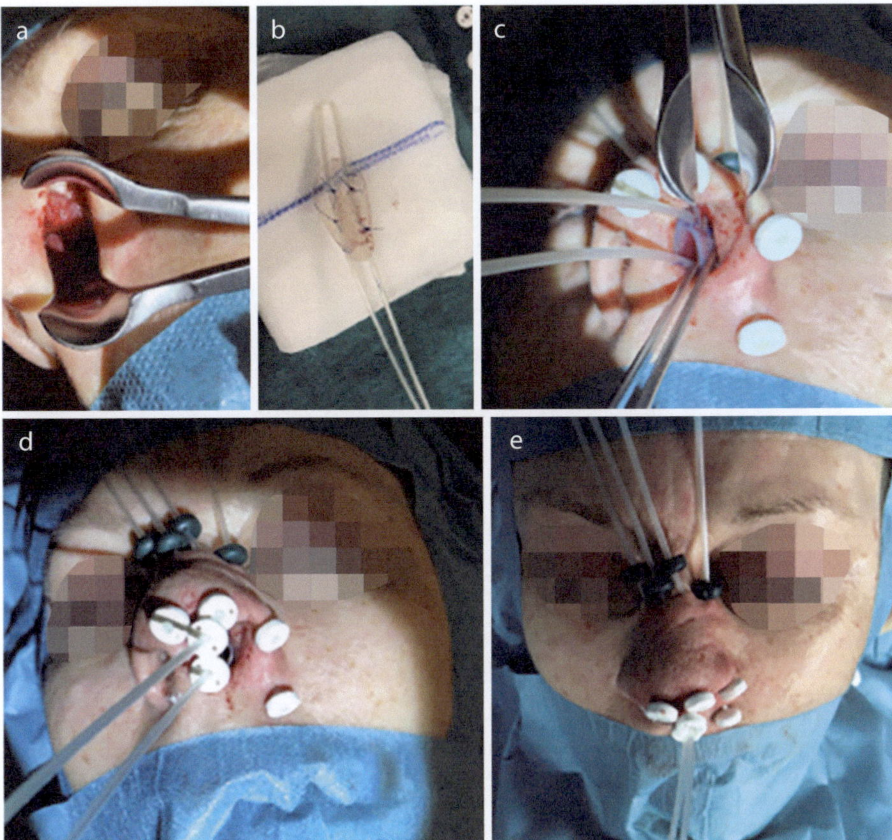

Fig. 13.10 A nose vestibule primary of the lateral wall showed a spread toward the nasal bones and the plane of the piriform opening (**a**) raising concerns about the possibility of a complete coverage of the CTV through a fully interstitial implant. In order to reach posteriorly at the level of the internal mucosal coverage of the nasal bones, plastic tubes were fixed on a silicon plate bended to adapt to the nasal wall itself (**b**). After the interstitial implant of four plastic tubes, placement of the silicon plate with two additional catheters allowed for the complete coverage of the CTV (**c**). Both the interstitial and endocavitary plastic tubes (**d**, **e**) were then further stabilized through buttons and stitches

immediately after the implant of interstitial tubes under endoscopic guidance. Such strategy could drastically improve reliability and stability of endocavitary implants and even lead to an enlargement of the indications to IRT for more posterior/nasal cavity proper lesions.

Also, the toxicity associated with endocavitary implants is higher, in fact we observed, as a typical sequela in correspondence to the hotspots on the mucosal surfaces, nasal wall synechiae, which are anyway easily treated by revision surgery 1 month after the end of irradiation (Fig. 13.12), but were never observed after fully interstitial dose delivery.

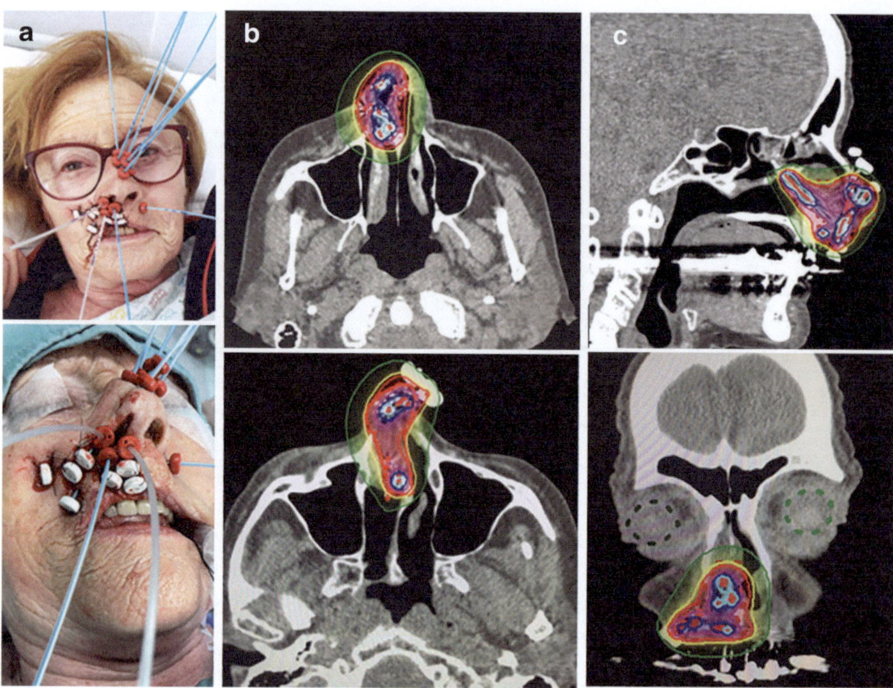

Fig. 13.11 An SCC arising from the inferior and medial (septal) walls of the nose vestibule showed a posterior spread, which made impossible a complete coverage of the target through interstitial tubes. Therefore, after placing interstitial tubes both along the nasal axis and in the superior lip to reach as much posterior as possible, other tubes were fixed on nasal packing, placed under endoscopic guidance and further stabilized with buttons on the skin (**a**). This allowed an optimal coverage of the target as shown on the axial (**b**), coronal, and sagittal (**c**) scans

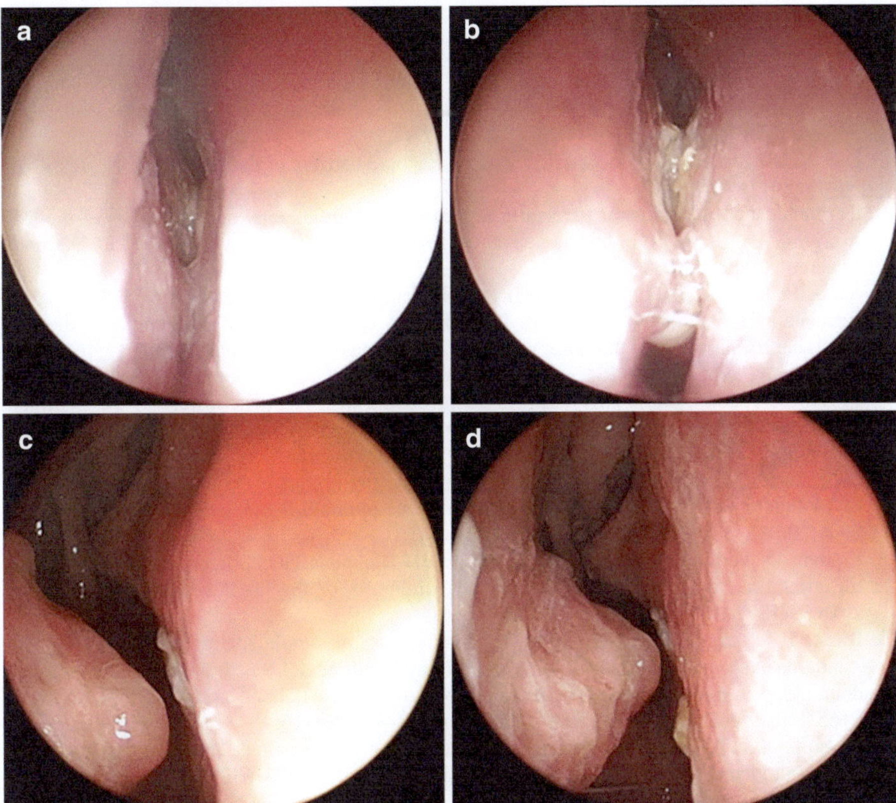

Fig. 13.12 Typical toxicity after endocavitary implant with the high dose on the mucosal surfaces, which may merge to form a synechia or synechiae, mostly turbinoseptal (**a**, **b**). These problems are easily treated by endoscopic approach using cold lysis and positioning of a silastic plate, with excellent anatomical and functional results (**c**, **d**)

13.5 Anesthesiology and Operating Theater Setting

The implants are best applied under general anesthesia, with orotracheal intubation being preferred, and laryngeal masks should be avoided to minimize the hindrance by the anesthesiology tube, which should be stabilized as far away as possible from the operating field. The implantation must be performed by the nose surgeon at the presence of experienced IRT radiation oncologists.

In selected cases of small anterior lesions, implantation can be performed under local anesthesia. Infiltration with local anesthetics, with or without adrenaline, of the subperichondrial planes, as in functional nose surgery, is fundamental to obtaining analgesia in case of local anesthesia and is helpful in facilitating the optimal catheter path along the planes also in general anesthesia.

The interaction between the surgeon and the IRT radiation oncologist at the implantation phase in the surgical theater is always recommended, also to improve the following cooperation in the CTV delineation and planning.

References

1. Bussu F, Tagliaferri L, Mattiucci G, et al. HDR interventional radiotherapy (brachytherapy) in the treatment of primary and recurrent head and neck malignancies. Head Neck. 2019;41:1667–75.
2. Mor N, Blitzer A. Functional anatomy and oncologic barriers of the larynx. Otolaryngol Clin N Am. 2015;48:533–45.
3. Caccialanza M, Piccinno R, Percivalle S, Rozza M. Radiotherapy of carcinomas of the skin overlying the cartilage of the nose: our experience in 671 lesions. J Eur Acad Dermatol Venereol. 2009;23:1044–9.
4. Sandell LJ. Novel functions for type II procollagen. Connect Tissue Res. 2014;55:20–5.
5. Caccialanza M, Piccinno R, Moretti D, Rozza M. Radiotherapy of carcinomas of the skin overlying the cartilage of the nose: results in 405 lesions. Eur J Dermatol. 2003;13:462–5.
6. Caccialanza M, Piccinno R, Gaiani F, Contini D. Relevance of dermatologic radiotherapy in the therapeutic strategy of skin epithelial neoplasms: excellent results in the treatment of lesions localized on eyelids and skin overlying the cartilage of the nose. G Ital Dermatol Venereol. 2013;148:83–8.
7. Caccialanza M, Bertani E, Piccinno R, Rozza M, Brambilla R, Percivalle S. Radiotherapy of T4 squamous cell carcinoma of the skin of nasal pyramid. J Eur Acad Dermatol Venereol. 2006;20:872–4.
8. Lipman D, Verhoef LC, Takes RP, Kaanders JH, Janssens GO. Outcome and toxicity profile after brachytherapy for squamous cell carcinoma of the nasal vestibule. Head Neck. 2015;37:1297–303.
9. Bussu F, et al. Multidisciplinary approach to nose vestibule malignancies: setting new standards Approccio multidisciplinare ai tumori maligni del vestibolo del naso: verso la definizione di nuovi standard Acta Otorhinolaryngologica Italica. 2021;41(Suppl. 1):S158–S165. https://doi.org/10.14639/0392-100X-suppl.1-41-2021-16.
10. Bussu F, et al. New standards for the management of nose vestibule malignancies Acta Oto-Laryngologica. 2023;143(3):215–22. https://doi.org/10.1080/00016489.2023.2179662.
11. Bussu F, Tagliaferri L, Mattiucci G, et al. Comparison of interstitial brachytherapy and surgery as primary treatments for nasal vestibule carcinomas. Laryngoscope. 2016;126:367–71.
12. Bussu F, Tagliaferri L, De Corso E, et al. Functional results of exclusive interventional radiotherapy (brachytherapy) in the treatment of nasal vestibule carcinomas. Brachytherapy. 2021;20:178–84.
13. Tagliaferri L, et al. Interventional radiotherapy as exclusive treatment for primary nasal vestibule cancer: single-institution experience Journal of Contemporary Brachytherapy 2020;12(5):413–19. https://doi.org/10.5114/jcb.2020.100373.
14. Levendag PC, Nijdam WM, van Moolenburgh SE, Tan L, Noever I, van Rooy P, Mureau MAM, Jansen PP, Munte K, Hofer SOP. Interstitial radiation therapy for early-stage nasal vestibule cancer: a continuing quest for optimal tumor control and cosmesis. Int J Rad Oncol Biol Phys. 2006;66:160–9.
15. Chargari C, Van Limbergen E, Mahantshetty U, Deutsch É, Haie-Méder C. Radiobiology of brachytherapy: the historical view based on linear quadratic model and perspectives for optimization. Cancer/Radiothérapie. 2018;22:312–8.
16. Czerwinski MD, van Leeuwen RGH, Kaanders JHA, Zwijnenburg EM, Lipman D, Takes RP, Verhoef CG. Image guided brachytherapy for cancer of the nasal vestibule: local control and cosmesis. Int J Rad Oncol Biol Phys. 2019;103:913–21.
17. Tagliaferri L, Bussu F, Rigante M, et al. Endoscopy-guided brachytherapy for sinonasal and nasopharyngeal recurrences. Brachytherapy. 2015;14:419–25.
18. Haynes WD, Ducote Haynes W, Tapley ND. Radiation treatment of carcinoma of the nasal vestibule. Am J Roentgenol. 1974;120:595–602.

Nasal Vestibule Cancer: Management of the Regional Lymph Nodes

14

Kimberley L. Kiong, William H. Morrison, Brandon Gunn, and Randal S. Weber

14.1 Background

Malignancies arising within the nasal vestibule most commonly include squamous cell carcinoma (SCC), basal cell carcinoma (BCC), and melanoma. Less commonly adnexal tumors arise in this location [1]. With the exception of BCC, all have the propensity to metastasize to the regional lymph node basins. This chapter will focus on management of the neck in patients with nasal vestibule cancers. Particular attention will be given to SCCs as the most common lesions that will metastasize to the regional lymphatics.

As discussed, clinical staging for nasal vestibule malignancies has not reached a consensus. Three staging systems, though not specific, have been used: the American Joint Committee on Cancer (AJCC) system for sinonasal cancer, the Wang's system [2], and the AJCC system for non-melanoma skin cancers. The discrepancy in staging systems used will thus confound the research and discussion on management of the neck depending on T staging, since this may differ from study to study. Regardless, these staging systems agree that bony invasion indicates advanced T stage and higher risk of lymph node metastases [1], thus portending a poorer prognosis.

K. L. Kiong
Department of Otorhinolaryngology-Head & Neck Surgery, Singapore General Hospital, Singapore, Singapore

W. H. Morrison · B. Gunn
Department of Radiation Oncology, M.D. Anderson Cancer Center, Houston, TX, USA
e-mail: whmorrison@mdanderson.org; GBGunn@mdanderson.org

R. S. Weber (✉)
Health Care Advancement, M.D. Anderson Cancer Center, Houston, TX, USA
e-mail: rsweber@mdanderson.org

© Springer Nature Switzerland AG 2023
F. Bussu (ed.), *Malignancies of the Nasal Vestibule*,
https://doi.org/10.1007/978-3-031-32850-3_14

14.2   Anatomy and Lymphatic Drainage

The nasal vestibule is defined as the part of the anterior nasal cavity extending from the anterior nares to the limen nasi. It is bounded by the columella, septum, and medial and lateral crus of the lower lateral cartilage, respectively. The nasal vestibule is lined by vibrissae bearing squamous epithelium with underlying sebaceous glands.

Lymphatic drainage of the nasal cavity is bidirectional, anterior and posterior. The anterior one third of the nasal cavity, including the nasal vestibule, drains primarily to the facial, submandibular, and parotid lymph nodes [3]. The second echelon of nodal drainage is to the superior deep cervical nodal basin (Fig. 14.1). Lymphatics in the posterior nasal cavity drain into the retropharyngeal and superior deep cervical nodes.

14.3   Incidence

At the time of diagnosis, the incidence of nodal metastasis is generally between 5% and 10% [4–7]. However, most studies do not report whether clinical examination or imaging was the basis upon which the status of the regional lymph nodes was determined. Given the retrospective nature of these reports, exact incidence of lymph node metastasis is uncertain.

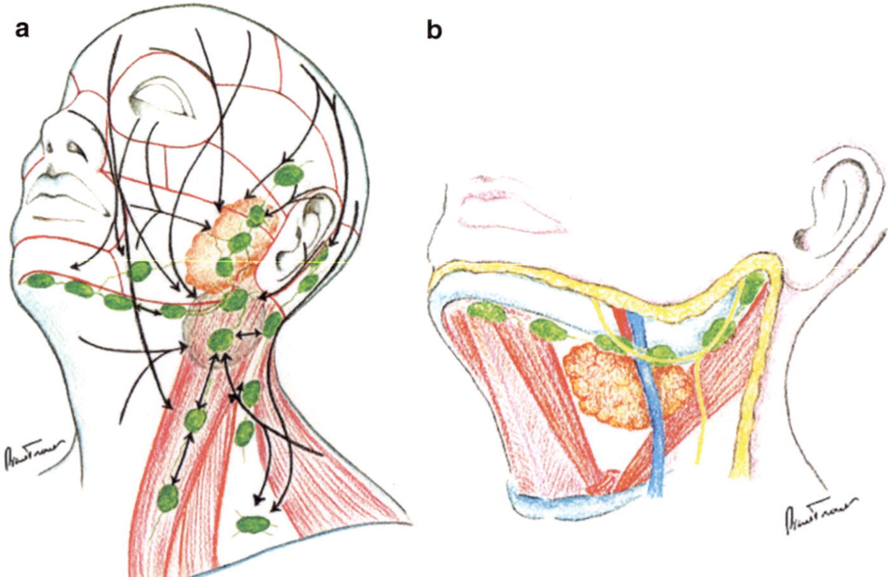

Fig. 14.1 (**a**) Pattern of superficial lymph nodes metastasis of head and neck skin squamous cell carcinoma. (**b**) Relationships between marginalis mandibulae, facial vessels, and upper level I nodes

In terms of delayed metastases, the largest nasal vestibule series to date reported a neck failure rate of 11% in 174 patients [7]. In their review of lymph node metastases in nasal vestibular SCC, Talmi et al. reported a range of 4–21% of delayed metastases to the neck [1]. One outlier quoted in this study was the paper by Fornelli et al. [8], reported a delayed nodal metastases rate of 41% among patients who were initially N0. Studies reporting the initial, delayed and overall rate of nodal metastases are shown in Table 14.1. Some studies have not differentiated between rates of delayed nodal metastases and recurrent neck disease after elective treatment of the neck; hence, we have excluded these in this part of our discussion as these represent different disease processes.

Schalekamp [9] analyzed 127 patients with nasal vestibule SCC and noted a total regional metastases rate of 16%, 20%, and 47% in patients with T1, T2, and T3 disease, respectively (classified with Wang's classification). Vital et al. also reported in their series that apart from one patient with a T2 tumor, all local recurrences or delayed regional lymph node metastasis occurred in patients with T4 tumors [14]. In these two papers, it was not stated if elective treatment of the neck was performed. In a more recent paper by Wray et al., they analyzed the neck control rates in their series of 94 patients with initial N0 necks [16]. Neck control at the completion of the study was achieved in 59 of 69 patients (86%) with T1–T2 cancers, compared with 39 of 47 patients (83%) with T4 cancers. Taking into account the use of elective neck treatment, they noted that in the 42 patients with de novo T1–T2 cancers, there were no failures in the four patients who underwent elective nodal irradiation (ENI). In 38 patients with de novo T1 and T2 cancers who did not receive ENI, there were three failures (8%). None of the patients with de novo T3–T4 cancers failed after ENI, but 5 of 23 (22%) patients with T3–T4 cancers failed in the neck when no ENI was performed. All in all, this suggests that advanced T stage tumors may have a higher incidence of nodal metastases and may support the use of ENI in this group.

Table 14.1 Rate of nodal metastases

Author	Study population	N+ initial (%)	N+ delayed (%)	N+ overall (%)
Wang [2]	36	–	–	10
Schalekamp and Hordijk [9]	127	4	20	24
Chobe et al. [10]	32	0	13	13
Levendag et al. [11]	63	6	6	12
Horsmans et al. [12]	66	7.5	6	13
Langendijk et al. [13]	56	0	12	12
Jeannon et al. [5]	84	9.5	4	13
Wallace et al. [6]	79	5	8	13
Agger et al. [7]	174	6	7	13
Vital et al. [14]	30	7	7	14
Vanneste et al. [15]	81	0	10	10
Wray et al. [16]	99	5	14	19

14.4 Evaluation of the Regional Lymph Node Basins

Initial workup should include a imaging of the neck and fine-needle aspiration (FNA) of any suspicious lymph nodes. Either ultrasound (US) and/or CT scan may be utilized to image the neck. CT scans may be utilized in evaluation of the primary site and neck and may show enlarged, rounded lymph nodes that suggest involvement by metastases. A CT is also useful in cases of gross extranodal extension, indicating which structures are involved for better surgical planning. On the other hand, US may pick up more subtle abnormalities in unenlarged lymph nodes, for example, a loss of fatty hilum, which may alert a clinician to possible nodal involvement. These scans are hence complementary.

14.5 Treatment of the Neck

14.5.1 Elective Neck Management

There is no consensus on elective treatment of the N0 neck in nasal vestibular SCC, with surgery or ENI. Proponents of elective neck treatment quote a lower rate of recurrent neck disease, while others quote a similar rate of nodal recurrence and also point out the potential side effects of surgery or irradiation of the neck, which often requires bilateral treatment. In general, elective treatment of the neck is indicated when the risk of regional metastasis is greater or equal to 20%. As such, given the morbidity of treatment, ENI is considered for T3 and T4 primary lesions.

Levendag et al. reported a series of 63 patients with T1 and T2 lesions, where ENI of bilateral necks (40 Gy) was performed in nine patients with T1 disease and 16 patients with T2 disease. Two regional failures developed in each of the groups that did and did not receive ENI. The authors thus recommended against elective treatment of the neck [11].

Wray et al. [16] noted in their series of 99 patients with SCC of the nasal vestibule that in the N0 patients with a controlled primary site and no ENI, the neck remained negative in 59 of 69 patients (86%). In the N0 patients with a controlled primary site who received ENI, the neck remained negative in 24 of 25 patients (96%). ENI was recommended in patients with locally recurrent, poorly differentiated, and/or T4 cancers. This was administered with an anterior field to deliver approximately 50 Gy in 25 fractions to one or both sides of the neck depending on the extent of the primary tumor. They further attempted to stratify their data with T stage and de novo versus recurrence status. It was observed that in the 42 patients with de novo T1–T2 cancers, all four patients who had ENI did not recur. However, in the 38 patients with T1-T2 cancers who did not receive ENI, there were three failures (8%). Of the eight patients with recurrent T1–T2 cancers, 0/2 (0%) receiving ENI failed while 2/6 (33%) who did not receive ENI failed. Furthermore, none of the patients with de novo T3–T4 tumors failed after ENI, but 5 of 23 (22%) patients with T3–T4 tumors failed in the neck when no ENI was performed.

In keeping with the above findings, Vanneste et al. also found that regional control was significantly worse for patients with a higher T classification [15]. Several other studies have suggested prognostic factors that may increase the risk for occult involvement of the regional lymphatics, including high tumor grade, large tumor volume, recurrent disease, and deep infiltration of structures with increased capillary lymphatics, such as the upper lip and columella [9, 17].

Also crucial in the discussion of whether the neck should be prophylactically treated would be the salvage rate of delayed nodal metastases. While the numbers requiring salvage therapy are small, available literature suggests a reasonable salvage rate of 80–90% [12, 15, 17], with regional control rates after 5 years in excess of 97% [13].

Therefore, given the potential for salvage therapy and the risks of elective neck treatment, we would not recommend for routine prophylactic treatment of the N0 neck. However, elective neck treatment can be considered in advanced T stage tumors (e.g., with extensive soft tissue or bony invasion) and/or other adverse prognostic factors such as recurrent disease.

Sentinel lymph node biopsy is standard of care for cutaneous melanomas of a significant depth. This practice has been expanded to other lesions of the head and neck, such as oral cavity SCC. There is also ongoing research for this practice in other sinonasal cancers, and this may prove to be a staging option in nasal vestibular SCCs in time to come [1].

14.5.2 Therapeutic Neck Management

As previously mentioned, the rate of clinically detected nodal metastases at initial presentation is less than 10%. Patients with node positive necks should receive either a neck dissection or therapeutic doses of radiation.

Wray et al. published a series of patients treated primarily with upfront radiation therapy; out of five patients with a clinically positive neck, neck control was achieved in three patients treated with RT alone. The remaining two patients had residual disease after RT and required a neck dissection [16].

The recommended surgery for neck disease is a Level I-III neck dissection, unless the nodal disease extends beyond these levels. In the series by Jeannon et al., therapeutic neck dissections performed in clinically N+ patients all yielded positive nodes in only level 1 [5]. While it has been noted that nasal vestibule malignancies may metastasize to the parotid nodes, the true incidence is unclear. Therefore, the authors do not recommend prophylactic parotidectomy in view of the potential morbidity of facial nerve injury.

The indications for adjuvant RT or chemoradiation post surgery are not well established in nasal vestibular SCC, due to the rarity of the disease. The practice has varied across different series, with some inclined to give adjuvant treatment to the neck in cases with traditional poor prognostic features, such as multiple lymph node involvement and extranodal extension. The role of chemotherapy in nasal vestibule SCC is even less established, with differences in opinion arising from the fact that these malignancies behave neither like mucosal SCCs of the sinonasal cavity, nor cutaneous SCCs of the external nose, but somewhere in between in terms of aggressiveness and survival. The small number of cases precludes prospective studies in this area, and conclusions will likely continue to be extrapolated from research in SCC of other regions in the head and neck.

14.6 Survival Outcomes

The largest series of 174 patients reports a 5-year disease-specific survival (DSS) of 74% and overall survival (OS) of 50% [7]. Other studies report a 5 year OS of 58–85% [1, 4, 11, 13].

It is well known that for mucosal SCCs in the head and neck region, the presence of lymph node metastases decreases survival rate by up to 50%. Similarly, for nasal vestibule malignancies, positive nodal disease portends a poorer prognosis. Horsmans et al. noted significantly poorer relapse-free, disease-specific and overall survival rates in patients with N+ disease at presentation [12].

Jeannon et al. analyzed the factors affecting survival in nasal vestibular SCC [5]. They found that 5-year OS for N+ patients was 40% compared with 65% for N-patients ($p = 0.001$, hazard ratio = 0.538). They also performed a multivariate analysis, which found that age (hazard ratio = 0.24), N stage (hazard ratio = 0.53), and Wang's classification (hazard ratio = 0.33) were significant prognostic factors for overall survival. In terms of disease-free survival, the following factors were significant predictors of poorer survival: N stage, grade, and depth of invasion. They also found that median survival for patients with nodal metastasis was 9 months.

Given the rarity of this disease, it is yet unknown if elective treatment of the neck has an impact on survival. As mentioned, most series find that there is a reasonable salvage rate for delayed neck metastases.

14.7 Follow-Up and Surveillance

While follow-up recommendations for surveillance interval and investigations are also not well established, some studies have also shown that as with other SCCs of the head and neck, the time of presentation of delayed nodal metastases is generally within the first 2 years [11]. They therefore suggest that US neck with possible FNA is warranted in the first 2 years of follow-up to pick up these neck recurrences early. It has also been observed that regional recurrences are associated with local recurrence [4, 13], emphasizing the importance of careful restaging when a local recurrence is detected.

14.8 Conclusion

In nasal vestibular carcinoma, the positive nodal rate at the time of diagnosis is less than 10%. Delayed nodal metastases occur at a rate of between 10% and 20%. While survival has been shown to be significantly reduced with the presence of positive nodal metastases, most cases of delayed nodal metastases can be successfully salvaged. As such, most literature recommends against elective treatment of the neck, except in cases with advanced T stage, recurrent or poorly differentiated tumors. We recommend careful initial staging and follow-up with a thorough clinical examination and imaging such as US neck to detect nodal metastases at a treatable stage.

References

1. Talmi YP, Ferlito A, Takes RP, et al. Lymph node metastasis in nasal vestibule cancer: a review. Head Neck. 2011;33:1783–8.
2. Wang CC. Treatment of carcinoma of the nasal vestibule by irradiation. Cancer. 1976;38:100–6.
3. Fletcher GH, Goepfert H, Jesse RH. Nasal and paranasal sinuses. In: Fletcher GH, editor. Textbook of radiotherapy. 3rd ed. Philadelphia, PA: Lea & Febiger; 1980. p. 408–25.
4. Mendenhall WM, Stringer SP, Cassisi NJ, Mendenhall NP. Squamous cell carcinoma of the nasal vestibule. Head Neck. 1999;21:385–93.
5. Jeannon JP, Riddle PJ, Irish J, O'Sullivan B, Brown DH, Gullane P. Prognostic indicators in carcinoma of the nasal vestibule. Clin Otolaryngol. 2007;32:19–23.
6. Wallace A, Morris CG, Kirwan J, et al. Radiotherapy for squamous cell carcinoma of the nasal vestibule. Am J Clin Oncol. 2007;30:612–6.
7. Agger A, von Buchwald C, Madsen AR, et al. Squamous cell carcinoma of the nasal vestibule 1993–2002: a nationwide retrospective study from DAHANCA. Head Neck. 2009;31:1593–9.
8. Fornelli RA, Fedok FG, Wilson EP, Rodman SM. Squamous cell carcinoma of the anterior nasal cavity: a dual institution review. Otolaryngol Head Neck Surg. 2000;123:207–10.
9. Schalekamp W, Hordijk GJ. Carcinoma of the nasal vestibule: prognostic factors in relation to lymph node metastasis. Clin Otolaryngol Allied Sci. 1985;10:201–3.
10. Chobe R, McNeese M, Weber R, Fletcher GH. Radiation therapy for carcinoma of the nasal vestibule. Otolaryngol Head Neck Surg. 1988;98:67–71.
11. Levendag PC, Pomp J. Radiation therapy of squamous cell carcinoma of the nasal vestibule. Int J Radiat Oncol Biol Phys. 1990;19:1363–7.
12. Horsmans JDJ, Godballe C, Jorgensen KE, Bastholt L, Lontoft E. Squamous cell carcinoma of the nasal vestibule. Rhinology. 1999;37:117–21.
13. Langendijk JA, Poorter R, Leemans CR, de Bree R, Doornaert P, Slotman BJ. Radiotherapy of squamous cell carcinoma of the nasal vestibule. Int J Radiat Oncol Biol Phys. 2004;59:1319–25.
14. Vital D, Morand G, Huber G, Struder G, Holzmann D. Outcome in squamous cell carcinoma of the nasal vestibule: a single center experience. Head Neck. 2015;37(1):46–51.
15. Vanneste BG, Lopez-Yurda M, Tan IB, Balm AJ, Borst GR, Rasch CR. Irradiation of localized squamous cell carcinoma of the nasal vestibule. Head Neck. 2016;38(Suppl 1):E1870–5.
16. Wray J, Morris CG, Kirwan JM, Amdur RJ, Werning JW, Dziegielewski PT, Mendenhall WM. Radiation therapy for nasal vestibule squamous cell carcinoma: a 40-year experience. Eur Arch Otorhinolaryngol. 2016;273(3):661–9.
17. McCollough WM, Mendenhall NP, Parsons JT, et al. Radiotherapy alone for squamous cell carcinoma of the nasal vestibule: management of the primary site and regional lymphatics. Int J Radiat Oncol Biol Phys. 1993;26:73–9.

Malignancies of the Nose Vestibule: Salvage Strategies

15

Corrado Rubino, Emilio Trignano, Noemi Spissu,
Carla Fonnesu, Claudia Crescio, Jacopo Galli,
and Francesco Bussu

15.1 Introduction

Squamous cell carcinoma (SCC) of the nasal vestibule is classically considered a rare condition, reported to account for about 1% of head and neck cancer, even if its incidence is most probably underestimated [1, 2]. Nevertheless, it is a peculiar condition, owing to the unique and fine anatomy of the area and the features of the epithelium where the neoplasm originates from. All these factors result in several peculiarities in both staging and treatment.

Surgery and radiotherapy alone (Wang T1 and T2 lesions), or in combination (Wang T3), are both reported for the treatment of primary lesions (see Chaps. 6–15).

It is still controversial which is the best treatment modality. Many papers report similar results in locoregional control and survival both with surgery and exclusive radiotherapy [3–6].

Recent works by Bussu and coworkers compare the results of surgical versus brachytherapy treatment in a close cooperation between surgeons and radiation

C. Rubino · E. Trignano · N. Spissu
Department of Medicine, Surgery and Pharmacy, University of Sassari, Sassari, Italy

Plastic Surgery Unit, Azienda Ospedaliera Universitaria, Sassari, Italy
e-mail: corubino@uniss.it; etrignano@uniss.it; Noemi.spissu@aouss.it

C. Crescio (✉) · C. Fonnesu
Otolaryngology Division, Azienda Ospedaliera Universitaria, Sassari, Italy
e-mail: claudia.crescio@aouss.it; carla.fonnesu@aouss.it

J. Galli
Istituto di Otorinolaringoiatria, Università Cattolica del Sacro Cuore, Rome, Italy
e-mail: jacopo.galli@unicatt.it

F. Bussu
Department of Medicine, Surgery and Pharmacy, University of Sassari, Sassari, Italy

Otolaryngology Division, Azienda Ospedaliera Universitaria, Sassari, Italy

© Springer Nature Switzerland AG 2023

F. Bussu (ed.), *Malignancies of the Nasal Vestibule*,
https://doi.org/10.1007/978-3-031-32850-3_15

oncologists; the authors report similar locoregional control and survival, but a higher patient satisfaction after brachytherapy. This result is mainly attributed to a better aesthetic result [4, 7–9].

Locoregional control after primary treatment is reportedly 83–86%. When the primary tumor is treated by brachytherapy (BT), the neck should be treated primarily by surgery (either in case of elective treatment, metastasis at diagnosis, delayed metastasis, see Chap. 14).

In case of nodal recurrence, the preferred and most validated treatment modality is surgery on N. In case of local recurrence, surgery remains the most validated modality, however, especially in cases which did not undergo previous irradiation (EBRT and/or BT/IRT), radiotherapy and in particular brachytherapy is a reasonable option to consider.

15.2 Regional Recurrence

Salvage of resectable (the vast majority of cases) nodal recurrences is therefore mostly surgical, through a comprehensive neck dissection. The most frequently involved level is Ib and in particular nodes along the facial vessels immediately below the marginalis mandibulae nerve (see Chap. 14).

We usually recommend adjuvant radiotherapy (combined with chemo in case of multiple nodes or extracapsular spread) after surgical salvage of neck recurrences (mostly delayed neck metastases) if the neck of the patient was not previously irradiated.

15.3 Local Recurrence

The issue of local recurrence of nose vestibule SCC is characterized by a very low amount of evidence being the event relatively rare in correctly staged and treated cases. In consideration of such lack of evidence and of a reportedly worse oncological outcome of brachytherapy in case of recurrences [7, 8], surgery remains the current standard, unless serious issues concerning cosmetic results and consequent refusal of the patient. In the last case, brachytherapy can be employed also in recurrences with analog criteria than in untreated SCC; otherwise, surgery should be preferred as it is reported to increase local control of the disease up to 96%, and therefore worthwhile, whenever possible. Such treatment poses unique problems in terms of demolition and reconstruction, owing to the complex anatomy of the area and to the pattern and location of the recurrence.

The strategy of salvage surgical procedures should involve an accurate diagnosis of the size, position and spread of the recurrent lesion, and a careful assessment of the scars and possible defects of previous surgery. Lastly, it is to consider the extent and magnitude of the residual radiation damage after external beam radiotherapy or brachytherapy and the reconstructive options already exploited.

Planning of reconstruction after excision consists of an analysis of the expected defect after lesion removal and the choice among the reconstructive options left after previous surgery.

Being ready for a reconstructive plan A and plan B is particularly important in salvage surgery, where the pattern of spread of the recurrent lesion may be unpredictable.

15.3.1 Preoperative Evaluation

Any persistent crusting nodularity or ulceration during follow-up should be suspected as recurrence and biopsied.

Once diagnosis is established, a CT scan or MRI can help clinical examination in evaluating soft tissue and/or bone extension, according to the Head and Neck Multidisciplinary Tumor Board (MDTB) decision.

The spread of the recurrent lesion is dependent on the site of recurrence.

Lesions recurring on the ala nasi often spread to the skin, becoming "through-and-through" lesions of the ala and/or to the tip of the nose, or toward the nasolabial area and can invade the bone of the pyriform opening.

Lesions recurring on the membranous septum spread to the cartilaginous septum up to the vomer and/or to the columella and the nasal spine.

Lesions recurring on the nostril sill spread to the upper lip up to maxillary bone.

Accurate evaluation of the extent of the neoplasm has to be performed, also taking into account the quality of the tissue around the lesion. Previous scars and clinically evident radiation tissue changes need to be noted, in order to possibly include them into the excision plan.

Precise photographic documentation has to be taken and recorded.

15.3.2 Surgical Planning

Planning of resection follows the analysis of recurrent lesion and surrounding scars and radiation damage, and therefore, it has to be individualized.

The resection must include the recurrent lesion, the scarred and/or radiation damaged surrounding soft tissue, and a healthy margin of at least 1 cm, if possible.

Bone needs to be included in the resection when contiguous or invaded by the lesion. The amount of resection depends on cancer invasion. Bone healthy margin cannot be assessed intraoperatively; therefore, a wide bone resection, if feasible, should be performed. According to the position of the lesion, nasal septum, nasal bones, the ascending branch of maxillary bone, the upper part of the upper maxilla, and the nasal spine may need to be removed with criteria analogous to what described in Chap. 8.

Intraoperative histopathologic control of soft tissues margins must always be planned.

15.3.3 Reconstructive Options

Reconstruction of defects after salvage surgery of the nasal vestibule is a challenging task, for the following reasons:

1. The demolitive surgery follows the pattern of the recurrent lesion and, therefore, the size and the geometry of the defects are often peculiar and unpredictable.
2. Bone margins cannot be assessed intraoperatively; therefore, the team has to decide whether reconstruction should be immediate, carrying the risk of hiding a further recurrence, or delaying reconstruction, leaving the patient with a disfiguring defect for at least 6 months, in subtotal nasal reconstruction.
3. Post-surgical scarring, radiation damage, or both may hinder some reconstructive options.

Potential scenarios for reconstruction after surgical salvage of nose vestibule recurrences.

In summary, the reconstructive surgeon faces these possibilities in salvage surgery of the nasal vestibule [10–18].

- Resection of a recurrent lesion of the vestibular lateral lining results in a full thickness defect of ala nasi, with or without involvement of the margin of the pyriform opening [18, 19].
- Resection of a recurrence of the medial vestibular skin produces a defect of the tip of the nose with varying degrees of lack of septal support, which may include, in different cases, a defect in nasal lining, nasal bones, nasal spine, and dorsal nasal skin.
- A recurrence of a lesion on the lining of the nasal sill may lead to a defect extending to the upper lip and/or to the maxillary bone.
- The sum of two or more of the above defects.

1. As to the first possibility, the reconstructive surgeon must, first of all, assess the quality of the skin of the nasolabial fold and the cheek. If no scars of signs of radiation damage to the skin are present, reconstruction of full thickness defects of ala nasi can be performed using nasolabial flaps. The lining is provided in salvage procedures using skin turnover flaps from the edge of the defect and folding the flap for the border of the ala. The flap is based on a superior pedicle, and a cartilage alar batten from auricular cartilage is useful as a support for the alar margin support, mainly in a second step after 3–4 weeks. In salvage procedures, the use of composite grafts from the auricle is not indicated because of decreased vascularity due to scarring or previous radiotherapy. If previous scars or extensive radiation damages or wider excisions preclude the use of nasolabial flaps, a paramedian forehead is the preferred choice.
2. The recurrence of cancers of the medial vestibule of the nose invades columella, the septum and, ultimately, the defect after salvage resections results in a loss of

the tip of the nose that may extend to wide portions of septum, sometimes involving part of nasal bones and dorsal nasal coverage. This means that the patient needs a subtotal nasal reconstruction. Provided that the paramedian forehead flaps have not been used yet and no scars or other damage preclude its use, forehead flaps are the best choice for such defects. It is important that the Head and Neck MDTB consider the possibility of a delayed reconstruction in cases of skeletal tumor invasion, (1) because it is not possible to have an intraoperative pathological evaluation of margins; (2) because the detection of early recurrence inside the nose is more difficult being hidden by reconstruction; and (3) in case of further recurrence, we have exploited already the best possible reconstruction. Therefore, in such cases a reconstruction delayed after 6 months is often a wise decision. Lining may rely only for limited needs on turnover skin flaps in salvage cases. If radiotherapy has been used for primary therapy, the remaining nasal lining cannot be used as flaps to provide lining for reconstruction. The same applies for cartilage and mucosal flaps to be used for skeletal support: they are not reliable if radiotherapy or heavy scarring is present. Therefore, our first choice in salvage procedures of subtotal nasal reconstruction is a delayed three-step paramedian forehead folded flap. Lining is provided by folding of the flap for the caudal lining and by a full thickness skin graft for the remaining part. Skeletal support, according to the needs, is provided by cartilage costal grafts for dorsum and for columellar support, alar batten, or tip graft by auricular cartilage. The timing of reconstruction depends on the necessity of dorsal and columellar support ("L" strut). In cases "L" strut is not needed, the forehead flap is elevated and transposed in the first step with folding of the distal flap; the flap is elevated at the tip for defatting, inserting alar cartilage grafts and skin graft for lining after 3–4 weeks and sutured, without section of the pedicle; the pedicle is sectioned and removed with final remodeling in the third step. In cases "L" strut is needed, the first step consists of harvesting costal cartilage and pre-laminating the flap with insertion of the grafts between the skin and galea plane in the forehead in a position corresponding to the dorsum and the columella in the flap; in the second step after 3–4 weeks, the flap is elevated and the two grafts are fixed to the dorsum, to the area of nasal spine and between them at nose tip in a "L" fashion; skin graft for lining and alar graft can be added at this time; section of the pedicle and remodeling are performed after other 4 weeks in the final step [20].

3. Recurrences of nasal vestibular cancers in the area of the nostril still lead to defects on the tissue of the upper lip base of the ala nasi and columella, with possible involvement of maxillary bone and nasal spine. Destruction of nasal tip and caudal septum can result from bigger lesions. In these situations, it is imperative a reconstruction of what is called the platform of the nose with cheek or nasolabial flaps for soft tissues and cartilage grafts for nasal spine. It is noteworthy that reconstruction of the nasal platform is to be performed before sub-total nasal reconstruction with forehead or other flaps; otherwise, the resulting reconstruction will lack tip projection and will show midline retrusion.

4. In reconstruction of composite wide defects extending to neighbor anatomic areas or involving two or all vestibular subunits, the surgeon should first consider

if the use of locoregional available flaps will suffice; if not, the use of a free forearm flap for lining, associated with cartilage grafts and a forehead flap for skin cover, may be planned if patient clinical conditions would allow that. The radial forearm free flap is harvested in the first stage folded and transposed to the nose to reconstruct the nasal lining, the nasal sill, and nostrils, a skin graft covers dorsum. During following stages, cartilage grafts for support and a paramedian forehead flap for skin reconstruction complete nasal reconstruction.

Examples of such reconstructive options are provided in Figs. 15.1, 15.2, 15.3, and 15.4.

An alternative to full thickness subtotal surgical reconstruction of the nose is the use of a custom-made nasal prosthesis [19, 21, 22] (see Chap. 9).

It is an important alternative to surgical reconstruction to be discussed with the patients. It does not preclude further surgery, if necessary, it has a good aesthetic outcome and allows easy follow-up for recurrences. On the other hand, the need to be removed for daily maintenance and the fact that changes in facial skin tone and atrophy may cause discomfort and embarrassment to the patient. Furthermore, in post irradiation recurrences, the quality of the bone may pose issues to the placement of osteointegrated implants, which are the best option for prosthesis fixation. Therefore, pros and cons of the various alternatives must be discussed thoroughly with the patient.

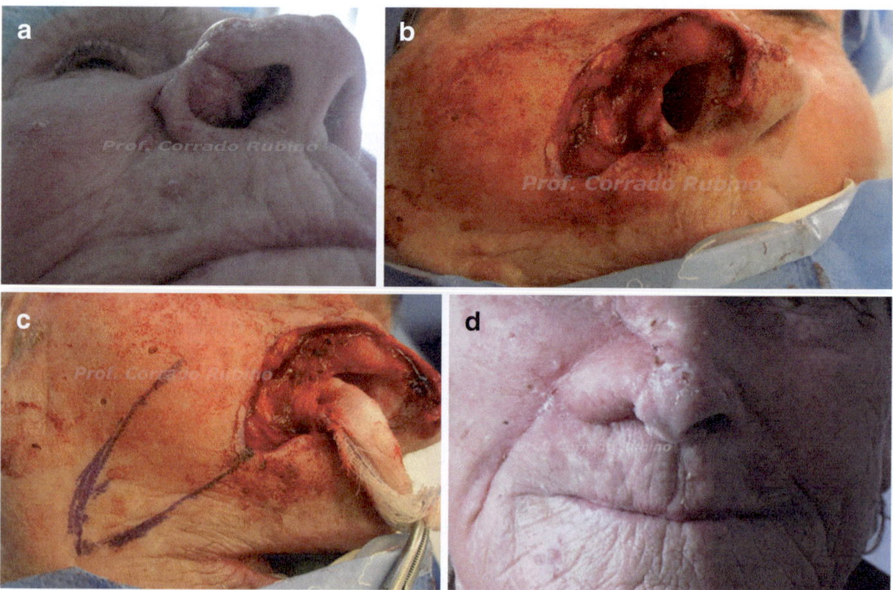

Fig. 15.1 (**a**) Recurrent neoplasm of the right nostril. (**b**) Defect after wide excision. (**c**) Marking of the right superior pedicle nasolabial flap. (**d**) Postoperative result after 6 months

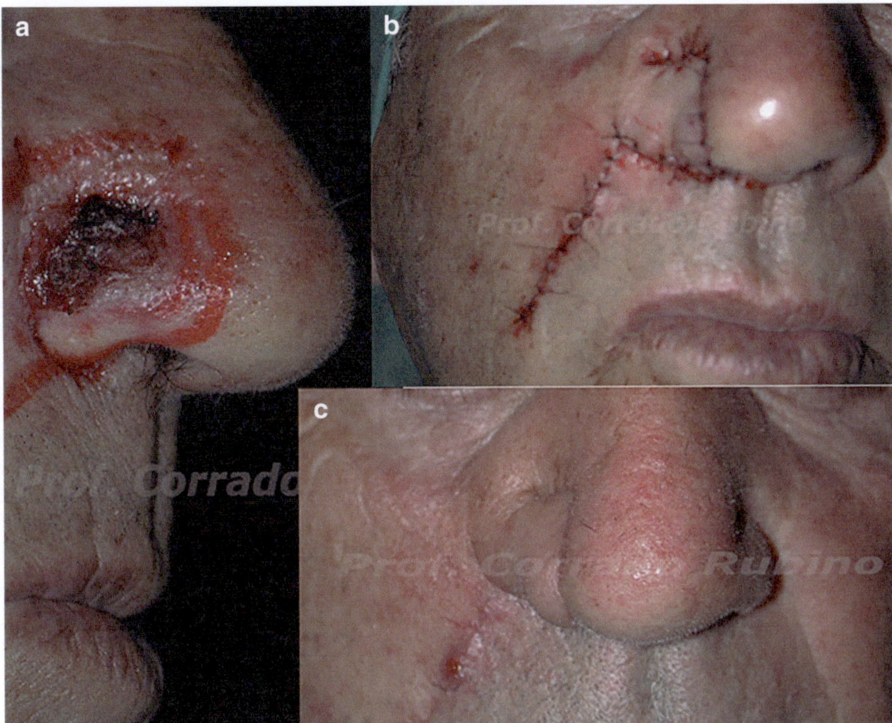

Fig. 15.2 (**a**) Recurrent neoplasm of the right nasal ala. (**b**) Reconstruction after pedicle nasolabial flap. (**c**) Postoperative result after 6 months

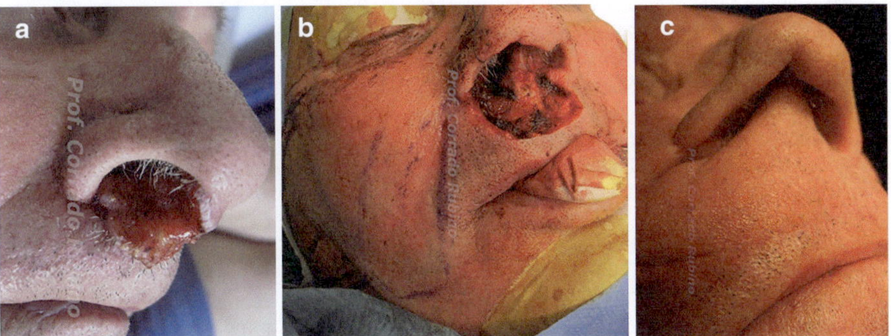

Fig. 15.3 (**a**) Infiltrative neoplasm of the right medial nasal vestibule. (**b**) Defect invading columella and cartilagineous septum and upper lip. Superior-based right nasolabial flap is marked. (**c**) Postoperative result after 1 year

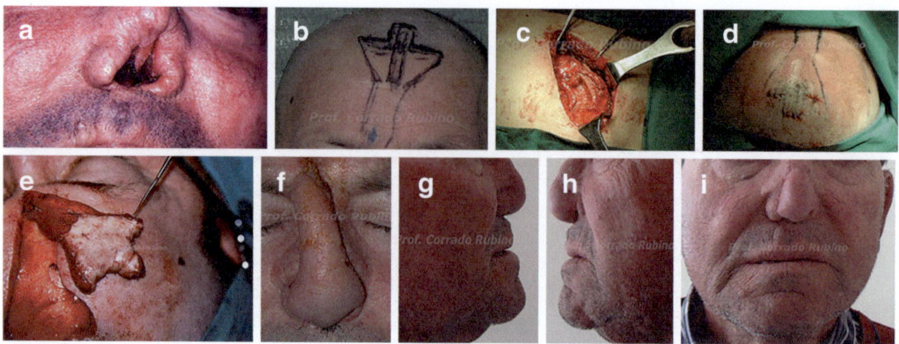

Fig. 15.4 (**a**) Subtotal resection after multiple treatments of neoplasm originated by left nose vestibule. (**b**) Planning of the first step showing the marking of the flap and the planned position of cartilagenous graft. (**c**) Costal cartilagenous graft harvesting. (**d**) Step I: result after insertion of cartilagenous graft into the forehead. (**e**) Step II: forehead flap harvested with the skin graft for lining. (**f**) The flap after 3 weeks after step 2. (**g**–**i**) Postoperative result 20 years after step III: resection of the pedicle and flap shaping

References

1. Bussu F, Tagliaferri L, Piras A, Rizzo D, Tsatsaris N, De Corso E, Parrilla C, Paludetti G. Multidisciplinary approach to nose vestibule malignancies: setting new standards. Approccio multidisciplinare ai tumori maligni del vestibolo del naso: verso la definizione di nuovi standard. Acta Otorhinolaryngologica Italica. 2021;41(Suppl. 1):S158–S165. https://doi.org/10.14639/0392-100X-suppl.1-41-2021-16.

2. Bussu F, Tagliaferri L, Crescio C, Rizzo D, Gallus R, Parrilla C, Fionda B, Lancellotta V, Mattiucci GC, Galli J. New standards for the management of nose vestibule malignancies. Acta Oto-Laryngologica. 2023;143(3):215–22. https://doi.org/10.1080/00016489.2023.2179662.

3. Czerwinski MD, van Leeuwen RGH, Kaanders J, Zwijnenburg EM, Lipman D, Takes RP, et al. Image guided brachytherapy for cancer of the nasal vestibule: local control and cosmesis. Int J Radiat Oncol Biol Phys. 2019;103(4):913–21.

4. Bussu F, Tagliaferri L, Mattiucci G, Parrilla C, Dinapoli N, Micciche F, et al. Comparison of interstitial brachytherapy and surgery as primary treatments for nasal vestibule carcinomas. Laryngoscope. 2016;126(2):367–71.

5. Zaoui K, Plinkert PK, Federspil PA. Primary surgical treatment of nasal vestibule cancer - therapeutic outcome and reconstructive strategies. Rhinology. 2018;56(4):393–9.

6. Langendijk JA, Poorter R, Leemans CR, de Bree R, Doornaert P, Slotman BJ. Radiotherapy of squamous cell carcinoma of the nasal vestibule. Int J Radiat Oncol Biol Phys. 2004;59(5):1319–25.

7. Bussu F, Tagliaferri L, De Corso E, Passali GC, Lancellotta V, Mattiucci GC, et al. Functional results of exclusive interventional radiotherapy (brachytherapy) in the treatment of nasal vestibule carcinomas. Brachytherapy. 2020;20:178.

8. Tagliaferri L, Fionda B, Bussu F, Parrilla C, Lancellotta V, Deodato F, et al. Interventional radiotherapy (brachytherapy) for squamous cell carcinoma of the nasal vestibule: a multidisciplinary systematic review. Eur J Dermatol. 2019;29(4):417–21.

9. Bussu F, Tagliaferri L, Mattiucci G, Parrilla C, Rizzo D, Gambacorta MA, Lancellotta V, Autorino R, Fonnesu C, Kihlgren C, Galli J, Paludetti G, Kovács G, Valentini V. HDR interventional radiotherapy (brachytherapy) in the treatment of primary and recurrent head and neck malignancies. Head Neck. 2019;41(6):1667–75.

10. Burget GC, Menick FJ. The subunit principle in nasal reconstruction. Plast Reconstr Surg. 1985;76(2):239–47.
11. Burget GC, Menick FJ. Nasal support and lining: the marriage of beauty and blood supply. Plast Reconstr Surg. 1989;84(2):189–202.
12. Burget GC, Menick FJ. Nasal reconstruction: seeking a fourth dimension. Plast Reconstr Surg. 1986;78(2):145–57.
13. Burget GC, Walton RL. Optimal use of microvascular free flaps, cartilage grafts, and a paramedian forehead flap for aesthetic reconstruction of the nose and adjacent facial units. Plast Reconstr Surg. 2007;120(5):1171–207; discussion 208–216.
14. Gary C, Burget FJM. Aesthetic reconstruction of the nose. St. Louis, MO: Mosby; 1994.
15. Menick F. Nasal reconstruction: art and practice. Philadelphia, PA: Saunders; 2008.
16. Menick FJ. A 10-year experience in nasal reconstruction with the three-stage forehead flap. Plast Reconstr Surg. 2002;109(6):1839–55; discussion 56-61.
17. Menick FJ, Salibian A. Microvascular repair of heminasal, subtotal, and total nasal defects with a folded radial forearm flap and a full-thickness forehead flap. Plast Reconstr Surg. 2011;127(2):637–51.
18. Qian C, Yaodong X, Xiaoming H, Shaochong F, Yiqing Z. Repair of full-thickness alar defects. Dermatol Surg. 2012;38(10):1639–44.
19. Malard O, Lanhouet J, Michel G, Dreno B, Espitalier F, Rio E. Full-thickness nasal defect: place of prosthetic reconstruction. Eur Ann Otorhinolaryngol Head Neck Dis. 2015;132(2):85–9.
20. Rubino C, Sanna M, Figus A, Farace F, Bocchiotti MA. Three-dimensional prelaminated forehead flap: two cases of composite nasal reconstruction. Rivista Italiana di Chirurgia Plastica. 2004;36:39–44.
21. Romo T III, Pearson JM. Nasal implants. Facial Plast Surg Clin North Am. 2008;16(1):123–32, vi.
22. Romo T III, McLaughlin LA, Levine JM, Sclafani AP. Nasal implants: autogenous, semisynthetic, and synthetic. Facial Plast Surg Clin North Am. 2002;10(2):155–66.

Setting New Standards for Nasal Vestibule Malignancies

16

Francesco Bussu, Luca Tagliaferri, Michal Czerwinski, Agata Rembielak, Claudia Crescio, Lia Verhoef, Gyorgy Kovacs, Jacopo Galli, and Vincenzo Valentini

16.1 Setting New Standards for Classification and Staging

Squamous cell carcinoma (SCC) of the nasal vestibule (NV) is usually considered to be a relatively rare cancer, accounting for about 1% of all head and neck malignancies [1]. A Danish group estimated an annual incidence of squamous cell of the

F. Bussu
Otolaryngology Division, Azienda Ospedaliera Universitaria di Sassari, Sassari, Italy

Department of Medicine, Surgery and Pharmacy, University of Sassari, Sassari, Italy

L. Tagliaferri · V. Valentini
UOC Radioterapia Oncologica, Dipartimento di Diagnostica per Immagini, Radioterapia Oncologica ed Ematologia, Fondazione Policlinico Universitario A. Gemelli, IRCCS, Rome, Italy
e-mail: luca.tagliaferri@policlinicogemelli.it; vincenzo.valentini@policlinicogemelli.it

M. Czerwinski · L. Verhoef
Radiation Oncology, Radboud University Medical Centre, Nijmegen, Netherlands
e-mail: Michal.Czerwinski@radboudumc.nl; Lia.Verhoef@radboudumc.nl

A. Rembielak
Clinical Oncology, The Christie NHS Foundation Trust, Manchester, UK
e-mail: agata.rembielak@nhs.net

C. Crescio (✉)
Otolaryngology Division, Azienda Ospedaliera Universitaria, Sassari, Italy
e-mail: claudia.crescio@aouss.it; ccrescio1@uniss.it

G. Kovacs
Gemelli-INTERACTS, Università Cattolica del Sacro Cuore, Rome, Italy
e-mail: gyorgy.kovacs@unicatt.it

J. Galli
Unit of Otorhinolaryngology, "A. Gemelli" University Hospital Foundation, IRCCS, Rome, Italy

Department of Head-Neck and Sensory Orngans, Università Cattolica del Sacro Cuore, Rome, Italy
e-mail: jacopo.galli@unicatt.it

© Springer Nature Switzerland AG 2023
F. Bussu (ed.), *Malignancies of the Nasal Vestibule*,
https://doi.org/10.1007/978-3-031-32850-3_16

nasal vestibule of 0.41 per 100,000 inhabitants [2, 3]. Nevertheless, we believe that this prevalence is largely underestimated because of two clear reasons:

- the frequent misdiagnosis and misclassification of these lesions as primary skin malignancies;
- in the WHO International Classification of Diseases for Oncology (ICD-O), nasal vestibule malignancies [4] are classified together and assigned the same topographic code (C30.0) as those of the rest of the nasal cavity (nasal cavity proper); therefore, their real prevalence cannot be extrapolated from most cancer registries.

1. The first issue derives from the peculiar pattern of spread of nasal vestibule cancers (see Chap. 3). They infiltrate the skin very early, following a path along the nasal cartilages. The external cutaneous part of the lesion is most easily noticed and often treated by non-ENT surgeons, leaving the root of the lesion in the nasal vestibule untreated. This can potentially result in multiple recurrences and an oncological and cosmetic disaster for the patient. Therefore, we recommend that all suspicious lesions of the (peri)nasal skin discovered by general practitioners, dermatologists, or plastic surgeons should be referred for an ENT evaluation, to exclude a nasal vestibule primary before treatment decisions are made.

   In fact, it should be obvious that the therapeutic approach to a primary nasal vestibule cancer is completely different than that to a primary skin cancer. This is particularly true in case of primary surgical treatment, which must always be radical: in case of a skin primary, nasal tip cartilages can often be spared with negative margins, and a full thickness ("through") resection is only necessary in locally advanced cases. On the contrary, when the primary tumor arises in the nasal vestibule, their typical spread along and between cartilages most often calls for a "through" resection also in early lesions, with the known reconstructive issues (see Chaps. 3, 8, and 9).

2. A single WHO topographic code for the nasal vestibule and nasal cavity proper is in our opinion no longer acceptable, as has been explained in the previous chapters. The most important reasons are in summary:
   (a) The abovementioned impossibility to accurately estimate the respective prevalence as well as prognosis of nasal vestibule and nasal cavity proper cancers using cancer registries mostly based on WHO codes.
   (b) The inherent huge differences between nasal vestibule and nasal cavity malignancies in terms of histopathology (see Chap. 2), clinical history, metastatic behavior, patterns of spread (see Chap. 3), and responsivity to different treatment modalities (see Chaps. 6–11).

However, defining a specific topographic code for the nasal vestibule would not be the only necessary change.

In fact, the current AJCC staging criteria for primary lesions of the nasal vestibule (T) are identical to the nasal cavity proper and ethmoid, but the distinct anatomical features and spreading patterns clearly make these criteria inadequate for tumors of the nasal vestibule [1, 2, 4–7]. For example, skin invasion through the nasal valve (mostly deep to alar and superficial to lateral nasal cartilage) is almost constant among SCC involving the lateral wall of the NV (see Chap. 3) and makes most of them cT4a according to AJCC. On the other hand, paradoxically, bony invasion, which, according to the AJCC, can be present even in cT1 ethmoid/nasal cavity lesions, is seen only in the bulkiest, most difficult to treat, vestibular SCC and predicts worse tumor control [1, 5–7]. Back in 1976, C. C. Wang outlined that "there is no acceptable classification for tumors of the nasal vestibule" and proposed a classification of primary lesions (T) specific for the nasal vestibule [8] (Table 16.1). The Wang classification gives a more appropriate relevance and weight to skin and bone invasion and has been reported to be a better prognostic tool than recent AJCC/UICC T-classifications. It remains broadly used in staging of nasal vestibule malignancies [1, 3, 5–7, 9]. In spite of that, the Wang classification can result difficult to apply in daily practice and to lower it down to AJCC/UICC classification as it is, mainly for three reasons (see Chap. 5):

- There are only three T classes (and not four, as is usual in the AJCC/UICC classification).
- Clear anatomical landmarks identifiable both clinically and radiologically are not defined.
- There is a lack of objective parameters in particular to discriminate between T2 and T3 (e.g., it is not clear what is meant with "massive lip invasion").

16.1.1 Rethinking the Classification and Staging of Nasal Vestibule Malignancies

Based on the above considerations, there is a need for a shared international standard for classification and staging of nasal vestibule malignancies (in particular SCC). We propose two changes to the current TNM based on the evidence mentioned above.

Table 16.1 Preliminary proposal of a new T-classification in nasal vestibule malignancies

T1	The lesion is limited to the nasal vestibule internal surface (skin and/or mucosa)
T2a	The lesion invades superficial structures outside the nasal cavity (skin and subcutaneous planes), in particular the upper lip, philtrum, the skin of the nose and/or nasolabial fold, but does not destroy cartilage, nor invade bony structures or structures beyond the plane of the pyriform aperture (septum, lateral wall, turbinates, etc.)
T2b	Disruption of cartilages is evident, without invasion of bony structures, nor structures beyond the plane of the pyriform aperture (septum, lateral wall, turbinates, etc.)
T3	The lesion extends beyond the pyriform aperture (septum, lateral wall, turbinates, etc.)
T4a	The lesion invades bony structures such as the hard palate, nasal bones, frontal process of the maxilla, the ethmoid, and the orbit
T4b	Tumor invades any of the following: orbital apex, dura, brain, anterior and middle cranial fossa, cranial nerves other than (V2), nasopharynx, or clivus

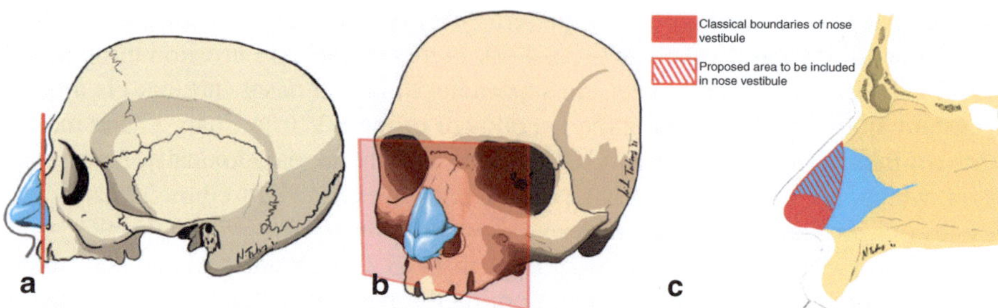

Fig. 16.1 The acknowledgement of the nasal vestibule as a distinct subsite of the nose is proposed, based on anatomical (**a**), radiological (**b**) and oncological criteria (**c**). The posterior boundary, easy to identify also on imaging, would be a tangential plane along the piriform opening. This will lead to the inclusion of a wider area in the "nasal vestibule" (**c**)

1. Clearly define the boundaries of nasal vestibule, which would encompass the portion of the nasal cavity extending from the pyriform opening to the nostrils (Fig. 16.1 see Chap. 1 [10, 11]). A specific WHO topographical code should be assigned to this subsite, distinct from nasal cavity proper. Nasal vestibule shall become the third subsite for nasal and paranasal malignancies in AJCC/UICC staging manual. ~~This would allow to better define the diagnosis and assess specific incidence of nasal vestibule malignancies;~~
2. Consequently, define specific AJCC T classification criteria for the nasal vestibule, distinct from the existing ones for nasal cavity (proper)/ethmoid and maxillary sinus, which are the two currently acknowledged subsites with specific staging criteria. Such criteria, mostly borrowed from the Wang staging system, will retain its improved predictive power. ~~This will allow to better predict prognosis and also to standardize treatment strategy, considering the peculiar aspects of malignancies of the nasal vestibule. Such criteria will be partly borrowed from the Wang classification.~~ A hypothetical draft of the new T classification is reported in Chap. 5 (Table 16.1) [10–12].

16.2 Current Treatment Options for Nasal Vestibule SCCs: Evidence Supporting Brachytherapy as the New Standard for Treatment of the Primary Lesion

16.2.1 Oncological Outcomes

Surgery, External Beam Radiotherapy (EBRT) and Interventional Radiotherapy (IRT, Brachytherapy, BT) are the currently employed therapeutic options in clinical practice [2, 9–19]. As discussed in Chap. 14, it must never be forgotten that the main issue in head and neck SCC is the neck, so a careful staging of the neck must be carried out, resorting also to fine needle biopsy (which in our opinion is particularly reliable when performed in a lump clinic, by an head and neck surgeon, under US guidance, and with rapid onsite evaluation by a cytopathologist) [13, 20] or to PET CT in doubtful cases. If neck treatment is indicated, it is rational to use the same treatment modality than for T (surgery or EBRT). If the treatment modality on the primary lesion is IRT, being it a very conformal, "local" treatment, a sort of radio-surgery of the primary lesion, it is in our opinion more rational to manage the neck by surgery performing neck dissection(s) when indicated (see Chap. 14). Postoperative radiotherapy for the neck might be indicated, basing upon the histopathology report (in these cases, a VMAT technique may be used, tapering the EBRT dose toward the brachy area, and covering also the moustache nodes). Recent papers focusing on the comparison between surgery and IRT [5] and on IRT alone [6, 21, 22] for the treatment of the primary lesion showed that brachytherapy is not inferior to surgery as for oncological results (OS over 90% in cT1 and cT2 according to Wang) and is most likely superior to EBRT [14]. Many older retrospective studies also support the findings of excellent local control of IRT [9, 18, 23, 24].

In addition, cosmetic and functional issues are of great importance for treatment selection particularly in this site.

16.2.2 Cosmetic Outcomes

The aesthetic appearance can be deeply impacted by any therapeutic procedure involving the nose and the nasal vestibule in particular, which is substantially the inner surface of the nose tip [1, 5, 7]. After ablative surgery, the reconstruction of the cartilaginous framework of the nasal tip, is notoriously extremely difficult for at least two reasons:

- These areas are the most exposed and readily visible parts of the entire body, where light and human eyes always land. Therefore, minimal imperfections, scars, color mismatches, and deformities can have a highly significant esthetical and social impact.
- It is practically impossible to faithfully restore the complex pattern of raised relieves and dips, created by the nasal cartilages and underlying maxillary and nasal bones on the nose tip, with surgery. Free flaps, which have drastically changed head and neck surgical oncology in the last few decades, are not making a resolutive impact here (see Chap. 8). According to several authors [2, 17, 25], in case of total or subtotal rhinectomy defects, bone anchored prosthesis remains the best option from an esthetical point of view (see Chap. 9).

Therefore, preserving the anatomical structures, and especially the osseocartilaginous framework, is the best option from a cosmetic point of view in midface and nasal vestibule malignancies [5, 17]. In addition, if we consider that nose cartilage itself generally tolerates radiation very well (if the trophic support by perichondrium is preserved), the preservation of the nose tip framework, with consequently markedly better cosmetic results, reported for high dose rate (HDR) IRT (Fig. 16.2) when compared to surgery (see Chap. 7) [5], can be easily explained. For the same reasons, also EBRT is considered a valid alternative option from an esthetic point of view [3, 15–17, 24, 26] and is currently probably the most frequently recommended primary treatment in Western countries [15, 26]. However, both oncological [14] (see functional outcomes) [21] of IRT are superior to EBRT in case of nasal vestibule malignancies.

16.2.3 Functional Outcomes

The nose is primarily part of the respiratory system, being the first section of the airway passed through by inhaled air. Thus, by evolution, the nose has developed

Fig. 16.2 A series of nasal vestibule cases implanted in different institutions between 2011 and 2022 by the same surgeon (FB) and treated by exclusive IRT on the primary lesion: the primary lesion, the pattern of spread (Before treatment) as well as the oncological and the cosmetic results (After treatment) are shown. *Patient 1*: A bulky lesion involving all the walls of the nasal vestibule and extensively spreading to the nasal and lip skin is shown before treatment. One year after exclusive IRT and bilateral prophylactic neck dissection (1 involved node on the right side, pT1), the cosmetic appearance is pretty satisfying considering that surgery would have required total rhinectomy enlarged to the superior lip and probably to the maxillary bone. The patients is still undergoing follow-up and is alive and well without evidence of disease 5 years after the primary treatment. *Patient 2*: A bulky lesion spreading between the cartilages and the nasal bones is shown before treatment. Bone was involved. After IRT, a complete response and an acceptable cosmetic result are shown, yet 6 months later the patient experienced progressive disease from a recurrence in the pterygoid fossa (perivascular spread?) and died from disease. *Patient 3*: "Classical" nasal vestibule SCC arising between the lateral and the medial wall and spreading to the subcutaneous tissue sliding between the alar and lateral cartilages is shown before treatment. Two years after IRT, cosmetic results appear good despite a slight retraction of the ala of the nasal. The patient is alive and free of disease 11 years after the primary treatment. *Patient 4*: Before treatment, the SCC carcinoma of the nasal vestibule arose from the anterior part of the septum, showing signs of initial invasion of the subcutaneous area on the nasal tip. Five months after IRT treatment, the cosmetic result is already good. One year after treatment, the patient is still alive and free of disease. *Patient 5*: The invasion of a nasal vestibule SCC spreading between the lateral cartilage and the nasal bones is shown before treatment. Forty months after IRT treatment, the patient is alive and free of disease. Cosmetic outcome is more than fair. *Patient 6*: A case of a primary SCC of the vestibular septum is shown before and 1 year after IRT treatment. The patient is alive and free of disease 10 years after treatment. *Patient 7*: A bulky lesion spreading extensively to the skin of the nasal tip from the lateral wall of the nasal vestibule is shown before treatment. One year after the IRT, the cosmetic outcome is extremely satisfying as surgery would have required total rhinectomy. The patient is alive and free of disease 8 years after the treatment. *Patient 8*: A lesion arising from the inferior and medial wall of the nasal vestibule and spreading to the superior lip is shown before treatment. Six months after IRT, the cosmetic results are very good. The patient is alive and free of disease 2 years after. *Patient 9*: Primary bilateral lesion of the medial wall of the vestibule and of the columella spreading to the nasal spine. Six months after IRT, the cosmetic results were acceptable. The patient experienced a small recurrence on the nasal spine, which was successfully salvaged and is alive and free of disease 8 years after the treatment

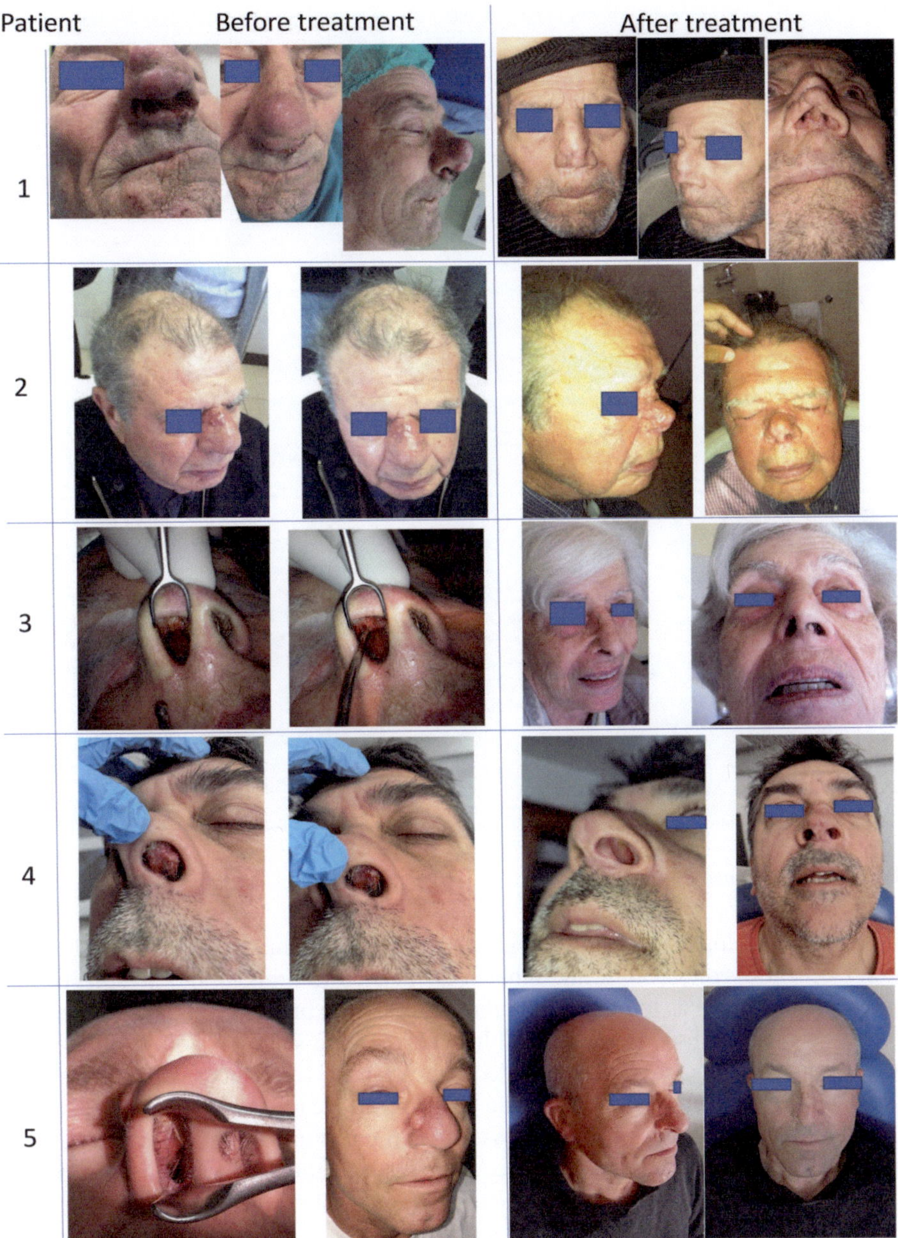

Patient
Before treatment
After treatment
1
2
3
4
5

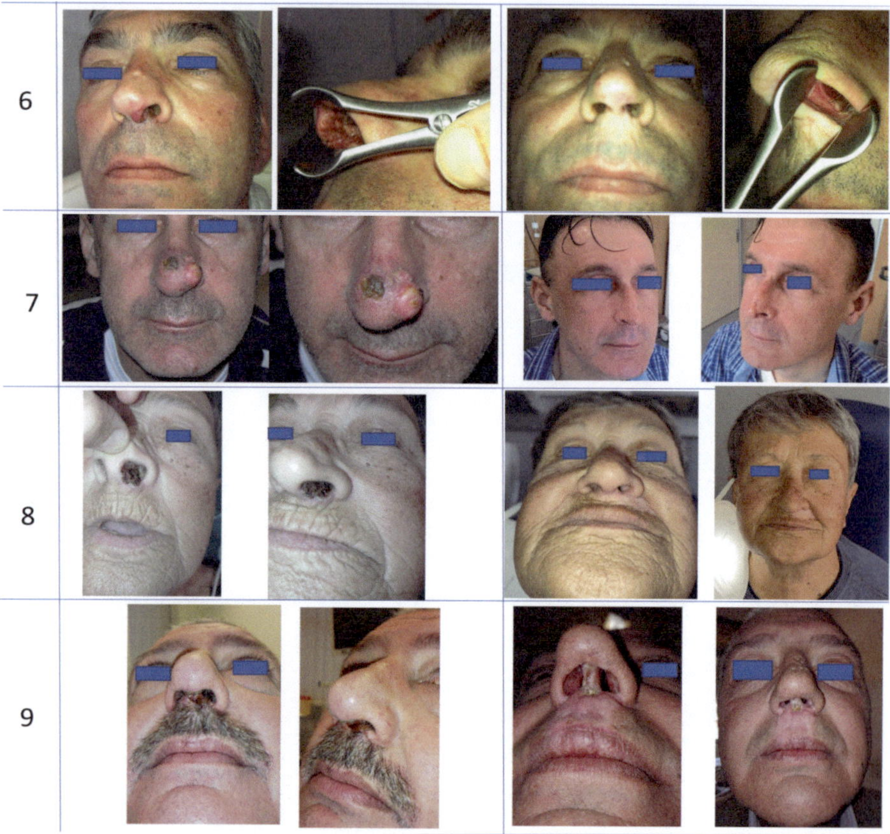

Fig. 16.2 (continued)

multiple physiologic strategies to regulate flow speed, temperature, and humidification (somehow conditioning the inhaled air headed to bronchi and alveoli) of the inspired air, as well as to tightly modulate its ability to protect itself and the respiratory system as a whole from external hazards. Among such physiologic strategies, we can distinguish maintenance of adequate intranasal resistances within the physiologic variations during the nasal cycle [27], the sneeze reflex [28], and the complex immunological and mechanical defense system constituted by nasal mucosa, with all its cellular components (both in the ciliated epithelium and in the stroma) and the mucus itself. One of the most characteristic and well-known expressions of this defensive system is the mucociliary clearance.

Disturbances in any of the above physiological functions may be secondary to gross anatomical variations, such as after oncological surgery, or to other pathological processes involving and affecting one or more of the above mechanisms, mainly at the level of the nasal mucosa, such as in the case of irradiation, which notoriously harbors acute and especially late toxicity.

With the knowledge that evidence supporting EBRT versus IRT is lacking from a cosmetic point of view, we recently compared both modalities in terms of outcomes in nasal function [21]. Nasal functions are notoriously affected by radiation [29–31], and many complaints from patients with a history of nasal radiotherapy, such as crusting [31], nose dryness [32], dysosmia [30, 33], and dysgeusia [30], are clearly linked to the disruption of physiological mechanisms by the mucosal toxicity of radiotherapy [32, 34, 35]. By performing specific tests, most of these physiological alterations have been recently confirmed after EBRT, but were not found after IRT [21], which was associated with a substantial preservation of nasal function and cytological findings. The rapid dose fall-off specific for IRT, which can also be exploited in the adjuvant/perioperative setting [36, 37], results in a drastic reduction of the irradiated mucosal surface inside the nasal/paranasal cavities and may be a decisive factor in this.

16.2.4 The New Standard

Such evidence, together with the confirmation of the oncological effectiveness, which of course remains the most relevant argument, supports the establishment of interstitial IRT as the new standard for the treatment of the primary lesion in cT1 and cT2 (according to the Wang classification) NV SCCs.

16.3 Implantation Technique for Nasal Vestibule Primaries

The aim of functional and especially cosmetic preservation in patients with nasal vestibule carcinoma can be achieved through the preservation of the cartilaginous framework of the nasal tip that has not yet been compromised by tumor growth. It is well known, also from laryngeal oncology [38], that cartilage itself is particularly resistant to tumor invasion since it is devoid of blood vessels and fed through the interstitium by direct diffusion from vascularized perichondrium [39], and that as blood vessels are brought in by ossification, the probability of direct invasion drastically increases. In the nose, the situation is more favorable, as nasal cartilages, unlike laryngeal- and thyroidal ones in particular, do not usually get ossified even in the elderly; therefore, direct invasion occurs in a late stage in nasal vestibule SCCs (see Chap. 3). This fact, combined with the resistance and low toxicity rates of radiotherapy on cartilages [5, 21, 40–43], can benefit the cartilage preservation and cosmetic results after irradiation of these malignancies.

However, a notorious long-term toxicity of IRT in the nasal vestibule is chondronecrosis and consequential septal (and in rare cases even alar) perforations [18]. These sequelae are reported more frequently after interstitial delivery than when using a endocavitary/mold technique [18], suggesting that chondronecrosis potentially occurs due to the mechanical damage and interruption of the mucoperichondrium (which feeds the cartilage) rather than by the radiation damage to cartilage itself. It is not surprising for nose surgeons who know very well that septal perforations, even in functional surgery of the nose, always derive from the interruption of mucoperichondrium. Starting from this awareness, we modified our implantation technique (see Chap. 13), basing on the principle of avoiding perforation of the mucoperichondrium, we support, as long as it is possible to obtain a proper coverage of the CTV, "fully" interstitial implantation, which is also more stable and therefore reliable. To support this, we entrust the implantation phase of nasal vestibule SCCs to skilled nasal surgeons who insert the plastic tubes along the subperichondral planes, the main dissection routes of functional and aesthetic surgery of the nose (Fig. 16.3). This anatomic implantation technique, systematically preserving the mucoperichondrium, resulted in no septal perforation whatsoever in our experience, with markedly better results than in previous series [18]. This "anatomic" implantation technique may conflict with the "classical" Paris system [44], which prioritizes an optimal dose distribution through tridimensional geometric rules. Adhering to the Paris system may be especially important, for example, using linear LDR sources, but the features of modern interventional radiotherapy (HDR stepping source technology combined with image guidance) allow for dose modulation that results in a very good dose distribution even after "anatomic" implantation.

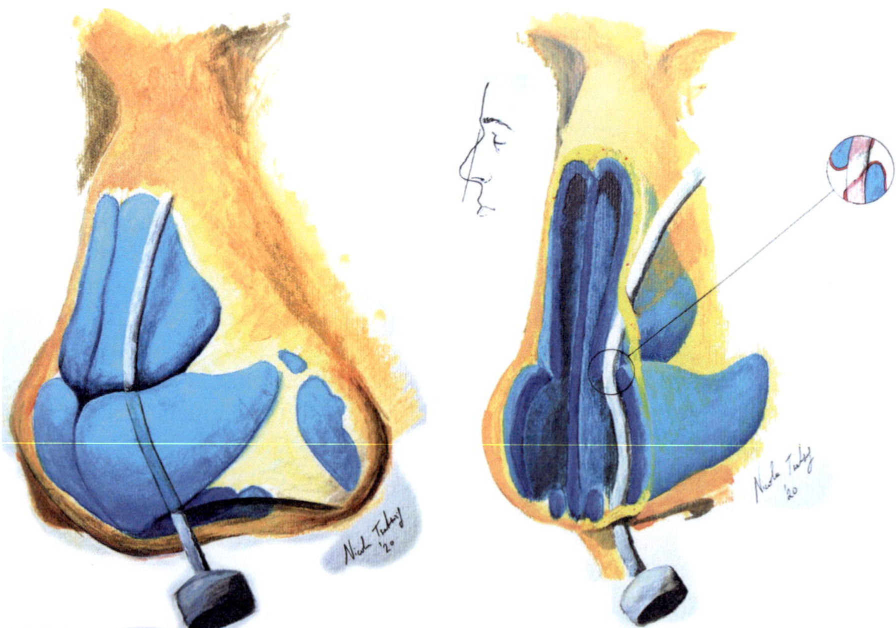

Fig. 16.3 The plastic tubes are ideally placed along the subperichondral route. Cartilages and perichondrium should not be disrupted, and the tubes should pass from the submucosal to the subcutaneous plane through the junction between the alar and lateral cartilages. Such an implant is particularly fit for primary tumor invading the skin. In substance, ideally, the implant should follow the same route as malignancy along cartilagineous surfaces

This approach achieves a low toxicity rate and high local control, which is not inferior to other brachytherapy series [5, 7, 9, 18, 21, 22].

Nevertheless, in order to emphasize these innovations, we strongly advocate to call this treatment modality for all the indications (and not only for nasal vestibule) "interventional radiotherapy", replacing the old term "brachytherapy" [45].

16.4 Conclusions: Toward New Standards

The abovementioned evidence and considerations all point to the need for a paradigm shift in various phases of nasal vestibule carcinoma management:

1. *Diagnosis and staging.* The nasal vestibule should be considered a distinct subsite in the nose, with its own refined T-classification, based on the Wang staging with some improvements (Table 16.1).
2. *Treatment choice.* IRT (administered with HDR) offers clear advantages in terms of oncological, cosmetic, and functional results and should be considered the new standard for early stage primary lesions; cT1-2, according to Wang, and cT1-2-3 according to the novel classification (Fig. 16.4). When neck treatment is

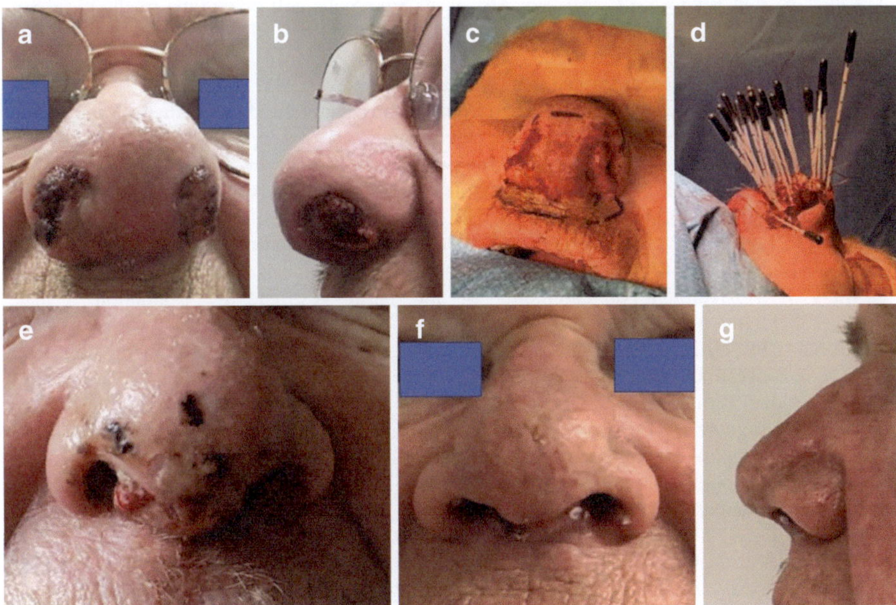

Fig. 16.4 A bulky (**a**, **b**) nasal vestibule cancer located in the columella (median wall), successfully treated by IRT (**c**, **d**) at the Radboud University Medical Centre Nijmegen, The Netherlands. Early (shortly after removal of the catheters **e**), and late (**f**, **g**) results are displayed. Cosmetic and functional outcomes are very satisfying

indicated (either elective or therapeutic), we recommend surgery for the neck (neck dissection) combined with IRT to the primary lesion. The role of sentinel node biopsy in high-risk cN0 nasal vestibule carcinoma is currently being evaluated [46].

When nodal risk factors such as extranodal extension are found, or in case regional recurrence, additional EBRT to the neck remains a viable option.

3. *IRT technique.* The most feared long-term toxicity of IRT in the nasal vestibule is chondronecrosis and consequential perforations due to mechanical damage to the perichondrium. This can be avoided using an anatomic implantation of plastic tubes, which should be placed along the subperichondral planes classically exploited in nasal surgery. The dose distribution can then be optimized by image-guided treatment planning and intensity modulation.

References

1. Jeannon JP, Riddle PJ, Irish J, O'sullivan B, Brown DH, Gullane P. Prognostic indicators in carcinoma of the nasal vestibule. Clin Otolaryngol. 2007;32(1):19–23.
2. Vital D, Morand G, Huber GF, Studer G, Holzmann D. Outcome in squamous cell carcinoma of the nasal vestibule: a single center experience. Head Neck. 2015;37(1):46–51.
3. Agger A, von Buchwald C, Madsen AR, et al. Squamous cell carcinoma of the nasal vestibule 1993-2002: a nationwide retrospective study from DAHANCA. Head Neck. 2009;31(12):1593–9.
4. Amin MB. AJCC: Cancer staging manual. 8th ed. New York, NY: Springer; 2017.
5. Bussu F, Tagliaferri L, Mattiucci G, et al. Comparison of interstitial brachytherapy and surgery as primary treatments for nasal vestibule carcinomas. Laryngoscope. 2016;126(2):367–71.
6. Tagliaferri L, Fionda B, Bussu F, et al. Interventional radiotherapy (brachytherapy) for squamous cell carcinoma of the nasal vestibule: a multidisciplinary systematic review. Eur J Dermatol. 2019;29(4):417–21.
7. Bussu F, Tagliaferri L, Mattiucci G, et al. HDR interventional radiotherapy (brachytherapy) in the treatment of primary and recurrent head and neck malignancies. Head Neck. 2019;41:1667.
8. Wang CC. Treatment of carcinoma of the nasal vestibule by irradiation. Cancer. 1976;38(1):100–6.
9. Levendag PC, Nijdam WM, van Moolenburgh SE, et al. Interstitial radiation therapy for early-stage nasal vestibule cancer: a continuing quest for optimal tumor control and cosmesis. Int J Radiat Oncol Biol Phys. 2006;66(1):160–9.
10. Bussu F, Tagliaferri L, Piras A, Rizzo D, Tsatsaris N, De Corso E, Parrilla C, Paludetti G. Multidisciplinary approach to nose vestibule malignancies: setting new standards. Approccio multidisciplinare ai tumori maligni del vestibolo del naso: verso la definizione di nuovi standard. Acta Otorhinolaryngologica Italica. 2021;41(Suppl. 1):S158–S165. https://doi.org/10.14639/0392-100X-suppl.1-41-2021-16.
11. Bussu F, et al. New standards for the management of nose vestibule malignancies. Acta Oto-Laryngologica. 2023;143(3):215–22. https://doi.org/10.1080/00016489.2023.2179662.
12. Evaluation of Staging Systems for Cancer of the Nasal Vestibule Cancers. 2023;15(11):3028. https://doi.org/10.3390/cancers15113028.
13. Petrone G, Rossi ED, Gallus R, Petrelli L, Marrone S, Rizzo D, Piras A, Garofalo G, Rindi G, Galli J, et al. Utility of ultrasound-guided fine needle aspiration cytology in assessing malignancy in head and neck pathology. Cytopathology. 2021;32:407–15. https://doi.org/10.1111/cyt.12955.

14. Czerwinski MD, Jansen PP, Zwijnenburg EM, Al-Mamgani A, Vergeer MR, Langendijk JA, Wesseling FWR, Kaanders JHAM, Verhoef CG. Radiotherapy as nasal preservation treatment strategy for cancer of the nasal vestibule: the Dutch experience. Radiother Oncol. 2021;164:20–6. https://doi.org/10.1016/j.radonc.2021.08.018. Epub 2021 Sep 4. PMID: 34487765.
15. Horsmans JD, Godballe C, Jorgensen KE, Bastholt L, Lontoft E. Squamous cell carcinoma of the nasal vestibule. Rhinology. 1999;37(3):117–21.
16. Guinot JL, Rembielak A, Perez-Calatayud J, et al. GEC-ESTRO ACROP recommendations in skin brachytherapy. Radiother Oncol. 2018;126(3):377–85.
17. Goepfert H. The vex and fuss about nasal vestibule cancer. Head Neck. 1999;21(5):383–4.
18. Lipman D, Verhoef LC, Takes RP, Kaanders JH, Janssens GO. Outcome and toxicity profile after brachytherapy for squamous cell carcinoma of the nasal vestibule. Head Neck. 2015;37(9):1297–303.
19. Koopmann M, Weiss D, Savvas E, Rudack C, Stenner M. Clinicopathological and immunohistochemical characteristics of surgically treated primary carcinoma of the nasal vestibule- an evaluation of 30 cases. Clin Otolaryngol. 2014;40:240.
20. Preoperative Diagnosis of Warthin Tumors Combining Cytological Clinical and Ultrasonographic Information within a Multidisciplinary Approach in a Lump Clinic Journal of Personalized Medicine. 2023;13(7):1075. https://doi.org/10.3390/jpm13071075.
21. Bussu F, Tagliaferri L, De Corso E, et al. Functional results of exclusive interventional radiotherapy (brachytherapy) in the treatment of nasal vestibule carcinomas. Brachytherapy. 2020;20:178.
22. Czerwinski MD, van Leeuwen RGH, Kaanders J, et al. Image guided brachytherapy for cancer of the nasal vestibule: local control and cosmesis. Int J Radiat Oncol Biol Phys. 2019;103(4):913–21.
23. Lancellotta V, Kovacs G, Tagliaferri L, et al. The role of personalized Interventional Radiotherapy (brachytherapy) in the management of older patients with non-melanoma skin cancer. J Geriatr Oncol. 2019;10(3):514–7.
24. Langendijk JA, Poorter R, Leemans CR, de Bree R, Doornaert P, Slotman BJ. Radiotherapy of squamous cell carcinoma of the nasal vestibule. Int J Radiat Oncol Biol Phys. 2004;59(5):1319–25.
25. Wagenblast J, Baghi M, Helbig M, et al. Craniofacial reconstructions with bone-anchored epithesis in head and neck cancer patients--a valid way back to self-perception and social reintegration. Anticancer Res. 2008;28(4C):2349–52.
26. Mendenhall WM, Stringer SP, Cassisi NJ, Mendenhall NP. Squamous cell carcinoma of the nasal vestibule. Head Neck. 1999;21(5):385–93.
27. Mirza N, Lanza DC. The nasal airway and obstructed breathing during sleep. Otolaryngol Clin N Am. 1999;32(2):243–62.
28. Nonaka S, Unno T, Ohta Y, Mori S. Sneeze-evoking region within the brainstem. Brain Res. 1990;511(2):265–70.
29. Kilic C, Tuncel U, Comert E, Kaya BV. The effect of radiotherapy on mucociliary clearance in patients with laryngeal and nasopharyngeal cancer. Eur Arch Otorhinolaryngol. 2015;272(6):1517–20.
30. Alvarez-Camacho M, Gonella S, Campbell S, Scrimger RA, Wismer WV. A systematic review of smell alterations after radiotherapy for head and neck cancer. Cancer Treat Rev. 2017;54:110–21.
31. Kamel R, Al-Badawy S, Khairy A, Kandil T, Sabry A. Nasal and paranasal sinus changes after radiotherapy for nasopharyngeal carcinoma. Acta Otolaryngol. 2004;124(4):532–5.
32. Surico G, Muggeo P, Mappa L, et al. Impairment of nasal mucociliary clearance after radiotherapy for childhood head cancer. Head Neck. 2001;23(6):461–6.
33. Holscher T, Seibt A, Appold S, et al. Effects of radiotherapy on olfactory function. Radiother Oncol. 2005;77(2):157–63.
34. Stringer SP, Stiles W, Slattery WH III, et al. Nasal mucociliary clearance after radiation therapy. Laryngoscope. 1995;105(4 Pt 1):380–2.

35. Riva G, Boita M, Ravera M, et al. Nasal cytological changes as late effects of radiotherapy for nasopharyngeal cancer. Am J Rhinol Allergy. 2015;29(2):e41–5.
36. Tagliaferri L, Bussu F, Rigante M, et al. Endoscopy-guided brachytherapy for sinonasal and nasopharyngeal recurrences. Brachytherapy. 2015;14(3):419–25.
37. Tagliaferri L, Bussu F, Fionda B, et al. Perioperative HDR brachytherapy for reirradiation in head and neck recurrences: single-institution experience and systematic review. Tumori. 2017;103(6):516–24.
38. Mor N, Blitzer A. Functional anatomy and oncologic barriers of the larynx. Otolaryngol Clin N Am. 2015;48(4):533–45.
39. Sandell LJ. Novel functions for type II procollagen. Connect Tissue Res. 2014;55(1):20–5.
40. Caccialanza M, Piccinno R, Percivalle S, Rozza M. Radiotherapy of carcinomas of the skin overlying the cartilage of the nasal: our experience in 671 lesions. J Eur Acad Dermatol Venereol. 2009;23(9):1044–9.
41. Caccialanza M, Piccinno R, Moretti D, Rozza M. Radiotherapy of carcinomas of the skin overlying the cartilage of the nasal: results in 405 lesions. Eur J Dermatol. 2003;13(5):462–5.
42. Caccialanza M, Piccinno R, Gaiani F, Contini D. Relevance of dermatologic radiotherapy in the therapeutic strategy of skin epithelial neoplasms: excellent results in the treatment of lesions localized on eyelids and skin overlying the cartilage of the nasal. G Ital Dermatol Venereol. 2013;148(1):83–8.
43. Caccialanza M, Bertani E, Piccinno R, Rozza M, Brambilla R, Percivalle S. Radiotherapy of T4 squamous cell carcinoma of the skin of nasal pyramid. J Eur Acad Dermatol Venereol. 2006;20(7):872–4.
44. Chargari C, Van Limbergen E, Mahantshetty U, Deutsch E, Haie-Meder C. Radiobiology of brachytherapy: the historical view based on linear quadratic model and perspectives for optimization. Cancer Radiother. 2018;22(4):312–8.
45. Tagliaferri L, Vavassori A, Lancellotta V, De Sanctis V, Barbera F, Fusco V, Vidali C, Fionda B, Colloca G, Gambacorta MA, Aristei C, Corvò R, Magrini SM. Can brachytherapy be properly considered in the clinical practice? Trilogy project: the vision of the AIRO (Italian Association of Radiotherapy and Clinical Oncology) Interventional Radiotherapy study group. J Contemp Brachyther. 2020;12(1):84–9. Epub 2020 Feb 28. PMID: 32190074; PMCID: PMC7073336.
46. Czerwinski MD, Verhoef CG, Kaanders JHAM Sentinel NOSE study: prospective registration study on the sentinel node procedure for bulky squamous cell carcinoma of the nasal vestibule. Identifier: NCT05637307. 2023. https://clinicaltrials.gov/ct2/show/NCT05637307?cond=sent inel+nose&draw=2&rank=1.

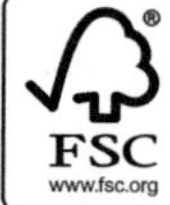

MIX
Papier aus verantwortungsvollen Quellen
Paper from responsible sources
FSC® C105338

If you have any concerns about our products,
you can contact us on
ProductSafety@springernature.com

In case Publisher is established outside the EU,
the EU authorized representative is:
Springer Nature Customer Service Center GmbH
Europaplatz 3, 69115 Heidelberg, Germany

Printed by Libri Plureos GmbH
in Hamburg, Germany